Pediatric
Epileptology

Pediatric Epileptology

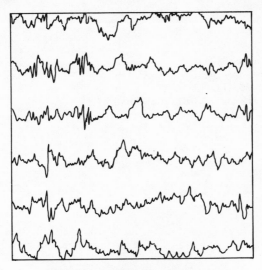

Classification and Management of Seizures in the Child

Fritz E. Dreifuss
with contributions

John Wright · PSG Inc
Boston   Bristol   London
1983

Library of Congress Cataloging in Publication Data
Main entry under title:

Pediatric epileptology.

   Bibliography: p.
   Includes index.
   1. Epilepsy in children.   I.   Dreifuss, Fritz E.
[DNLM: 1.   Epilepsy--In infancy and childhood.   WL 385
T674]
RJ496.E6T66 1983   618.92'853   83-1257
ISBN 0-7236-7039-0

Published simultaneously by:
John Wright • PSG Inc, 545 Great Road, Littleton,
Massachusetts 01460, U.S.A.
John Wright & Sons Ltd, 823–825 Bath Road,
Bristol BS4 5NU, England

First Printing 1983
Second Printing 1984

Printed in the United States of America

International Standard Book Number: 0-7236-7039-0

Library of Congress Card Number: 83-1257

DEDICATION

To our families for their encouragement and to those whose efforts
sustain the Epilepsy Movement.

CONTRIBUTORS

FRITZ E. DREIFUSS, MB, FRCP, FRACP
Professor of Neurology
School of Medicine, University of Virginia
Director, Comprehensive Epilepsy Program
Charlottesville, Virginia

JONAS H. ELLENBERG, PhD
Section on Mathematical Statistics
Office of Biometry and Field Studies
National Institute of Neurological and Communicative Disorders and Stroke
Bethesda, Maryland

CAROL APPOLONE FORD, MSSW
Research Instructor in Neurology
Bowman Gray School of Medicine
Winston-Salem, North Carolina

JOHN M. FREEMAN, MD
Associate Professor of Neurology and Pediatrics
The Johns Hopkins University School of Medicine
Baltimore, Maryland

PATRICIA GIBSON, MSSW
Assistant Professor of Neurology
Associate Director, Comprehensive Epilepsy Program
Bowman Gray School of Medicine
Winston-Salem, North Carolina

SOO IK LEE, MD
Professor of Neurology
School of Medicine, University of Virginia
Director, Electroencephalographic Laboratory
Charlottesville, Virginia

KARIN B. NELSON, MD
Cerebral Palsy and Other Motor Disorders Section
National Institute of Neurological and Communicative Disorders and Stroke
National Institute of Health
Bethesda, Maryland

MICHAEL E. NEWMARK, MD
Associate Professor
University of Louisville, School of Medicine
Chief, Neurological Service
Veterans Administration Medical Center
Louisville, Kentucky

J. CHRIS SACKELLARES, MD
Assistant Professor of Neurology
University of Michigan School of Medicine
Ann Arbor, Michigan

SUSUMU SATO, MD
Neurologist, Epilepsy Branch
Neurological Disorders Program
National Institute of Neurological and Communicative Disorders and Stroke
Bethesda, Maryland

CONTENTS

ACKNOWLEDGMENTS

We wish to acknowledge with gratitude the assistance of Deanna Kirby, for 15 years devoted to electroencephalography in epilepsy research, and of Diane Payne and Violet Cleveland in the preparation of the manuscript.

INTRODUCTION

The features of the epilepsies in childhood are sufficiently distinctive to deserve separate treatment. Neonatal seizures, infantile spasms, febrile convulsions, and the absence seizure syndrome are specific childhood seizure types. The causes of the epilepsies in childhood differ from those in adult epilepsy, with the preponderance of seizures falling into the primary generalized or idiopathic group. The effects of anticonvulsant drugs differ in children, particularly in their effects on cognitive function. The biopsychosocial aspects of epilepsy in childhood are infrequently commented upon in standard texts. In childhood, particular opportunity exists for prevention of epilepsy by early detection and treatment.

Important advances in epileptology have occurred in the past several years, and these were the temporal determinants for the appearance of this book. The Commission for the Control of Epilepsy and Its Consequences explored the epilepsies in depth from basic scientific research to day-to-day management of the consequences of seizures and touched upon prevention, medical services, social adjustment and mental health, education and employment, independence and equality, living arrangements, and the development of comprehensive epilepsy services and programs. The classification of epileptic seizures was revised in the light of modern investigation of seizures and results of the application of modern pharmacotherapy. Intensive monitoring became commonplace and led to the widespread application of improved differential diagnosis of episodic neurologic disturbances. New pharmacologic agents have begun to be more abundantly developed. Techniques for the evaluation of new drugs have improved and the rational application of the science of neuropharmacology has improved the outlook for patients previously deemed to be suffering from intractable epilepsy.

In the past two years, recent advances in knowledge have been discussed in several major symposia including the topics of classification of seizure types and syndromes, genetics of the epilepsies, results stemming from the large perinatal study particularly as they pertain to neonatal seizures and to febrile convulsions. A major consensus conference on febrile convulsions was held. The results of collaborative epilepsy studies led to new knowledge of absence seizures and of the prognosis of various types of epilepsy. An international conference on status epilepticus led to an updated review of its etiology, biochemistry, pathophysiology, and treatment.

Improved investigative methodology has led to increased studies of the infantile spasms and the Lennox-Gastaut syndrome, two of the most intractable forms of childhood seizures.

All these recent developments form the major topics in the book, which is a collection of treatises incorporating the current knowledge in an in-depth review of the individual topics.

The book is divided into introductory chapters dealing with classification, genetics, and electrophysiology, followed by a review of the generalized and partial seizures. Among the latter, particular pediatric syndromes and etiologies are stressed. Seizures characteristic of the pediatric age group including neonatal seizures, febrile seizures, and the reflex epilepsies receive special attention. The third series of chapters consists of a discussion of the management of patients with epilepsy with major emphasis on the subjects of pharmacologic management and the development of Comprehensive Epilepsy Programs. The psychosocial implications of the epilepsies are addressed.

Each of the contributors has made major contributions in the realm of his or her topic and has produced a worthy source of reference for anyone interested in the art and science of the study of epilepsy, for so long the paradigm of disorders of the central nervous system.

CHAPTER 1

Classification of Seizures and the Epilepsies

Fritz E. Dreifuss

HISTORY OF CLASSIFICATION OF SEIZURES AND EPILEPSIES

The present classification of seizures and epilepsies has evolved over a long time. Classifications are essential for grouping together conditions with similar manifestations; in this manner we can learn more about the conditions, thereby creating more knowledge about each condition and at the same time disseminating knowledge. Lack of clarity long impeded advances in knowledge about epilepsy. Attempts of modern authors to apply modern concepts to the writings of neurologic sages such as Hippocrates were not helpful; Galen, too, surely did not conceive of idiopathic, symptomatic, focal, or partial epilepsies in the same way as we do (Temkin 1971). By lending historical dignity to their writings in regard to classification, confusion can arise (Masland 1974). Calmeil in 1824 introduced classifications based on severity of attacks, and this classification method was soon elaborated by Delasiauve (1854), who used the terms *idiopathic* to describe seizures in which there was no anatomically demonstrable lesion, *symptomatic* for seizures in which there was a demonstrable lesion in the brain, and *sympathetic* to describe seizures due to the effects on the brain of diseases elsewhere in the body. In 1861, Reynolds stated, "Perhaps no disease has been treated with more perfect empiricism on the one hand, or more rigid rationalism on the other than has epilepsy. Unfortunately, both methods have often and completely failed; the former, as it must do, in a certain proportion of cases; the latter, in the still larger number because the theories upon which it has rested, have often been abundantly wrong.

Hughlings Jackson (1931) first expressed the idea that a classification should take into consideration anatomical lesions, physiological disturbances of function, and pathological processes. He first introduced the concept of generalized and partial seizures; the former he called "genuine epilepsy" and the latter "convulsions beginning unilaterally." Because of their disturbance of the state of consciousness, he spoke of absence seizures and generalized tonic-clonic seizures as "highest level seizures," and he recognized that partial seizures resulted from a focal discharge of the cerebral gray matter. Jackson was the first to introduce a truly anatomical concept when he spoke of "uncinate fits." The Montreal School (Penfield and Jasper 1954) elaborated the concept of focal seizures, so-called centrencephalic seizures, and unlocalized seizures; the first being the result of demonstrable lesions, the second "idiopathic," and the third the result of systemic disease. They also distinguished within groups the attack pattern, the electroencephalographic findings, the radiographic findings, and the pathological findings. Symonds (1955) pointed out that patients with focal seizures might be clinically indistinguishable from those with "central seizures" (such as one sees in absence and complex partial attacks on occasion and recommended that the EEG be made part of the classification.

CLASSIFICATION OF EPILEPTIC SEIZURES

Between 1964 and 1969, the International League against Epilepsy, through the Commission on Classification, developed a classification whose main aim was universal acceptance. The League realized the great importance to communication of unanimity of terminology (Gastaut 1970, 1973). The first International Classification was published in 1969 and represented a milestone in attempts at classification of epileptic seizures. At the same time, an outline of another classification of the epilepsies was proposed (Merlis 1970). This classification of epileptic seizures was primarily descriptive and the classification of the epilepsies was an early attempt at syndromic delineation. Both classifications were characterized by the distinction between seizures that are generalized from the beginning and those that are partial or focal in onset and become generalized secondarily.

The development and diversification of objective methods for documenting seizures (including prolonged EEG recording and the use of video tape, which allows for capture and availability for review of seizures) has allowed further elaboration with more accurate description of individual epileptic seizures types—as it were, the pigments of which the painting of the epilepsies is composed.

The descriptive purity of these component seizures is mandated now by more than theoretical considerations. The development of new and more specific drugs has reinforced the necessity for the development of more accurate diagnosis and quantification. Accurate prognostication of different seizure types is important because increased knowledge about the side effects of medication have raised questions regarding which seizures should be treated for what length of time. Prognostic and therapeutic imperatives have teamed with the availability of modern technology in the upgrading of the system of classification for both research and utilitarian purposes. The publication of the revised classification proposal (Commission on Classification and Terminology 1981) represented a further advance because it incorporated for the first time a glossary of terms used in the classification to ensure universal unanimity of interpretation of the terminology.

This most recent proposed classification introduces two major departures from previous schemes. The first is the separation of partial seizures into simple and complex, depending on whether or not consciousness is disturbed. The second is the ability to describe the evolution of a seizure longitudinally and sequentially. Thus, a seizure may begin as a simple seizure and may evolve into a complex, partial seizure. Descriptive accuracy is improved by removing the need for procrustean exertion in fitting the attack into a descriptive niche. Under this scheme, unclassifiable epilepsies would include those where seizures are too rare to enable clinical analysis.

With increasing technological sophistication using videotape analysis and simultaneous EEG recording, we have a better opportunity to build a universally acceptable classification of the epilepsies by developing a uniformity that was not possible on the basis of clinical observation of fleeting events. Any classification will aid in mobilizing newer concepts, and these in turn will lead to further modification of the classification. This is particularly true of the epilepsies of childhood; cerebral maturation plays a large part in the spread of the discharge or clinical manifestation and in the alteration of seizures with the passing of the years.

I. PARTIAL (FOCAL, LOCAL) SEIZURES

Partial seizures are those in which, in general, the first clinical and electroencephalographic changes indicate initial activation of a system of neurons limited to part of one cerebral hemisphere. A partial seizure is classified primarily on the basis of whether or not consciousness is impaired during the attack. When consciousness is not impaired, the seizure is classified as a simple partial seizure. When consciousness is impaired, the seizure is classified as a complex partial seizure. Impairment of consciousness may be the first clinical sign, or simple partial seizures may evolve into complex partial seizures. In patients with impaired consciousness, aberrations of behavior (automatisms) may occur. A partial seizure may not terminate but instead may progress to a generalized motor seizure. Impaired consciousness is defined as the inability to respond normally to exogenous stimuli by virtue of altered awareness and/or responsiveness (see following section, Definition of Terms).

There is considerable evidence that simple partial seizures usually have unilateral hemispheric involvement and only rarely have bilateral hemispheric involvement; complex partial seizures, however, frequently have bilateral hemispheric involvement.

Partial seizures can be classified into one of the following three fundamental groups: a) simple partial seizures; b) complex partial seizures; c) partial seizures evolving to generalized tonic-clonic convulsions (GTC).

A. Simple Partial Seizures

CLINICAL SEIZURE TYPE: Simple partial seizures: consciousness not impaired.

EEG SEIZURE TYPE: Local contralateral discharge starting over the corresponding area of cortical representation (not always recorded on the scalp).

EEG INTERICTAL EXPRESSION: Local contralateral discharge.

1. With motor signs
   a. focal motor without march
   b. focal motor with march (Jacksonian)
   c. versive
   d. postural
   e. phonatory (vocalization or arrest of speech)
2. With autonomic symptoms (including epigastric sensation, pallor, sweating, flushing, piloerection, and pupillary dilatation)
3. With somatosensory or special sensory symptoms (simple hallucinations, eg, tingling, light flashes, buzzing)
   a. somatosensory
   b. visual
   c. auditory
   d. olfactory
   e. gustatory
   f. vertiginous
4. With psychic symptoms (disturbance of higher cerebral function). These rarely occur without impairment of consciousness and are more commonly seen as complex partial seizures.
   a. dysphasic
   b. dysmnesic (eg, déjà vu)

    c. cognitive (eg, dreamy states, distortions of time sense)
    d. affective (fear, anger and other emotional states)
    e. illusions (eg, macropsia)
    f. structured hallucinations (eg, music, scenes)

B. Complex Partial Seizures

CLINICAL SEIZURE TYPE: Complex partial seizure: with impairment of consciousness; may sometimes begin with simple symptomatology.

EEG SEIZURE TYPE: Unilateral or, frequently, bilateral discharge, diffuse or focal in temporal or frontotemporal regions.

EEG INTERICTAL EXPRESSION: Unilateral or bilateral, generally asynchronous focus; usually in the temporal regions.

  1. Simple partial onset followed by impairment of consciousness
    a. with simple partial features (A1–A4) followed by impaired consciousness
    b. with automatisms
  2. With impairment of consciousness at onset
    a. with impairment of consciousness only
    b. with automatisms

C. Partial Seizures Evolving to Generalized Tonic-Clonic Seizures (GTC)

CLINICAL SEIZURE TYPE: GTC with partial or focal onset.

EEG SEIZURE TYPE: Discharges like those for complex partial seizures, becoming secondarily and rapidly generalized.

  1. Simple partial seizures (A) evolving to GTC
  2. Complex partial (B) evolving to GTC
  3. Simple partial seizures evolving to complex partial seizures evolving to GTC

II. GENERALIZED SEIZURES (CONVULSIVE OR NONCONVULSIVE)

Generalized seizures are those in which the first clinical changes indicate initial involvement of both hemispheres. Consciousness may be impaired and this impairment may be the initial manifestation. Motor manifestations are bilateral. The ictal electroencephalographic patterns initially are bilateral and presumably reflect neuronal discharge that is widespread in both hemispheres.

A. Absence Seizures
  1. Typical absence seizures (b-f may be used alone or in combination)
    a. impairment of consciousness only
    b. with mild clonic components
    c. with atonic components
    d. with tonic components
    e. with automatisms
    f. with autonomic components

CLINICAL SEIZURE TYPE: Absence seizure.

EEG SEIZURE TYPE: Usually regular and symmetrical 3-Hz activity, but may be 2- to 4-Hz spike-and-slow-wave complexes and may have multiple spike-and-slow-wave complexes. Abnormalities are bilateral.

EEG INTERICTAL EXPRESSION: Background activity is usually normal, although paroxysmal activity (such as spikes or spike-and-slow-wave complexes) may occur.

This activity is usually regular and symmetrical.
2. Atypical absence seizures: may have
   a. changes in tone that are more pronounced
   b. onset and/or cessation that is not abrupt
EEG SEIZURE TYPE: More heterogeneous; may include irregular spike-and-slow-wave complexes, fast activity, or other paroxysmal activity. Abnormalities are bilateral but often irregular and asymmetrical.
EEG INTERICTAL EXPRESSION: Background usually abnormal; a proxysmal activity (such as spikes or spike-and-slow-wave complexes) frequently irregular and asymmetrical.

B. Tonic-Clonic Seizures
EEG SEIZURE TYPE: Rhythm at 10 or more cycles per second, decreasing in frequency and increasing in amplitude during tonic phase, interrupted by slow waves during clonic phase.
EEG INTERICTAL EXPRESSION: Polyspike-and-wave discharges, or spike-and-wave discharges, or sometimes sharp-and-slow-wave discharges.

C. Myoclonic Seizures
CLINICAL SEIZURE TYPE: Myoclonic jerks (single or multiple).
EEG SEIZURE TYPE: Polyspike-and-wave discharges, or sometimes spike-and-wave or sharp-and-slow-wave discharges.
EEG INTERICTAL EXPRESSION: Same pattern as in ictal period.

D. Clonic Seizures
EEG SEIZURE TYPE: Fast activity (10 cycles per second or more) and slow waves; occasional spike-and-slow-wave patterns.
EEG INTERICTAL EXPRESSION: Spike-and-wave or polyspike-and-wave discharges.

E. Tonic Seizures
EEG SEIZURE TYPE: Low-voltage, fast activity or a fast rhythm (9–10 cycles per second or more) decreasing in frequency and increasing in amplitude.
EEG INTERICTAL EXPRESSION: More or less rhythmic discharges of sharp and slow waves, sometimes symmetrical.

F. Atonic Seizures
EEG SEIZURE TYPE: Polyspikes and wave discharges or flattening or low-voltage fast activity.
EEG INTERICTAL EXPRESSION: Polyspikes and wave activity.

III. UNCLASSIFIED EPILEPTIC SEIZURES
Includes all seizures that cannot be classified because of inadequate or incomplete data and some that defy classification in hitherto described categories. This includes some neonatal seizures, eg, rhythmic eye movements, chewing, and swimming movements.

ADDENDUM
1. Repeated epileptic seizures occur under a variety of circumstances:

a. as fortuitous attacks, coming unexpectedly and without any apparent provocation

b. as cyclic attacks, at more or less regular intevals (eg, in relation to the menstrual cycle or to the sleep–waking cycle)

c. as attacks provoked by 1) nonsensory factors (fatigue, alcohol, emotion) or 2) sensory factors, and sometimes referred to as "reflex seizures"

2. Prolonged or repetitive seizures (status epilepticus). The term "status epilepticus" is used whenever a seizure persists for a sufficient length of time or is repeated frequently enough that recovery between attacks does not occur. Status epilepticus may be divided into partial (eg, Jacksonian) or generalized (eg, absence status or tonic-clonic status). When very localized motor status occurs, it is referred to as epilepsia partialis continua.

DEFINITION OF TERMS

In this section each seizure type will be described so that the criteria used will not be in doubt.

Partial Seizures

The fundamental distinction between simple partial seizures and complex partial seizures is the presence or the impairment of the fully conscious state.

Consciousness has been defined as "that integrating activity by which Man grasps the totality of his phenomenal field" (Evans 1972) and incorporates it into his experience. It corresponds to *Bewusstsein* and is thus much more than "Vigilance," for were it only vigilance (which is a degree of clarity) then only confusional states would be representative of disordered consciousness.

Operationally, in the context of this classification, *consciousness* refers to the degree of awareness and/or responsiveness of the patient to externally applied stimuli. *Responsiveness* refers to the ability of the patient to carry out simple commands or willed movement, and *awareness* refers to the patient's contact with events during the period in question. A person aware and unresponsive will be able to recount the events that occurred during an attack and his inability to respond by movement or speech. In this context, unresponsiveness is other than the result of paralysis, aphasia, or apraxia.

A. Partial Seizures

1. WITH MOTOR SIGNS. Any portion of the body may be involved in focal seizure activity, depending on the site of origin of the attack and the motor strip. Focal motor seizures may remain strictly focal, or they may spread to contiguous cortical areas and produce a sequential involvement of body parts in an epileptic "march." The seizure is then known as a Jacksonian seizure. Consciousness is usually preserved; however, the discharge may spread to structures whose participation is likely to result in loss of consciousness and generalized convulsive movements. Other focal motor attacks may be versive, with the head turning to one side, usually the side contraversive to the discharge. If speech is involved, involvement includes speech arrest or, occasionally vocalization. When aphasia occurs, it is transitory. Occasionally a partial dysphasia is seen in the form of epileptic palilalia with involuntary repetition of a syllable or phrase.

Following focal seizure activity there may be a localized paralysis in the previously involved region. This is known as Todd's paralysis and may last from minutes to hours.

When focal motor seizure activity is continuous, it is known as epilepsia partialis continua.

2. WITH AUTONOMIC SYMPTOMS. Vomiting, pallor, flushing, sweating, piloerection, pupil dilatation, boborygmi, and incontinence may occur as simple partial seizures.

3. WITH SOMATOSENSORY OR SPECIAL SENSORY SYMPTOMS. Somatosensory seizures arise from those areas of cortex subserving sensory function. The sensation accompanying these seizures is usually described as pins and needles or a feeling of numbness. Occasionally a disorder of proprioception or spatial perception occurs. Like motor seizures, somatosensory seizures also may march and also may spread at any time to become a complex partial or generalized tonic-clonic seizure as in seizures with motor signs. Special sensory seizures include visual seizures that vary in elaborateness (depending on whether the primary or association areas are involved) from flashing lights to structured visual hallucinatory phenomena, including persons and scenes (see section A4f). Like visual seizures, auditory seizures may also run the gamut from crude auditory sensations to such highly integrated functions as music (see section A4f). Olfactory sensations, usually in the form of unpleasant odors, may occur.

Gustatory sensations may be pleasant or odious taste hallucinations. They vary in elaboration from crude (salty, sour, sweet, bitter) to sophisticated. They are frequently described as "metallic."

Vertiginous symptoms include sensations of falling in space, floating, as well as rotatory vertigo in a horizontal or vertical plane.

4. WITH PSYCHIC SYMPTOMS (disturbance of higher cerebral function). These symptoms usually occur with impairment of consciousness (ie, complex partial seizures).

a. *Dysphasia:* this was discussed in the section on seizures with motor signs.

b. *Dysmnesic symptoms:* these symptoms include a distorted memory experience such as a distortion of the time sense, a dreamy state, a flashback, or a sensation as if a naive experience had been experienced before (known as déjà vu) or as if a previously experienced sensation had not been experienced (known as jamais vu) may occur. When this refers to auditory experiences, these are known as déjà entendu or jamais entendu. Occasionally, as a form of forced thinking, the patient may experience a rapid recollection of episodes from his past life, known as panoramic vision.

c. *Cognitive disturbance may be experienced:* these include dreamy states, distortions of the time sense, sensations of unreality, detachment, or depersonalization.

d. *Affective symptoms:* a sensation of extreme pleasure or displeasure, as well as fear and intense depression with feelings of unworthiness and rejection, may be experienced during seizures. Unlike the symptoms of psychiatrically induced depression, these symptoms tend to come in attacks lasting for a few minutes. Anger or rage is occasionally experienced, but unlike temper tantrums, epileptic anger is apparently unprovoked and abates rapidly. Fear or terror is the most frequent symptom; it is sudden in onset, is usually unprovoked, and may lead to running away. Frequently associated with the terror are objective signs of autonomic activity, including pupil dilatation, pallor, flushing, piloerection, palpitation, and hypertension.

Epileptic or gelastic seizure laughter should not, strictly speaking, be classified under affective symptoms because the laughter is usually without affect and is hollow. Like other forms of pathological laughter, it is often unassociated with true mirth.

e. *Illusions:* these symptoms take the form of distorted perceptions in which objects may appear deformed. Polyoptic illusions such as monocular diplopia, distortions of size, macropsia, or micropsia, or of distance may occur. Similarly, distortions of sound, including microacusia and macroacusia, may be seen. Depersonalization, as if the person were outside his body, may occur. Altered perception of size or weight of a limb may be noted.

f. *Structured hallucinations:* hallucinations may occur as manifestations or perceptions without a corresponding external stimulus and may affect somatosensory, visual, auditory, olfactory, or gustatory senses. If the seizure arises from the primary receptive area, the hallucination would tend to be rather primitive. In the case of vision, flashing lights may be seen; in the case of auditory perception, rushing noises may occur. With more elaborate seizures involving visual or auditory association areas with participation of mobilized memory traces, formed hallucinations occur; these may take the form of scenery, persons, spoken sentences, or music. The character of these perceptions may be normal or distorted.

B.   Seizures with Complex Symptomatology

1. AUTOMATISMS. (These may occur in both partial and generalized seizures. They are described in detail here for convenience). In the *Dictionary of Epilepsy* (Gastaut 1973), automatisms are described as "more or less coordinated, adapted (eupractic or dyspractic), involuntary motor activity occurring during the state of clouding of consciousness either in the course of or after an epileptic seizure, and usually followed by amnesia for the event. The automatism may be simply a continuation of an activity that was going on when the seizure occurred, or, conversely, a new activity developed in association with the ictal impairment of consciousness. Usually, the activity is commonplace in nature, often provoked by the subject's environment, or by his sensations during the seizure; exceptionally, fragmentary, primitive, infantile, or antisocial behavior is seen. From a symptomatological point of view the following are distinguished, a) eating automatisms (chewing, swallowing); b) automatisms of mimicry, expressing the subject's emotional state (usually of fear) during the seizure; c) gestural automatisms, crude or elaborate, directed toward either the subject or his environment; d) ambulatory automatisms; e) verbal automatisms."

Ictal epileptic automatisms usually represent the release of automatic behavior under the influence of clouding of consciousness that accompanies a generalized or partial epileptic seizure (confusional automatisms). They may occur in complex partial seizures as well as in absence seizures. Postictal epileptic automatisms may follow any severe epileptic seizure, expecially a tonic-clonic one, and are usually associated with confusion.

Although some investigators regard masticatory or oropharyngeal automatisms as arising from the amygdala or insula and opercular regions, these movements are occasionally seen in the generalized epilepsies (particularly absence seizures) and are not of localizing help. The same is true of mimicry and gestural automatisms. In the latter, fumbling with the clothes, scratching, and other complex motor activity may occur both in complex partial and absence seizures. Ictal speech automatisms are occasionally seen. Ambulatory seizures again may occur either as prolonged automatisms of absence (particularly prolonged absence continuing) or of complex partial seizures. In the latter, patients may occasionally continue to drive a car, though they may contravene traffic light regulations.

There seems to be little doubt that automatisms are a common feature of different types of epilepsy. Although they do not lend themselves to simple anatomical interpretation, they appear to have in common a discharge involving various areas of the limbic system. Crude and elaborate automatisms do occur in patients with absence as well as complex partial seizures. Of greater significance are the precise descriptive history of the seizures, the age of the patient, and the presence or absence of confusion. The EEG is of cardinal localizational importance here.

2. DROWSINESS OR SOMNOLENCE. This symptom implies a sleep state from which the patient can be aroused to make appropriate motor and verbal responses. In stupor, the patient may make some spontaneous movement and can be aroused, by painful or other vigorously applied stimuli, to make avoidance movements. The patient, in confusion, makes inappropriate responses to his environment and is disoriented as regards place or time or person.

3. AURA. Aura is a term frequently used in the description of epileptic seizures. According to the *Dictionary of Epilepsy* (Gastaut 1973), this term was introduced by Galen to describe the sensation of a breath of air that is felt by some subjects prior to the onset of a seizure. Others have referred to the aura as the portion of the seizure experienced before loss of consciousness occurs. This loss of consciousness may be the result of secondary generalization of the seizure discharge or of alteration of consciousness imparted by the development of a complex partial seizure.

The aura is that portion of the seizure that occurs before consciousness is lost and for which memory is retained afterward. It may be that, as in simple partial seizures, the aura is the whole seizure. Where consciousness is subsequently lost, the aura is, in fact, the signal symptom of a complex partial seizure.

An aura is a retrospective term that is described after the seizure is ended.

Generalized Seizures

A. Absence Seizures

The hallmarks of the absence attack are sudden onset, interruption of ongoing activities, a blank stare, and possibly a brief upward rotation of the eyes. If the patient is speaking, speech is interrupted; if walking, he stands transfixed; if eating, the food will stop on its way to the mouth. Usually the patient will be unresponsive when spoken to. The attack lasts from a few seconds to half a minute and evaporates as rapidly as it commenced.

1. ABSENCE WITH IMPAIRMENT OF CONSCIOUSNESS ONLY. The preceding description fits the description of a simple absence attack in which no other activities take place during the attack.

2. ABSENCE WITH MILD CLONIC COMPONENTS. The onset of the attack is indistinguishable from the preceding description, but clonic movements may occur in the eyelids, at the corners of the mouth, or in other muscle groups. The clonic movements may vary in severity from almost imperceptible movements to generalized myoclonic jerks. Objects held in the hand may be dropped.

3. ABSENCE WITH ATONIC COMPONENTS. A diminution in tone of muscles subserving posture as well as the limbs may occur and may lead to dropping of the arms and relaxation of the grip. Rarely, tone is sufficiently diminished to cause falling.

4. ABSENCE WITH TONIC COMPONENTS. During the attack, tonic muscular contraction may occur and cause increased muscle tone; contraction may affect the extensor muscles or the flexor muscles symmetrically or asymmetrically. If the patient is standing, the head may be drawn backward and the trunk may arch. This may lead to retropulsion. The head may tonically draw to one side or the other.

5. ABSENCE WITH AUTOMATISMS (see also prior discussion on automatisms). Purposeful or quasi-purposeful movements that occur in the absence of awareness during an absence attack are frequent and may range from lip licking and swallowing to fumbling with clothes or aimless walking. If spoken to, the patient may grunt or turn to the sound; when touched or tickled, the patient may rub the site. Automatisms are quite elaborate and may often consist of combinations of the previously described movements or they might be so simple as to be missed by casual observation. Mixed forms of absence frequently occur.

B. Tonic-Clonic Seizures

The generalized tonic-clonic seizures are the most frequently encountered of the generalized seizures and are often known as grand mal. Some patients experience a vague, ill-described warning, but the majority lose consciousness without any premonitory symptoms. There is a sudden sharp tonic contraction of muscles; when this involves the respiratory muscles, there is a cry or moan. The patient falls to the ground in the tonic state, occasionally injuring himself in falling. He lies rigid on the ground; during this stage, tonic contraction inhibits respiration and cyanosis may occur. The tongue may be bitten and urine may be passed involuntarily. This tonic stage then gives way to clonic convulsive movements that last for a variable period of time. During this stage, small gusts of respiration may occur between the convulsive movements, but usually the patient remains cyanotic and saliva may froth from the mouth. At the end of this stage, deep inspiration occurs and all the muscles relax. He then frequently goes into a deep sleep. When he awakens, he feels quite well apart from soreness and, frequently, headache. Grand mal convulsions may occur in childhood and in adult life and are not as frequent as absence seizures. Frequency may vary from one a day to one every three months and, occasionally, to one every few years. Very short attacks without postictal drowsiness may occur on occasion.

C. Myoclonic Seizures

Myoclonic jerks (single or multiple) are sudden, brief, shocklike contractions that may be generalized or confined to the face and trunk, or to one or more extremities, or even to individual muscles or groups of muscles. Myoclonic jerks may be rapidly repetitive or relatively isolated. They may occur predominantly around the hours of going to sleep or awakening from sleep. They may be exacerbated by volitional movement (action myoclonus). At times they may be regularly repetitive.

D. Clonic Seizures

Generalized convulsive seizures occasionally lack a tonic component and are characterized by repetitive clonic jerks. Although the frequency diminishes, the amplitude of the jerks does not. The postictal phase is usually short. Some generalized convulsive seizures commence with a clonic phase, which passes into a tonic phase (as described next) and leads to a "clonic-tonic-clonic" seizure.

E. Tonic Seizures

To quote Gowers (1901), a tonic seizure is "a rigid, violent muscular contraction, fixing the limbs in some strained position. There is usually deviation of the eyes and of the head towards one side, and this may amount to rotation involving the whole body and may actually cause the patient to turn around, even two or three times. The features are distorted; the color of the face, unchanged at first, rapidly becomes pale and then flushed and ultimately livid as the fixation of the chest by the spasms stops the movement of respiration. The eyes are open or closed; the conjunctiva is insensitive; the pupils dilate widely as cyanosis comes on. As the spasm continues, it commonly changes in its relative intensity in different parts, causing slight alterations in the position of the limbs."

Tonic axial seizures with extension of head, neck, and trunk may also occur.

F. Atonic Seizures

A sudden diminution in muscle tone occurs; the attack may be fragmentary and lead to dropping of the head with slackening of the jaw or to dropping of a limb, or it may involve a loss of all muscle tone and lead to slumping to the ground. When these attacks are extremely brief, they are known as "drop attacks." If consciousness is lost, this loss is extremely brief. The sudden loss of postural tone in the head and trunk may lead to injury by projecting objects. The face is particularly subject to injury. In the case of more prolonged atonic attacks, the slumping may be progressive in a rhythmic, successive-relaxation manner.

(So-called drop attacks may be seen in conditions other than epilepsy, such as brain stem ischemia and narcolepsy cataplexy syndrome.)

Unclassified Epileptic Seizures

This category includes all seizures that cannot be classified because of inadequate or incomplete data; it includes some seizures that by their nature defy classification in the previously defined broad categories. Many seizures occurring in the infant (eg, rhythmic eye movements, chewing, swimming movements, jittering, and apnea) will be classified here until such time as further experience with videotape confirmation and electroencephalographic characterization entitles them to subtyping in the extant classification.

Epilepsia Partialis Continua

This name has been assigned to simple partial seizures with focal motor signs without a march. The focal motor signs usually consist of clonic spasms, which remained confined to the part of the body in which they originate. However, the spasms may persist with little or no intermission for hours or days at a stretch. Consciousness is usually preserved, but postictal weakness is frequently evident.

Postictal Paralysis (Todd's Paralysis)

This refers to the transient paralysis that may occur following some partial epileptic seizures with focal motor components or with somatosensory symptoms. Postictal paralysis has been ascribed to neuronal exhaustion caused by the increased metabolic activity of the discharging focus, but it may also be attributable to increased inhibition in the region of the focus, a process that may account for its appearance in nonmotor somatosensory seizures.

CLASSIFICATION OF THE EPILEPSIES

The limitation of the classification of epileptic seizures to description of individual seizure varieties has perforce excluded the consideration of syndromic concatenations characterized by syndromes whose terminology is used daily in communication between colleagues and as diagnostic entries in hospital records and that form the subject of clinical trials and other investigations. In 1970, a preliminary proposal for an International Classification of the Epilepsies included three major divisions: generalized epilepsies, partial epilepsies, and unclassified epilepsies, with separation of the generalized epilepsies into primary generalized epilepsies, secondary generalized epilepsies, and undetermined generalized epilepsies (Merlis 1970). This is obviously just a beginning, and it lends itself to a subclassification by type of seizure, cause, proposed anatomy, precipitating factors, age of onset, severity and chronicity of seizures, and diurnal and circadian cycling. The concept of what constitutes primary generalized epilepsy and what constitutes secondary generalized epilepsy has to be further defined. It is not clear at this time which massive infantile spasms belong in which group; similarly, the individual cases of the Lennox-Gastaut syndrome cannot be assigned to a group. It is clear that both of these rubrics encompass different statistical populations. It may well be that the genetically determined, or idiopathic, forms represent primary generalized epilepsies and that the symptomatic forms represent secondary generalized epilepsies. Janz (1969) anticipated the dilemma by classifying epilepsies into small attacks and large attacks. The small attacks were subdivided into those that were age limited (these represented the generalized epilepsies) and those that were not age limited (these represented partial or focal epilepsies). Under the large attacks, he spoke of those that were associated with waking/sleeping and of those that were independent of either (diffuse epilepsies). This unfortunately disregards the secondary generalized attacks that make up a portion of both the small and the large attacks as defined (Wolf 1979).

A strictly syndromic classification might be envisioned as follows:

Age Related, Generalized Epilepsies
  Neonatal convulsions
  Infantile spasms (West syndrome)
  Febrile seizures
  Astatic-myoclonic seizures (Lennox-Gastaut)
  Absence epilepsy
  Juvenile epileptic myoclonus ("impulsive petit mal")
  Reflex epilepsies (eg, photically induced)
  Generalized tonic-clonic epilepsies (grand mal)

Age Related, Partial Epilepsies
  Neonatal convulsions
  Unilateral (hemicorporeal) seizures
  Astatic-myoclonic seizures (Lennox-Gastaut syndrome) with partial
    seizures
  Sylvian (Rolandic) seizures
  Epilepsia partialis continua
  Simple partial seizures
  Complex partial seizures

Partial seizures secondarily generalized
Occasional seizures of known cause
Stress-induced epilepsies
Sleep deprivation seizures
Alcohol withdrawal convulsions
Drug withdrawal convulsions
Convulsions due to toxic exposure (exogenous or endogenous)

Under this scheme, unclassifiable epilepsies would include those where seizures are too few and far between to enable critical analysis.

It is clear that considerable work remains to be done in building a universally acceptable classification of the epilepsies. With increasing knowledge, the categories may change, and the classification in itself will aid in mobilizing those concepts that will lead to its modification.

Meanwhile, the classification of epileptic seizures is a forward step in the development of a uniform medium for the exchange of information between members of the international community of epileptologists.

BIBLIOGRAPHY

Calmeil LF: *De l'epilepsie, étudiée sous le rapport de son siège et de son influence sur la production de l'aliénation méntale*, thesis. Paris, 1824.

Commission on Classification and Terminology, International League against Epilepsy: Proposed revisions of clinical and electroencephalographic classification of epileptic seizures. *Epilepsia* 1981;22:480–501.

Delasiauve LJF: *Traité de l'Epilepsie*. Paris, 1854.

Evans P: Henry Ey's concepts of the organization of consciousness and its disorganization: An extension of Jacksonian theory. *Brain* 1972;95:413–440.

Galen, cited by Temkin O: *The Falling Sickness: A History of Epilepsy from the Greeks to the Beginnings of Modern Neurology*, ed 2. Baltimore, Johns Hopkins Press, 1971.

Gastaut H: Clinical and electroencephalographical classification of epileptic seizures. *Epilepsia* 1970;11:103–113.

Gastaut H: *Dictionary of Epilepsy. Part 1: Definitions*. Geneva, World Health Organization, 1973.

Gowers WR: *Epilepsy and Other Chronic Convulsive Diseases*. London, Churchill, 1901.

Jackson JH: On epilepsy and epileptiform convulsions, in Taylor J (ed): *Selected Writings of J Hughlings Jackson*. London, Hodder & Staughton, 1931, vol 1.

Janz D: *Die Epilepsien. Spezielle Pathologie and Therapie*. Stuttgart, Georg Thieme Verlag, 1969.

Masland RL: The classification of the epilepsies, in Vinken PJ, Bruyn GW (eds): *Handbook of Clinical Neurology*. Amsterdam, North-Holland Publishing Co, 1974, vol 15.

Merlis JK: Proposal for an international classification of the epilepsies. *Epilepsia* 1970;11:114–119.

Penfield W, Jasper H: *Epilepsy and the Functional Anatomy of the Human Brain*. Boston, Little Brown & Co, 1954.

Reynolds JR: *Epilepsy: Its Symptoms, Treatment and Relations to Other Chronic Convulsive Diseases*. London, J Churchill, 1861.

Symonds CP: Classification of the epilepsies. *Br Med J* 1955;1:1235–1238.

Wolf P: Nomenklatur and Klassifikation epileptischer Anfälle and Syndrome. *Nervenarzt* 1979;50:547–554.

CHAPTER 2

Genetics of the Epilepsies

Michael E. Newmark

Physicians since antiquity have postulated a significant inheritance of epilepsy. As quoted by Temkin (1971), Hippocrates in the fifth century BC hypothesized that epilepsy was inherited as a specific disorder of the brain, which in susceptible individuals overflows with phlegm that clogs the veins and causes convulsions. Medieval Arabic and later Renaissance physicians commonly accepted inheritance as an etiology for epilepsy. In 1757 the Swedish government passed a law forbidding an epileptic individual to marry; and as late as the twentieth century, the Nazi regime sterilized epileptic patients in an effort to eliminate the disorder. Although several of these laws have since been repealed, the question of the inheritance of epilepsy has remained. For epileptics who plan to have children and for relatives of epileptic individuals, the question of the inheritance of epilepsy is a very real and significant one.

Despite the long history of a postulated inheritable etiology, reliable clinical data have not been obtained. Several reasons for some of the underlying confusion are given in the following list:

1. A single definition of epilepsy has not been universally accepted. If single seizures or febrile seizures are included in the definition of epilepsy, the baseline rate of epilepsy in a community, as well as the familial seizure rates, will change considerably.
2. Seizures may occasionally be misdiagnosed, and nonseizure episodes such as syncope, headache, or other paroxysmal disorders might be included. Absence attacks and complex partial seizures are occasionally very difficult to document.
3. The family history may not be accurate. Sufficient medical information may not be available or families may attempt to conceal a potentially embarrassing disease by not reporting it. Even if the information is supplied, studies vary according to the number of relatives and the closeness of the relationship. Several medical conditions unrelated to epilepsy, such as an infection or a severe metabolic disorder, may be accompanied by seizure.
4. As will be discussed later, epilepsy may be a symptom of several inheritable diseases, both metabolic and degenerative. If patients with these diseases are included in a small sample of accurately diagnosed epileptic patients, the inheritance of epilepsy may be exaggerated.
5. Multiple contributing factors must be analyzed to understand the

development of a seizure disorder. Seizures may arise from a number of causes, and the different causes must be considered separately.

6. As mentioned in other chapters, a considerable variety of seizure types exist, with each type possibly reflecting independent disorders. Each seizure type should be considered independently.

7. Finally, although a genetic tendency toward epilepsy may exist, seizures may not occur unless additional factors such as stress, hormonal change, or other environmental or physical triggers are present. As Metrakos and Metrakos (1961b) have suggested, individuals may have an inheritable epilepsy trait with identifiable electroencephalographic abnormalities but may not have clinical seizures. With some seizures, including absence and photically induced seizures, the age and sex of an individual are significant for the development of clinical attacks. Unless these developmental changes are considered, the diagnosis of epilepsy or the epilepsy trait might be inaccurate.

Despite the aforementioned problems, several basic trends concerning the genetics of epilepsy can be observed. In the following review, indirect evidence, animal models of epilepsy, and clinical data based on genetic patient studies will be presented.

INDIRECT EVIDENCE

Several studies have suggested that inheritance of epilepsy may be important. The studies may be grouped into those that have specifically investigated the inheritance pattern of patients with seizures and those that indirectly suggest the inheritance of epilepsy. Concerning the latter, several EEG patterns have been shown to be inherited. The generalized spike-and-wave complex, the photoparoxysmal response, and the mid-temporal-central spike have been associated with specific seizure symptoms and will be discussed later. Other electroencephalographic features that have not been as closely associated with epilepsy have also been described and suggest that some aspects of cerebral electrical organization may be partially inherited.

Using the gross visual appearance of the EEG, Lennox et al (1945) investigated electroencephalographic tracings of nonepileptic twins. Eighty-five percent of the electroencephalograms of monozygotic twin pairs were considered to be identical; in contrast, 5% of the electroencephalograms from the 19 dizygotic twin pairs were identical. Similarly, the visual-evoked and auditory-evoked potentials have a higher correlation between monozygotic twin pairs than between dizygotic ones (Dustman and Beck 1965, Rust 1975). Using frequency spectrum analysis, Lykken et al (1974) found that 96% of monozygotic twins have identical frequency patterns when compared with their co-twin's records.

Nonepileptiform EEG patterns have been described in a familial pattern. The 14-and 6-per-second positive spike pattern, a nonspecific EEG pattern, is present in approximately 50% of the siblings of individuals with this pattern (Rodin 1964, Petersen and Akesson 1968). In the Rodin series, a significantly lower rate of parents compared with siblings suggests that this pattern is age dependent.

Another familial inheritable pattern primarily present in 3- to 4-year-old children and consisting of monomorphic 4- to 6-per-second waves localized to the parietal regions has been described by Doose and Gerken (1972). In this study, 30% of the siblings of affected children were also found to have the theta rhythms, a rate approximately twice that of control children. Gerken and Doose (1972) have also described a familial occipital delta rhythm, which was most frequently present in children under 10 years of age and which was observed in a higher percentage of siblings of probands than in siblings of control patients. Both the occipital delta and the parietal theta rhythms are not highly correlated with seizures.

ANIMAL STUDIES

Several animal species have a high prevalence of seizures (Table 2-1). The audiogenic seizure-induced mouse, which has been extensively studied in its genetic, pharmacologic, and biochemical features (Seyfried 1979), is especially significant. This species of mouse experiences violent generalized seizures, which often lead to death and which are induced by a variety of noises from jangling keys to electric doorbells, may be classified as either nonseizing or seizing. Using recombinant inbred strains of mice, the inheritance pattern of sound-sensitive mice has been suggested by Seyfried et al (1980) to consist of a multiple gene effect that is additive upon the animal. Prominent environmental factors were also identified. Although the mechanisms of the increased sensitivity in these animals has not been fully explained, major neurologic dysfunction is present in several subcortical structures, including brain stem, spinal cord, and cerebellum. Biochemical abnormalities that have been identified include reduced ATPase activity, decreased phenylalanine hydroxylase activity, and abnormalities in CNS myelin. In addition, agents that reduce catecholamine levels increase the seizure sensitivity of these animals, whereas elevated γ-aminobutyric acid (GABA) levels reduce the sensitivity. The importance

Table 2-1
Animal Species with Increased Seizure Risk

Animal	Seizure Stimulus
Brown Swiss cattle	Spontaneous
Beagle	Spontaneous or photically induced
Mouse	Audiogenic
Mongolian gerbil	Spontaneous
Chicken	Photically induced, spontaneous
Deer mouse	Waltzing, audiogenic
British Alsatian	Spontaneous
Mouse-up	See-saw motion
Rabbit	Audiogenic
Rat	Audiogenic
Baboon (Papio papio)	Spontaneous or photically induced
Swine	Spontaneous
Irish setters	Spontaneous
Guinea pig	Audiogenic
Keeshonds	Spontaneous
Syrian golden hamsters	Spontaneous

18

of the audiogenic seizure-induced mouse to human epilepsy is still unclear, but the documentation that a form of epilepsy is inherited through multiple genes may have clinical significance.

Another mouse epilepsy model, the tottering mouse, has been analyzed by Noebels (1979). The partial seizures are inherited as an autosomal recessive pattern from a mutation in chromosome 8. This animal displays spontaneous partial motor seizures shortly after it develops an ataxic gait. The metabolic changes induced by the seizures, including increased local glucose utilization, have been outlined with deoxyglucose autoradiographs and are consistent with the clinical studies using this procedure.

A third animal that has been associated with both spontaneous and photically induced seizures is the photosensitive baboon, *Papio papio* (Newmark and Penry 1979). Although definite pedigrees have not been established with *Papio papio*, several social groups of baboons that are thought to interbreed with each other have been identified to be highly photosensitive. The mechanism of seizure in the photosensitive baboon has not been established, but numerous neurochemical alterations have been identified.

HEREDITARY DISEASES ASSOCIATED WITH EPILEPSY

Many inheritable disorders affecting the central nervous system have also been associated with seizures. Most of these disorders are quite rare, but occasionally they may be significant for small populations. The inheritable disorders associated with epilepsy have been reviewed by Gastaut (1969) and Skre (1975).

The most common of the diseases with autosomal dominant inheritance are tuberous sclerosis, porphyria, and neurofibromatosis. Other important, but rare, disorders associated with autosomal dominant phenotypes include Huntington's chorea, Sturge-Weber syndrome, endocrinomatosis, neuronal ceroid lipofuscinosis, and hemifacial atrophy. Several of these disorders are associated with obvious central nervous system lesions, including tumors (as in tuberous sclerosis and neurofibromatosis) or vasculopathies (as in Sturge-Weber syndrome). The association of epilepsy with Huntington's disease may be significant because of the abnormal dopaminergic findings in this disorder. The observations that several antiepileptic agents produce extrapyramidal toxicity and that phenothiazine agents may affect the seizure threshold further suggest a relationship of dopamine metabolism and epilepsy.

Numerous autosomal recessive disorders have been associated with seizures. These disorders have included disorders of amino acid, carbohydrate, and lipid metabolism; mucopolysacchridosis; and other metabolic disorders including disorders of copper metabolism, the porphyrias, and pyridoxine dependency. Several disorders including homocystinuria, phenylketonuria, and mucopolysaccharidosis may be diagnosed because of a characteristic appearance, typical metabolic findings in the urine or blood, or typical clinical symptoms in addition to the seizures. Other rare neurologic disorders, including leukodystrophies and Krabbe's disease (globoid cell leukodystrophy), metachromatic leukodystrophy, or gangliosidosis may be associated with seizures. Epilepsy, however, is a minor part of the disorder, as profound neurologic dysfunction usually dominates the symptomatology.

Hereditary ataxias and related disorders including Charcot-Marie-Tooth disease, Roussy-Levy disease, and hereditary spastic paraplegia are important neurologic syndromes that have been associaed with seizures. Gayral and Gayral (1969) observed that epilepsy was present in 9% of patients with an hereditary ataxia, including several in whom it was the primary neurologic symptom. Friedreich's ataxia has been specifically investigated by Andermann et al (1976), who described an increased prevalence of seizures among affected individuals with this disorder. The investigators concluded that epilepsy may be inherited either secondarily to the brain abnormalities caused by the ataxia gene itself or epilepsy may be inherited separately.

The progressive myoclonic epilepsies have been carefully investigated, and several inheritable forms have been described. Because the underlying defect or defects are not known, the syndrome of progressive myoclonic epilepsy may eventually be divided into a group of disorders rather than a specific disease. Essentially four types have been described: 1) the Unverricht variety characterized by recessive inheritance, severe course with early death, and Lafora bodies in the liver; 2) the Lundborg type characterized by recessive inheritance and a slower course; 3) the Hartung variety associated with autosomal dominant inheritance, variable course, and sensory neural hearing loss (Stern and Eldridge 1973); 4) an unclassifiably variable group (Vogel et al 1965, Vogel 1969). Both the fast and slow forms (the Unverricht and Lundborg types) may be present in the same family (Buscaino et al 1973). Diebold has classified an additional subtype, identified by degenerative changes of the central nervous system, slow progression, and an autosomal recessive inheritance, but this category is not clearly different from the Lundborg variation.

Metabolic disorders have been suggested in a variety of other myoclonic syndromes. Klein et al (1968) reported myoclonic epilepsy and retinitis pigmentosa in a family in which one member was found to have PAS-positive inclusions in several organs. In another patient (Guazzi et al 1973) with a progressive myoclonic syndrome, biopsy of her liver revealed evidence of a mucopolysaccharidosis. Finally, Chiofalo et al (1974) have studied several patients with a progressive myoclonic syndrome who had elevated plasma iron levels and iron present in several organs, including the central nervous system.

DIRECT EVIDENCE

The clinical data on the inheritance of epilepsy have often been inconsistent, but some generalizations may be offered. First, there are specific seizure types, most frequently the generalized seizures, which are inheritable to at least a small degree. A few seizure types, particularly febrile and photically induced seizures, are highly inheritable, with a large percentage of offspring and first degree relatives having the same disorder. On the other hand, except for benign rolandic epilepsy, the partial seizures do not appear to be strongly inherited and, in many instances, do not display an increased seizure risk among relatives.

Febrile Seizures

Febrile seizures frequently occur in the relatives of probands with febrile seizures, and a positive family history for individuals with febrile seizures ranges from 10% to 50% (Newmark and Penry 1980) (see Table 2-2). Frantzen et al (1970) found that 8.2% of the parents and 10.9% of the siblings of 2908 children with febrile seizures had a history of febrile seizures. In another study, 18% of 570 siblings of almost 1000 probands had febrile seizures (Ounsted et al 1966). In both studies, the seizure rate in siblings was high, but specific analysis could not be performed because of the lack of a control population. Tsuboi (1977) compared the relatives of probands with febrile seizures with a control population. In this important study, siblings of 450 children with febrile seizures were compared with the siblings of 620 randomly selected control children. The probands and the control children, who were 3 years of age, constituted 91% of the population of the area that was studied—a particular geographic region in Fuchu, Tokyo. Correcting for age, febrile seizures were present in 29.7% of siblings of probands with febrile seizures. The incidence of febrile seizures was only 6.2% among siblings of control children. Significantly, the incidence among siblings of probands reached 45% when two family members had febrile seizures. The incidence among siblings was higher also if one parent had a history of febrile seizures (36.5%) and lowest if neither parent had a history of febrile seizure (18%). The authors interpreted the findings to be most compatible with a multifactoral inheritance. A simple autosomal dominant inheritance was less likely because of the relatively low morbidity among siblings and parents, a morbidity that should reach 50% if this were the inherited pattern. However, as the authors mention, a simple autosomal dominant character might be explained if reduced penetrance is considered. The inheritance pattern may also differ from family to family.

Table 2-2
Febrile Seizures: Clinical Genetic Studies

Investigator	Percentage of Probands with Positive Family History	Percentage of Affected Siblings
Frantzen et al (1970)	50	10.9
Graveleau (1974)	21	
Herlitz (1941)	9.5	15.9
Hrbek (1957)	31	
Kagawa (1975)		19.9
Lennox (1949)	50	
Lupu et al (1971)	17	
Millichap et al (1960)	30	
Mollica et al (1973)	46	
Ounstead et al (1966)	41	17.9
Schiottz-Christiensen (1972)	14	
van den Berg (1974)		11.5

In addition to these family studies, there have been two major twin studies. Schiottz-Christiensen (1972) studied both monozygotic and dizygotic twins between the ages of 6 and 21 years with a history of febrile seizures. The co-monozygotic twins had a seizure rate of 31% in contrast with a 13.5% rate for the co-dizygotic twins. A prominent sex factor was observed: the female monozygotic twin pairs had the highest concordance rate (58%). In a second study conducted by Lennox-Buchthal (1971), monozygotic twins had a concordance rate of febrile seizures of 68%, in contrast with the 13% rate of dizygotic twins. If a pure autosomal dominant inheritance pattern existed for febrile seizures, the seizure frequency among monozygotic twins should be twice that of dizygotic twins. The findings in these studies, therefore, are not entirely consistent, as the first study supports an autosomal dominant pattern, whereas the second supports a polygenic inheritance. In any case, it is apparent that the development of febrile seizure is not a completely inheritable pattern, as some monozygotic twins do not develop the disorder. Tsuboi (1977a) has suggested that the inheritability of liability from febrile seizures is 75%; most patients will develop the disease on an inheritable basis, but others may be significantly influenced by the environment.

A recent investigation of the possible inheritance of febrile seizures has been conducted by Tay (1979). In this study of parents of children with febrile seizures and of control children, the dermatoglyphic patterns of the families were investigated. Dermatoglyphic patterns have a polygenic inheritance, and the final pattern is determined by the 19th week of gestation. Any environmental factor that may affect the dermatoglyphic abnormalities must, therefore, appear in early uterine life. Children with fewer than four febrile seizures had a high incidence of abnormal dermatoglyphic changes, which were also present in their parents but not in the control children or in the children with more than four febrile seizures. The authors concluded that two forms of febrile seizures exist: one form with a genetic factor, and a second, more severe form, without a genetic factor.

Photically Induced Seizures

A second major inheritable group of seizures are the photically induced seizures. Increased photosensitivity in relatives of photosensitive probands had been reported by many investigators (Newmark and Penry 1979). In many published pedigree studies (Schaper 1961, Haneke 1963, Aoki 1969), photically induced seizures have appeared in several generations of families. Additionally, all but 1 co-twin of 12 monozygotic twin pairs of patients with photically induced seizures had a photically induced EEG abnormality. For the one patient who did not exhibit a photoparoxysmal response EEG testing on another occasion demonstrated the abnormal photic response (Jeavons and Harding 1975). Watson and Marcus (1962) examined the relatives of 60 photosensitive probands; 50% of the mothers, 17% of the fathers, 45% of the siblings, and 32% of the offspring exhibited photoparoxysmal responses. Similarly, Schaper (1961) found that 43% of the 54 siblings of 57 probands were photosensitive. In both studies the EEG abnormalities are more common than the actual environmentally induced, photically induced seizures, which are quite rare. EEG photosensitivity in a man without photically induced seizures is shown in Figure 2-1.

An age factor is prominent in the development of photically induced EEG abnormalities and may affect genetic studies. Doose et al (1969) compared 160 siblings of 99 photosensitive children with a control group of 265 nonepileptic children. Photically induced spike-wave complexes were seen in 26% of the 145 siblings under 16 years of age, compared with only 6.8% of the control children. The highest percentage of abnormalities was in the 11- to 15-year-old age group, in which almost 30% of the children were affected. A sex factor may also be present, as more girls are photosensitive than boys. In another study by Doose and Gerken (1973a), 23% of the siblings of 208 photosensitive probands had a photoparoxysmal response, compared with 11% of the siblings of nonphotosensitive probands. If 15- to 16-year-old sisters of photosensitive probands are selected, over half showed photically induced EEG abnormalities.

22

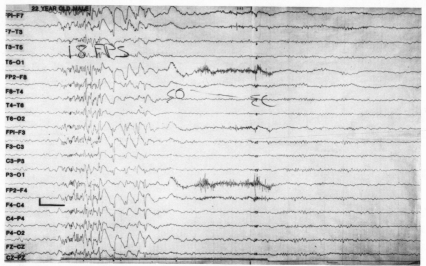

Figure 2-1 Response of a 22-year-old man without a history of photically induced seizures. The abnormal EEG response does not outlast the flicker stimulus (bottom channel).

Despite the frequent presence of EEG abnormalities, the seizure rate among the siblings of photosensitive probands is not high. In clinical analysis of 30 photosensitive siblings of nonepileptic, photosensitive probands, none of the siblings had developed a seizure (Doose and Gerken, 1973b). Although longitudinal studies have not yet been performed, it is likely that the photosensitivity will diminish as the siblings age. A slightly higher risk of seizure than in controls is present among photosensitive relatives of photosensitive probands who have seizures (Doose et al 1969), but the higher seizure rates in these relatives may be more closely associated with the associated seizures of the probands and not with photosensitivity.

Other sensory-evoked seizures may be inheritable, including eye-closure seizures, reading epilepsy, some startle-induced attacks, movement-induced dystonia, and paroxysmal choreoathetosis. These rare, but interesting, seizures are discussed in the chapter on sensory-evoked seizures.

Generalized Seizures

There have been several genetic studies of the generalized seizures, including studies of generalized tonic-clonic seizures and absence. Eisner et al (1960) and Tsuboi and Endo (1977) have conducted studies of large numbers of probands with generalized tonic-clonic seizure. In the Tsuboi and Endo study, 433 offspring of 130 probands with generalized tonic-clonic seizures, with or without an aura, were studied. The prevalence of either afebrile or febrile seizures in the offspring was 9.2%; the prevalence of afebrile seizures alone was 2.3%. Among the offspring of patients with generalized tonic-clonic seizures without an aura, 16.8% had either febrile or afebrile seizures and 4.7% had afebrile seizures alone. Because almost half the offspring were under the age of 10, these rates are underestimates and will increase upon later testing. A similar trend was observed by Eisner et al (1959): 5.26% of the close relatives (ie, siblings or parents) of the generalized tonic-clonic probands had afebrile seizures, in contrast with the considerably lower incidence of afebrile seizures (1.75%) in the control population. If the relatives of probands with afebrile seizure onset before the age of 4 are studied separately, a much higher epilepsy rate (8.3% compared with 1.45% in the control group) is seen.

This trend for higher seizure rates in probands with early onset seizure was also observed by Alstrom (1950) and Lennox (1947), who described a quadrupling of the seizure rate of relatives of probands with seizure onset before the age of 5, when compared with the relatives of probands with seizure onset after 20. These observations may be partially explained by three factors: 1) families of patients with early onset seizures may be more aware of the signs of seizures and may recognize the symptoms in other family members earlier; 2) probands with late onset seizures may not be able to obtain an accurate family history; 3) patients with late onset seizures are more likely to have seizures acquired from brain injury, attacks that are less likely to be inheritable.

Absence seizures have also been correlated with a positive family epilepsy history. Most studies, including those by Doose and Gerken (1972b), Eisner et al (1959), Jeras and Tividar (1973), and Matthes (1969), included all seizure types in the relatives, not specifically observed. Using these broad criteria, the seizure rate among the relatives varied from 3% to 10%, the higher rate being present in the siblings of female absence patients in the Doose and Gerken study. In a study that specifically investigated absence seizures in relatives of absence probands (Matthes and Weber 1968), 3% of the 232 siblings of 129 probands had absence seizures. In most studies, the closeness of the relationship is important in the determination of seizure rates of family members. More distant relatives have a lower seizure rate, a trend that may be secondary to either less accurate histories or to a genetic factor. As the seizure rate also drops for distant relatives in control populations, methodological considerations should be strongly evaluated.

Other seizure types have been associated with an increased familial history of epilepsy. From a review of the literature, Lacy and Penry (1976) have found that 1.5% of the 548 probands with infantile spasms have a family history of infantile spasms and that 8.5% have a family history of epilepsy. Degen et al (1972), in a study of the siblings and parents of patients with infantile spasms, found a family history of epilepsy in 10.8% of the probands. Because infantile spasms are a collection of disorders with multiple etiologies, some of which are genetic, the significance of a familial increase of epilepsy is unclear.

The Lennox-Gastaut syndrome, a condition that includes generalized and partial seizure types, has been examined by several investigators. Eisner et al (1959) did not find an increased risk for seizures in the families of probands with this syndrome, but other investigators have found a small, but significant, risk. Gastaut et al (1968) found a family history of epilepsy in 14% of probands after 25 years of following; Blume et al (1973) found a family history of epilepsy in 25% of probands; Doose et al (1970) found a family history of epilepsy in 56% of 50 probands. Five percent of the siblings' parents and grandparents had a seizure history in this latter study. Nevertheless, because of the lack of investigation of seizure rates of specific family members in the other studies, the significance of these increased rates is not known.

Generalized Seizures—EEG Studies

In addition to the preceding clinical epilepsy studies, generalized EEG epilep-

24

togenic abnormalities have also been analyzed. The photoparoxysmal response to flickering light is an inheritable pattern that is present in a high percentage of female siblings of photosensitive probands. The 3-per-second spike-and-wave complex, shown in Figure 2-2, has also been studied: 2.5% of 194 parents of absence probands and 10% of the siblings had generalized spike-and-wave complexes, as reported by Matthes and Weber (1968) and Matthes (1969).

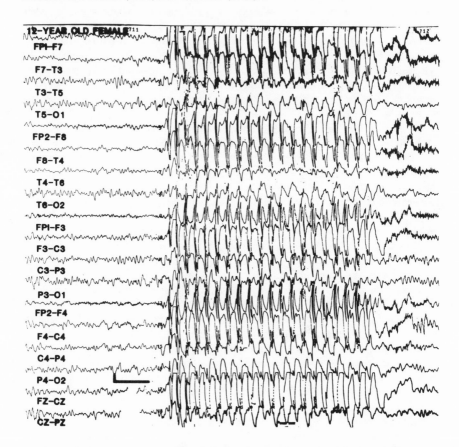

Figure 2-2 Three-hertz, generalized, spike-and-wave complexes in a girl with absence seizures.

In a series of reports by Metrakos and Metrakos (1961ab, 1969) and Metrakos et al (1966), the centrencephalic EEG pattern (defined as repetitive, generalized, spike-and-wave complexes) has been investigated. In the Metrakos studies, the centrencephalic pattern appeared in almost 50% of the siblings of the most susceptible age group (between 4 and 16 years). Seventy-eight percent of the parents and 37% of the siblings demonstrated this pattern. The specificity of the Metrakos studies is reduced by the high prevalence of abnormalities in the control population: 8.7% of controls had centrencephalic tracings and 15% had epileptiform activity in a population that did not have a high clinical seizure rate.

Partial Seizures

Patients with partial seizures and focal EEG abnormalities have usually not demonstrated as high a prevalence of a family history of epilepsy as patients with generalized abnormalities. Reports of studies of patients with partial seizures have revealed a prevalence of a positive family history that varies from 1% to over 50%. The wide range of prevalence of positive family histories may be explained by the variable ages of probands and relatives, the different seizure types, variable etiologies for the seizures, as well as possible inaccuracies in some of the family histories. Comparison with appropriate controls has rarely been performed. Reports of seizure rates in specific relatives have been only slightly more consistent, ranging from 1% (Penfield and Paine 1955) to approximately 10% (Ounsted et al 1966). Muller et al (1973) reported a seizure rate of 3% in 275 parents and 200 siblings of the proband children with partial seizures, a rate that contrasted with a 2% rate in control parents and siblings. The highest rates have been reported by Ounstead et al (1966), who identified a 15% seizure rate in siblings of probands with complex partial seizures and a 30% seizure rate in siblings of probands who had suffered status epilepticus. In this study, febrile seizures were common and status epilepticus was often associated with fever. The association of febrile seizures, inheritance, and complex partial seizure may be significant.

Andermann (1972), who has carefully investigated complex partial seizures in close relatives, found a seizure rate of 1.3%, which was only slightly higher than the control rate. Including single seizures, the seizure rate in relatives was 3.5%, a finding only slightly higher than the control rate of 2.9%. Eisner et al (1959) reported similar findings among relatives of patients with elementary partial seizures. The close relatives of the probands had a seizure rate of approximately 2.5%, a rate indistinguishable from that of the control population. However, in another report, Holowach et al (1958) found a history of epilepsy in 28% of the close relatives of 95 children with Jacksonian seizures. Blom et al (1972) and Shu (1975) have investigated the families of patients with the relatively benign seizure disorders associated with centrotemporal spikes and found a prevalence of a positive family history of 25%.

Thus, partial seizures in children may be slightly inheritable, but the evidence supporting this conclusion is not strong and the genetic influence is less than that in generalized seizures. Seizures associated with centrotemporal spikes and those arising after childhood febrile seizures are the more likely forms of partial seizures to be inheritable.

Partial Seizures—EEG Studies

The available EEG studies of focal probands have stressed anterior temporal and midtemporal spike foci. Andermann (1972) examined the relatives of 60 probands that underwent seizure surgery in Montreal. Although the relatives frequently had abnormal EEGs, almost 21% of the control population had abnormal tracings; and the significance of the findings is unclear. In studies of the midtemporal or centrotemporal spikes by Bray and Wiser (1964, 1965ab), similar discharges were present in 36% of the siblings and offspring of the probands and in 19% of the parents. Both rates were considerably higher than that found in controls. In another study by Heijbel et al (1975), 34% of the siblings but only 3% of the parents had centrotemporal spikes. Not all the patients in these studies had a history of seizures, so the significance of this EEG finding for epilepsy has not been completely established.

Seizures with Known Etiology

Seizures secondary to a known cause have not shown as strong a hereditary pattern as seizures without a known cause (see Table 2-3). Almost all studies of patients having seizures with a known cause have not compared the findings with control populations.

Table 2-3
Seizures of Known Cause: Clinical Genetic Studies

Investigator	Seizure Cause	Relatives	Percentage of Affected Relatives
Cobb (1932)	Head injury	Not specified	1.4
Conrad (1937)	Not specified	Offspring	1.62
Eisner et al (1959)	Not specified	Not specified	2.2
Harvald (1951)	Not specified	Siblings	1.2
Harvald (1954)	Not specified	Close relatives	1.0
Lennox (1951)	Not specified	Close relatives	1.8
Meyer et al (1976)	Ethanol withdrawal	Close relatives	1.3
Rimoin and Metrakos (1963)	Convulsive disorder and hemiplegia	Close relatives	2.04

Hemiplegic children with seizures have been reported to have a high percentage of affected relatives with seizures than do hemiplegic children who are free of seizures (Rimoin and Metrakos 1963). In another study, seizures associated with smallpox vaccinations had a familial pattern (Doose et al 1968), but this finding may be partially secondary to the precipitation of febrile seizures, which, as mentioned earlier, may be inheritable.

The inheritability of seizures induced by trauma has been vigorously debated (Pampus and Seidenfaden 1974). Walker (1962) investigated American soldiers who received significant head injuries in World War II and found positive family histories of epilepsy more frequently for patients who developed seizures than for those who did not. Evans (1962) similarly reported a family history of epilepsy in 7% of 80 posttraumatic seizure patients compared with a family history of epilepsy in 2% of those patients who did not develop seizures. Hoeppner et al (1973) have proposed a mechanism for the increased family history by suggesting that posttraumatic seizures are secondary to genetic factors that also cause exaggerated, hypertrophied scar and keloid formation.

MECHANISM

The mechanism of the inheritance of epilepsy is still unclear. No single metabolic abnormality has been associated with a specific seizure type, although a number of metabolic disorders have, as previously mentioned, been associated with seizures. Goodman et al (1980) have suggested that taurine transport may be abnormal in patients with seizures. In their studies of 41 patients, plasma taurine concentrations were relatively elevated and urinary taurine output was relatively reduced in comparison with control. Not all epileptic patients had elevated taurine concentrations or reduced taurine output, but approximately one-half of the patients demonstrated these findings. However, some epileptic patients had low plasma taurine and high taurine excretion, and approximately 12% of normal, nonepileptic individuals had the high plasma taurine concentrations more typically present in the epileptic patients. The relationship of antiepileptic medication to taurine metabolism is unclear, and conclusions about the significance of taurine metabolism for the inheritance of epilepsy are not yet possible.

Other investigators have used HLA antigen analysis to help investigate seizure patients. Initial reports were performed by Smeraldi et al (1975), who observed an increased HLA-7 prevalence in patients with the Lennox-Gastaut syndrome. Eeg-Olofsson et al (1982) have investigated HLA antigens in children with different types of seizures. These authors have found that in children with centrotemporal spikes (benign epilepsy of childhood) both the probands and parents have a relatively decreased prevalence of haplotype A1, B8. In addition, a similar but less significantly, reduced prevalence was found in children with absence seizures. The authors concluded that this HLA haplotype was a marker for a protecting gene; no evidence for a "disease" gene was found. The number of studies with HLA typing and seizures, however, has been quite low, and the usefulness of this genetic tool will not be determined until further studies can be performed.

CONCLUSION

Whether the genetics of epilepsy is important is a highly interesting question that has not been answered. A few seizures have been well correlated with an increased familial risk, but the mechanisms of inheritance and genetic patterns have largely been unavailable. It is reasonable, however, to expect that future developments with HLA typing, the identification of biochemical markers of disease, improved diagnostic criteria for EEG abnormalities and epilepsy, as well as improved epidemiological techniques, will bring a greater understanding of the inheritance of epilepsy.

BIBLIOGRAPHY

Alstrom CH: A study of epilepsy in its clinical, social and genetic aspects. *Acta Psychiatr Neurol Scand* (suppl) 1950;63:1–284.
Andermann ED: *Focal Epilepsy and Related Disorders: Genetic, Metabolic, and Prognostic Studies*, thesis. McGill University, Montreal, 1972.
Andermann ED, Remillard GM, Goyer C, et al: Genetic and family studies on Friedreich's ataxia. *Can J Neurol Sci* 1976;3:287–301.
Aoki Y: A clinical-electroencephalographic study on photosensitive epilepsy, with special reference to visual evoked potential. *Folia Psychiatr Neurol Jpn* 1969;23:103–119.
Blom S, Heijbel J, Bergfars PG: Benign epilepsy of children with centro-temporal electroencephalographic foci. Prevalence and followup study of forty patients. *Epilepsia* 1972;13: 609–619.
Blume WT, David RB, Gomez MR: Generalized sharp and slow wave complexes. Associated clinical features and long term followup. *Brain* 1973;96:289–306.
Bray PF, Wiser WC: Evidence for a genetic etiology of temporal-central abnormalities in focal epilepsy. *N Engl J Med* 1964;271:926–933.
Bray PF, Wiser WC: Hereditary characteristics of familial temporal-central focal epilepsy. *Pediatrics* 1965a;36:207–211.

Bray PF, Wiser WC: The relation of focal to diffuse epileptiform EEG discharges in genetic epilepsy. *Arch Neurol* 1965b;13:222–238.

Buscaino GA, Guazzi GC, Barbieri FA, et al: Ultrastructural and histochemical studies on the Unverricht Lundborg syndrome. Description of a family from the south of Italy. *Acta Neurol* 1973;28:291–322.

Chiofalo N, Fuentes A, Muranda M: Progressive myoclonus epilepsy associated with a disorder of iron metabolism. *Neurochiruga* 1974;32:71–77.

Cobb S: Special article. Causes of epilepsy. *Arch Neurol Psychiatr* 1932;27:1245–1263.

Conrad K: Erbanlage und epilepsie. IV. Ergebnisse einer nachkommenschaftsuntersuchung an epileptikern. *Z Gesamte Neurol Psychiatr* 1937;159:521–581.

Degen R, Arnold H, Brahn H: The genetics of infantile spasms. *Schweiz Arch Neurol Neurochir Psychiatr* 1972;110:189–203.

Doose H, Gerken H: The genetics of EEG anomalies. *Handbook of Electroencephalogr Clin Neurophysiol* 1972a;15:14–18.

Doose H, Gerken H: On the genetics of EEG-anomalies in childhood. IV. Photoconvulsive reaction. *Neuropaediatrie* 1973a;4:162–171.

Doose H, Gerken H: Possibilities and limitations of epilepsy prevention in siblings of epileptic children, in Parsonage MJ (ed): *Prevention of Epilepsy and Its Consequences*, proceedings of the Fifth European Symposium on Epilepsy, London, England, July 17–19, 1973b, pp 32–35.

Doose H, Eckel U, Volzke E: Convulsions after smallpox vaccination. *Z Kinderheilk* 1968; 103:214–236.

Doose H, Gerken H, Leonhardt M, et al: Centrencephalic myoclonic-astatic petit mal. Clinical and genetic investigations. *Neuropaediatrie* 1970;2:59–78.

Doose H, Gerken H, Volzke G, et al: Investigations of the genetics of photosensitivity. *Electroencephalogr Clin Neurophysiol* 1969;27:625.

Dustman RE, Beck EC: The visually evoked potentials in twins. *Electroencephalogr Clin Neurophysiol* 1965;19:570–575.

Eeg-Olofsson O, Safwenberg J, Wigertza T: HLA and epilepsy: An investigation of different types of epilepsy in children and their families. *Epilepsia* 1982;23:27–34.

Eisner V, Pauli LL, Livingston S: Hereditary aspects of epilepsy. *Bull Johns Hopkins Hosp* 1959;105:245–271.

Eisner V, Pauli LL, Livingston S: Epilepsy in the families of epileptics. *J Pediatr* 1960;56: 347–354.

Evans JH: Post-traumatic epilepsy. *Neurology (Minneap)* 1962;12:665–674.

Frantzen E, Lennox-Buchthal M, Nygaard A, et al: A genetic study of febrile convulsions. *Neurology* 1970;20:909–917.

Gastaut H: On genetic transmission of epilepsies. *Epilepsia* 1969;10:3–6.

Gastaut H, Tassinari CA, Roger J, et al: Juvenile epileptic encephalopathy associated with diffuse slow spike wave activity ("atypical petit mal"; Lennox syndrome). *Recenti Prog Med* 1968;45:117–146.

Gayral L, Gayral J: Epilepsy and hereditary spinocerebellar degeneration. *J Genet Hum* 1969; 17:127–136.

Gerken H, Doose H: On the genetics of EEG anomalies in childhood. II. Occipital 2-4/s rhythms. *Neuropaediatrie* 1972;3:437–454.

Goodman HO, Connolly BM, McLean W, et al: Taurine transport in epilepsy. *Clin Chem* 1980;26:414–419.

Graveleau D: Febrile convulsions. *Concours Med* 1974;96:5773–5785.

Guazzi GC, Ghetti B, Barbieri F, et al: Myoclonus epilepsy with cherry red spot in adult: A peculiar form of mucopolysacchridosis. A clinical, genetical, chemical, and ultrastructural study. *Acta Neurol* 1973;28:542–548.

Haneke K: Iber drei Falle latenter und manifester photogener Epilepsie in einer Familie. *Kinderaerztl Prax* 1963;31:149–156.

Harvald B: On the genetic prognosis of epilepsy. *Acta Psychiatr Neurol* 1951;26:339–357.

Harvald B: *Heredity in Epilepsy. An Electroencephalographic Study of Relatives of Epileptics.* Copenhagen, Ejnar Munksgaard, 1954.

Heijbel J, Blom S, Rasmuson M: Benign epilepsy of childhood with centrotemporal EEG foci: A genetic study. *Epilepsia* 1975;16:285–293.

Herlitz G: Studient uber die sogennanten initialen Fieberkramphe bei Kindern. *Acta Paediatr Scand* 1941;29(suppl 1):1–142.

Hoeppner T, Morrel F, Hoeppner JA: Skin scarring and post-traumatic epilepsy. *Neurology (Minneap)* 1973;23:437.

Holowach J, Thurston DL, O'Leary J: Jacksonian seizures in infancy and childhood. *J Pediatr* 1958;52:670–686.

Hrbek A: Febrile convulsions in childhood. *Ann Paediatr Basel* 1957;188:162–182.

Jeavons PM, Harding GFA: *Photosensitive Epilepsy. A Review of the Literature and a Study of 460 Patients.* London, William Heinenmann Medical Books, 1975.

Jeras J, Tividar I: *Epilepsies in Children.* Hanover, New Hampshire, University Press of New England, 1973.

Kagawa K: A genetic study of febrile convulsions. *Brain Dev* 1975;7:369–384.

Klein D, Mumenthaler M, Kraus-Ruppert R, et al: A large family of Valais affected with progressive myoclonic epilepsy and with retinitis pigmentosa. Clinical, genetic, and pathologic study. *Humangenetik* 1968;6:237–252.

Lacy JR, Penry JK: *Infantile Spasms.* New York, Raven Press, 1976.

Lennox MA: Febrile convulsions in childhood. A clinical and electroencephalographic study. *Am J Dis Child* 1949;78:868–882.

Lennox WG: The genetics of epilepsy. *Am J Psychiatry* 1947;103:457–462.

Lennox WG: The heredity of epilepsy as told by relatives and twins. *JAMA* 1951;146:529–536.

Lennox WG, Gibbs EL, Gibbs FA: The brain-wave pattern, an hereditary trait. Evidence from 74 "normal" pairs of twins. *J Hered* 1945;36:233–243.

Lennox-Buchthal M: Febrile and nocturnal convulsions in monozygotic twins. *Epilepsia* 1971; 12:147–156.

Lupu I, Macovei Lupu M, Cocinschi R, et al: Febrile infantile convulsions. Electroclinical contributions. *Electroencephalogr Clin Neurophysiol* 1971;30:360–361.

Lykken DT, Tellegen A, Thorkelson K: Genetic determination of EEG frequency spectra. *Biol Psychol* 1974;1:245–259.

Matthes A: Genetic studies in epilepsy, in Gastaut H, Hasper H, Bancaur J, Waltregny A (eds): *The Physiopathogenesis of the Epilepsies.* Springfield, IL, Charles C Thomas Publisher, 1969, pp 26–30.

Matthes A, Weber H: Clinical and electroencephalographic family studies in pyknolepsies. *Dtsch Med Wochenschr* 1968;93:429–435.

Metrakos JD, Metrakos K: Genetic studies in clinical epilepsy, in Jasper HH, Ward AA, Pope A (eds): *Basic Mechanisms of the Epilepsies.* Boston, Little Brown & Co, 1969, pp 700–708.

Metrakos JD, Metrakos K, Polizos P, et al: Genetics and ontogenesis of the centrecephalic EEG. *Electroencephalogr Clin Neurophysiol* 1966;21:404.

Metrakos K, Metrakos JD: Genetics of convulsive disorders. II. Genetics and electroencephalographic studies in centrencephalic epilepsy. *Neurology* 1961a;11:414–483.

Metrakos K, Metrakos JD: Is the centrencephalic EEG inherited as a dominant. *Electroencephalogr Clin Neurophysiol* 1961b;13:289.

Meyer JG, Holzinger H, Urban K: Epileptic seizures in alcoholic predelirium. Clinical and electroencephalographic studies on the differentiation of genetic conditioned attack predisposition and epilepsy. *Nervenarzt* 1976;47:375–379.

Millichap JG, Madsen JA, Alldort LM: Studies in febrile seizures. V. Clinical and electroencephalographic study in unselected patients. *Neurology (Minneap)* 1960;10:643–653.

Mollica F, Mazzone D, Pavone L: The familial incidence of febrile convulsions. *Clin Pediatr (Phila)* 1973;28:1–8.

Muller K, Arnold H, Bruhn B, et al: Familial predisposition in focal epilepsy. *Schweiz Arch Neurol Neurochir Psychiatr* 1973;113:45–55.

Newmark ME, Penry JK: *Photosensitivity and Epilepsy. A Review.* New York, Raven Press, 1979.

Newmark ME, Penry JK: *Genetics of Epilepsy. A Review.* New York, Raven Press, 1980, p 122.

Noebels JL: Analysis of inherited epilepsy using single locus mutations of mice. *Fed Proc* 1979;38:2405–2410.

Ounsted C, Lindsay J, Norman R: Biological factors in temporal lobe epilepsy, in *Clinics in Development Medicine #22.* London, The Spastics Society Medical Education and Information in association with William Heinemann Medical Books, Ltd, 1966.

Pampus I, Seidenfaden I: Posttraumatic epilepsy. *Fortschr Neurol Psychiatr* 1974;42:329–384.

Penfield W, Paine K: Results of surgical therapy for focal epileptic seizures. *Can Med Assoc J* 1955;73:516–531.

Petersen I, Akesson HO: EEG studies of siblings of children showing 14 and 6 per second positive spikes. *Acta Genet* 1968;18:163–169.

Rimoin DL, Metrakos JD: The genetics of convulsive disorders in the families of hemiplegics. Proceedings of the Second International Congress of Human Genetics 1963;3:1655–1658.

Rodin EA: Familial occurrence of the 14 and 6/sec positive spike phenomenon. *Electroencephalogr Clin Neurophysiol* 1964;17:566–570.

Rust J: Genetic effects of the cortical auditory evoked potential: A twin study. *Electroencephalogr Clin Neurophysiol* 1975;39:321–327.

Schaper G: Familiares workommen der Photosensibilitat, in Janzen R (ed): *Klinische Elektroencephalographie, 7. Kongress der Deutschen EEG-Gesellschaft.* Berlin, Springer-Verlag, 1961, pp 129–133.

Schiottz-Christiensen E: Genetic factors in febrile convulsions. An investigation of 64 same sexed twin pairs. *Acta Neurol Scand* 1972;48:538–546.

Seyfried TN: Audiogenic seizures in mice. *Fed Proc* 1979;38:2399–2404.

Seyfried TN, Tu RK, Glaser GH: Genetic analysis of audiogenic seizure susceptibility. C57BL/6J × DBA/2J recombinant inbred strains of mice. *Genetics* 1980;94:197–210.

Shu S: Polyphasic spike or spike and wave complexes occurring in the Rolandic region in children. *J Nagoya Med Assoc* 1975;97:141–146.

Skre H: A study of certain traits accompanying some inherited neurological disorders. *Clin Genet* 1975;8:117–135.

Smeraldi E, Scorza-Smeraldi R, Cazzullo CL, et al: A genetic approach to the Lennox-Gastaut syndrome by the "major histocompatibility complex" (MHC), in Janz D (ed): *Epileptology.* Proceedings of the Seventh International Symposium on Epilepsy. Berlin (West), June 1975, Thieme, Berlin, 1975, pp 33–37.

Stern RS, Eldridge R: Clinical and genetic study of the progressive myoclonic epilepsies. *Neurology (Minneap)* 1973;23:420.

Tay JS: Dermatoglyphics in children with febrile convulsions. *Br Med J* 1979;1:660.

Temkin O: *The Falling Sickness. A History of Epilepsy from the Greeks to the Beginnings of Modern Neurology,* ed 2. Baltimore, Johns Hopkins Press, 1971.

Tsuboi T: Genetic aspects of febrile convulsions. *Hum Genet* 1977;38:169–173.

Tsuboi T, Endo S: Incidence of seizures and EEG abnormalities among offspring of epileptic patients. *Hum Genet* 1977;36:173–189.

van den Berg BJ: Studies on convulsive disorders in young children. IV. Incidence of convulsions among siblings. *Dev Med Child Neurol* 1974;16:457–464.

Vogel F: The EEG of genetically different types of inherited myoclonic epilepsy. *Electroencephalogr Clin Neurophysiol* 1969;26:444.

Vogel F, Hafner H, Iebold K: Genetic studies on progressive myoclonus epilepsies. *Humangenetik* 1965;1:437–475.

Walker AE: Post-traumatic epilepsy. *World Neurol* 1962;3:185–194.

Watson CW, Marcus EM: The genetics and clinical significance of photogenic cerebral electrical abnormalities, myoclonus and seizures. *Trans Am Neurol Assoc* 1962;87:251–253.

CHAPTER 3

Electroencephalography in Infantile and Childhood Epilepsy

Soo Ik Lee

The electroencephalogram in infants and children normally varies in parallel with growth, development, and maturation of the brain. As the brain grows rapidly during intrauterine life and the infantile period, with neuronal migration, myelination, and synapse formation, age-related EEG changes are remarkable and are commensurate with the baby's conceptional age. Normal EEG patterns continue to change or mature throughout the rest of the patient's childhood.

Clinical manifestations of epilepsy vary with the patient's age, and different types of clinical seizures could be the variable, age-related expression of the same underlying cause. Neonatal seizures are more often subtle, multifocal, and tonic. Infantile spasms occur mostly during the latter half of infancy and continue to approximately 4 years. Absence seizures commonly begin in early childhood and are uncommon in adults, as is epileptic encephalopathy of childhood, or Lennox-Gastaut syndrome. Sylvian seizures are most common in early childhood and are hardly seen after the age of 15. Typical grand mal seizures are never observed in newborns; they occur after development of synchronizing mechanisms between the cerebral hemispheres. The age-related epileptic patterns are related not only to maturation of the brain but also to underlying etiological factors that have an age-specific occurrence.

The EEG is a physiological measure of the normal and the diseased brain; it reflects maturational changes of the cerebral function and age-related pathological alterations. The EEG manifestations of infantile and childhood epilepsy largely depend on the type of seizures, the patient's age, and the underlying cause. In this chapter, electroencephalograms in infantile and childhood epilepsy are treated in their chronological order, and salient electroencephalographic and clinical features and their correlations are discussed.

Electroencephalographic examination is essential in the initial evaluation of seizure disorders in patients of any age; it also is extremely valuable in the management and follow-up of epilepsy. Electroencephalograms provide supportive evidence for clinical diagnosis of epilepsy by demonstration of epileptic discharges, although normal EEGs do not exclude the presence of a seizure disorder. Fortunately, epileptic discharges are more readily recordable in infantile or childhood epilepsy. Electroencephalograms are valuable in the classification of epilepsy and in the selection of specific anticonvulsant drugs in given patients because they show the originating focus or foci of characteristic epileptic patterns. Electroencephalograms are particularly useful in childhood epilepsy because of the variable expression of epileptic activity, such as hypsarrhythmia, classic 3-Hz spike-and-wave

34

discharges, the protean nature of neonatal seizure activity, slow spike-and-wave discharges, and rolandic spikes. Electroencephalograms offer little direct information regarding pathological changes but are still able to provide suggestive evidence for the underlying cause, such as focal delta activity in space-occupying lesions or focal destructive processes, generalized polymorphic delta activity in diffuse encephalopathies, periodic discharges (either focal in herpes encephalitis or generalized in SSPE), focal spikes in focal atrophic or very slowly progressive lesion, and focal suppression in acute or extensive damage of the brain tissue (Figure 3-1). Electrocephalograms are of prognostic value as to control of the seizures, intellectual development of the patient, or quality of life in certain types of seizures. They are useful in the follow-up of epileptic patients for detection of altered epileptic pattern, changes in site and number of epileptic foci, progression of underlying organic changes, or development of new lesions. They can be used to judge the efficacy of therapy in certain types of seizures, and long-term recording or intensive monitoring procedures can be effectively used for this purpose. They are useful in differentiating pseudoseizures from genuine ones, even though one has to recognize the limitations of surface recording.

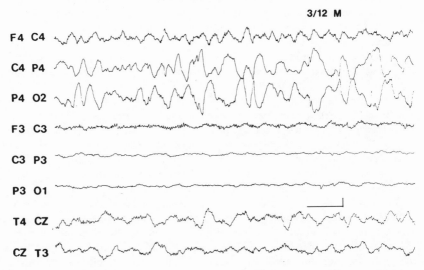

Figure 3-1 Focal delta and spike activity at the right parietal area and suppression of the left hemispheric activity. The 3-month-old boy had evacuation of bilateral subdural hematoma 8 days before this EEG; he had left hemiparesis and right-sided focal seizure. Calibration in all figures in this chapter: 50 μV and 1 second.

The routine EEG does not always demonstrate epileptic activity. In Ajmone Marsan and Zivin's (1970) study, only 56% of the patients showed epileptic activity in their first EEG; an additional 26% showed epileptic activity on subsequent recordings. The authors identified factors related to occurrence of epileptic discharges in EEG; these factors include 1) sampling effect or value of multiple recordings; 2) age of the patient—the younger the patient the better the possibility of recording epileptic activity; 3) type of seizure—absence and temporal lobe seizures more often demonstrating epileptic discharges; 4) frequency of seizures—the patients with more frequent seizures being more likely to show positive EEG; and 5) medication effect. Therefore, a normal EEG in a patient with clinical evidence of a seizure disorder does not exclude a diagnosis of seizure disorder, and repeat recordings should be requested. If the resting EEG fails to demonstrate epileptic activity, activation procedures (such as hyperventilation, photic stimulation, sleep or sleep deprivation, and pharmacological activation) increase positive yield. Special electrodes, such as nasopharyngeal and sphenoidal electrodes, enhance recording of epileptic activity of mesiobasal temporal or orbital frontal origin. Long-term recording, telemetry, and video-monitoring techniques increase the chance of recording epileptic discharges, particularly ictal activity, and help to provide clinical and electrographic correlation of epileptic and nonepileptic spells.

NEONATAL SEIZURES

Neonatal seizures are commonly observed in the newborn units and are distinguishable in their clinical and EEG manifestations from seizures of childhood and adults. The clinical seizures frequently observed at this age may be classified as subtle, focal clonic, multifocal clonic, tonic, or myoclonic seizures (Volpe 1973), or as focal clonic, fragmentary or migratory, tonic, myoclonic, or minimal seizures (Lombroso 1978, Rose and Lombroso 1970). Some of these seizure types are difficult to differentiate from clinical manifestations of active sleep, a jittery baby born to a mother who abused drugs, simple jaw tremor, or apneic episodes. On the other hand, some seizures may be manifested only by changes of respiration, heart rate, or skin color. Fortunately, neonatal seizures are often accompanied with EEG changes that are readily recordable, hence increasing the utility of EEG in the diagnosis of neonatal seizures. Furthermore, etiological diagnosis can be enhanced by administration of certain therapeutic agents, such as glucose, calcium, or pyridoxine, during EEG monitoring (Rose and Lombroso 1970, Werner et al 1977, Lombroso 1978). Electrographic seizures are rare before 32 weeks of conceptional age but become common by term. Electroencephalograms are of significant prognostic value for quality of subsequent life in neonatal seizures.

The electroencephalograms of neonatal seizures are quite different or bizarre compared with those of childhood and adult epilepsy. The seizure discharges during the ictal stage can be brief trains or longer runs of rhythmic activity of any frequency— delta, theta and alpha—or rhythmic sharp waves, spikes, or mixed sharp and slow waves. They are almost always focal or multifocal rather than generalized. Generalized or diffuse discharges may occur, but wave-to-wave bisynchrony is hardly seen and unilateral diffuse paroxysmal discharges can be observed. Classic, generalized, spike-and-wave activity is never seen and hypsarrhythmia is extremely rare (Ellingson 1979). Even in the seizures due to metabolic encephalopathies, such as hypoxia, hypoglycemia, or hypocalcemia, focal or multifocal epileptic discharges are more common rather than diffuse ones. Repetitive focal seizure activity could be observed in focal organic lesions such as congenital anomaly, but focal or multifocal epileptic activity in the neonatal period does not necessarily signify the presence of multiple or focal structural changes. The location of discharging foci may change on serial follow-up EEGs. It is not unusual to observe two, or even three, independent focal electrographic or ictal seizure discharges, which occur simultaneously or overlap one another. The wave forms of the ictal discharges are protean and variable even in the same recording session (Figure 3-2a and b).

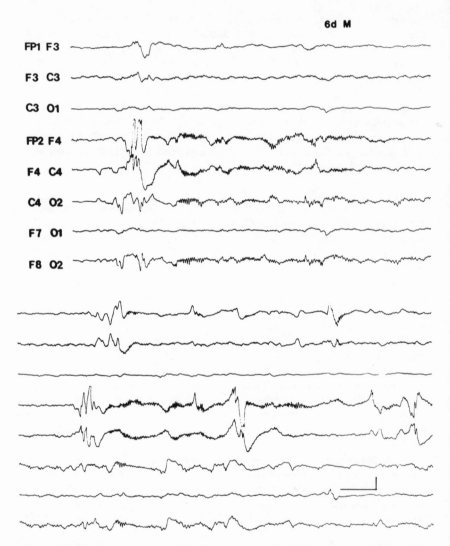

6d M

FP1 F3

F3 C3

C3 O1

FP2 F4

F4 C4

C4 O2

F7 O1

F8 O2

Figure 3-2A Neonatal seizure in a 6-day-old boy who had perinatal asphyxia. Pattern shows independent, bilateral, multiphasic, sharp waves followed by low-amplitude fast activity. Both Figure 3-2A and B illustrate protean multifocal seizure discharges in neonatal seizures.

Lombroso (1978) classified EEGs of neonatal seizures into the following five categories:

1. Normal EEG, which carries a good prognosis.

2. Unifocal EEG pattern, which is characterized by high-voltage trains of sharp waves originating locally and only slowly involving other areas around the focus and which occasionally appears in the homotopic areas of the opposite hemisphere. These are accompanied by concordant peripheral manifestations—usually clonic

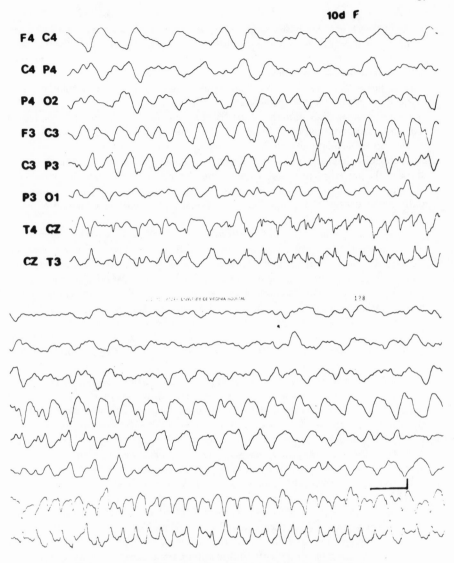

Figure 3-2B Neonatal multifocal (Cz, C3, C4) independent electrographic seizure discharges in a 10-day-old girl.

movement of the contralateral parts of the body. Well-organized background activity is present in the preictal or interictal EEGs. The pattern carries equivocal prognosis, and the patients with normal interictal background generally do better. According to one study (Monod and Dreyfus-Brisac 1972), 50% of the patients were normal, 30% were left with serious neurologic problems, and 20% died.

3. Multifocal EEG, which has an abnormal background activity interictally. During the ictal stage, the epileptic discharges may originate from one area and may

spread to another area, or discharges of one frequency may start over one part of the brain and reappear at a different part of the brain. On some occasions, the discharge may occur simultaneously and independently in different parts of the brain. Such EEG patterns are accompanied with clinical fragmentary, myoclonic, minimal, or tonic types of seizures. The combination of these EEG and clinical manifestations frequently indicates a poor prognosis.

4. Paroxysmal EEG pattern, which is characterized by the presence of higher voltage paroxysmal bursts of irregular discharges separated by a period of almost isoelectric or very low amplitude EEG, approaching suppression-burst pattern. The interictal EEG has an abnormal background. Clinical seizures are quite similar to those of the preceding category, showing fragmentary, myoclonic, tonic, or minimal seizures. This pattern carries a poor prognosis, and some of the patients with this pattern may evolve into a hypsarrhythmic pattern later, with development of infantile spasms.

5. Low-voltage or a flat EEG pattern consisting of a low-voltage, sometimes almost isoelectric, pattern interrupted here and there by a few flurries of disorganized activity of discharges, which may be low in amplitude and slow in frequency and which often occur over one part of the brain but sometimes reappear in another part. This pattern occurs in children with severe brain insult such as hypoxia, intraventricular hemorrhage, bacterial meningitis, subdural hematoma, and profound dysgenetic malformations. The pattern usually carries a poor prognosis.

As it is suggested in the preceding discussion, interictal background activity is more closely related to prognosis than are seizure discharges (Monod and Dreyfus-Brisac 1972, Werner et al 1977, Lombroso 1978, Tharp 1980). A summary by Werner et al (1977) of previous studies revealed that 1) seizure activity with interictal "flat," paroxysmal (burst-suppression), or slow backgrounds carries a grave prognosis; 2) rhythmic activity in the theta band superimposed on a low-voltage background carries a grave prognosis; 3) slow activity on a low-voltage background is correlated with an unfavorable outcome when recorded in the first month of life in the term infant; 4) multifocal spikes on a depressed background carries a grave prognosis; 5) absence of sleep organization for 2 to 3 days in association with seizures may be indicative of an unfavorable prognosis. These findings indicate that, in addition to ictal EEGs, one has to record interictal tracings to come up with an understanding of the total picture. According to some authors (Monod and Dreyfus-Brisac 1972), the clinical seizures that are not accompanied with epileptic EEG changes bear the worst prognostic significance, and the electrographic seizure without clinical seizures are of poor prognosis in 89% of patients. In the latter circumstance, one has to be careful that subtle or atypical clinical seizure manifestations are not overlooked as is frequently the case in fragmentary, minimal, or subtle seizures. Electroclinical parallelism in neonatal seizure carries a favorable prognosis compared to the aforementioned cases, and 28% of the patients had normal development.

Interictal paroxysmal discharges such as repetitive spikes may occur unilaterally or bilaterally in neonatal seizures. Spikes in neonatal seizures have long duration and a slow rate and must be differentiated from the normal sharp transients of premature infants and neonates. Spikes occurring in groups in a repetitive fashion or spikes occurring during the low-amplitude phase of the alternating pattern (trace alternant) or discharges occurring during active sleep are more significant (monod and Dreyfus-Brisac 1972, Engel 1975). In premature infants and neonates, the significance of some isolated spikes or sharp waves is not clear and they must be interpreted conservatively. Some authors claim that rolandic positive spikes, which are observed uniquely in neonates, are manifestations of intraventricular hemorrhage (Cukier et al 1972, Werner et al 1977, Ellingson 1979), but they also are observed in other clinical conditions (Tharp 1980).

HYPSARRHYTHMIA AND INFANTILE SPASMS

Hypsarrhythmia [hypsi (Greek), "high" or "lofty"] was first described by Gibbs and Gibbs (1952). It is a specific EEG pattern characterized by profoundly disorganized mixtures of continuous high-amplitude slow waves with spikes and sharp waves of varying amplitude and morphology. The spikes and sharp waves do not have a constant relationship with slow waves; they originate from multiple independent areas of both hemispheres (Figure 3-3). The pattern tends to become bisynchronous and intermittent during sleep. It is an age-related pattern; onset of this pattern usually occurs during the second half of the first year, mostly after 2 months of age, and is rare after the age of 5. It is accompanied by clinical massive infantile spasms in approximately 90% of the cases (Jeavons and Bower 1974, Lacy and Penry 1976, Kurokawa et al 1980). Friedman and Pampiglione (1971) demonstrated that 26% of their patients with hypsarrhythmia had other forms of seizures; this group of patients had poor prognosis. Not all patients with infantile spasms demonstrate hypsarrhythmia in their EEG, particularly in the early stage of the illness. Electroencephalograms may be normal during the first few months of life; the patterns may then develop minor focal abnormalities (such as focal sharp waves), then multifocal spikes, and finally evolve into typical hypsarrhythmia (Watanabe et al 1973). With clinical seizures, the EEG may show generalized high-amplitude sharp and slow wave discharge or "electrodecremental" activity (Bickford and Klass 1963) with or without preceding high-amplitude paroxysmal slow waves or sharp-and-slow-wave

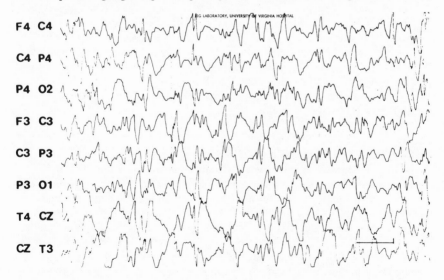

Figure 3-3 Hypsarrhythmia in an 18-month-old girl with infantile spasms. From Dreifuss and Lee (1981). Reproduced with permission from Medical Examination Publishing Co.

complexes. The electrodecremental activity consists of a sudden attenuation of all activity, which may or may not be overlapped with low-amplitude fast activity in the 20-Hz range. The sharp-and-slow-wave complexes are usually associated with single myoclonic jerks, whereas electrodecremental activity tends to be accompanied by longer lasting massive flexion spasms (Bickford and Klass 1963).

Hypsarrhythmia is often due to severe insult to the developing brain in approximately 60% of the cases and may occur de novo in the remainder; the latter cases carry a better prognosis (Lacy and Penry 1976). A large variety of etiological factors have been described and include tuberous sclerosis (Pampiglione and Moynahan 1976), anoxic insult, mongolism, microcephaly, trauma, pyridoxine dependency or deficiency, phenylketonuria, encephalitis or meningitis, and congenital anomaly (Kurokawa et al 1980, Jeavons and Bower 1974). "Hemihypsarrhythmia" involving one hemisphere was described in association with hemimegalencephaly (Tjiam et al 1978) and Aicardi's syndrome, ie, a combination of multiple congenital malformations and infantile spasms (Aicardi et al 1969). The characteristic EEG pattern in Aicardi's syndrome was described as "multifocal epileptiform abnormalities occurring on a burst-suppression pattern showing complete asynchrony between the two hemispheres." Six months after onset of the symptoms, the EEG tends to show multiple epileptic foci with a severely disorganized background (Fariello et al 1977).

Hypsarrhythmia has unfavorable prognostic significance for intellectual development, even though it may improve or disappear with treatment, or spontaneously, as the patient becomes older. The hypsarrhythmic pattern may improve and become normal or it may change into other epileptic patterns, such as multifocal spikes and slow spike-and-wave discharges (Watanabe et al 1973, Friedman and Pampiglione 1971, Jeavons et al 1973). With clinical improvement of infantile spasms accompanying ACTH therapy, hypsarrhythmia also improves or disappears. Total sleep and REM periods significantly decrease in infantile spasms, and REM sleep increases with ACTH treatment (Hrachovy et al 1981). Electroencephalograms are generally of little value in identifying underlying causes or in predicting outcome for patients with hypsarrhythmia. In rare cases of pyridoxine dependency or deficiency, one may see prompt improvement after intravenous administration of pyridoxine (Saunders and Westmoreland 1979). Lombroso and Fejerman (1977) described an unusual group of patients who were 3 to 8 months old and who demonstrated clinical infantile spasms with a normal EEG; these patients recovered completely without an intellectual dysfunction.

CLASSIC 3-HZ SPIKE-AND-WAVE
DISCHARGES AND ABSENCE SEIZURES

The first description of the classic 3-Hz spike-and-wave pattern and its clinical correlation with absence seizures was made by Gibbs et al (1935). The discharge suddenly occurs, usually from a normal background, as generalized, bisynchronous, high-amplitude spike-and-wave (Figure 3-4). The frequency of the spike-wave complex is usually 3 Hz, but tends to be faster (3.5–4 Hz) at the beginning of the discharge and is slower (2–2.5 Hz) at the end. The activity is generalized and has the highest potential field at the frontal regions in most patients, although amplitude dominance at the posterior head region can be observed in younger children. The discharge can be multiple spikes or multiple-spike-waves at the beginning (Figure 3-5). Weir (1965) carefully studied the morphology of spike-wave complexes in the

EEG tracings of 200 patients and concluded that it was complex. It seemed that the most common sequence of events in the individual spike-wave complex consists of a small (25–50 μV), short-duration (10 msec), negative spike, followed by a prominent positive transient from which the second larger amplitude, longer duration (30–90 msec), negative spike takes origin. These are superimposed on a more consistently present, positive transient that occurs 5–10 msec before the first negative peak and that may last from 100 to 150 msec and blend into the final negative slow wave, which lasts from 200 to 500 msec. The first negative spike is maximal at the centrotemporal regions in one-half of the cases and anywhere else in the others. The second negative spike is maximal at the frontal regions and the final negative slow wave is maximal at the frontoparietal areas. The discharge lasts for a variable interval and abruptly ceases with little postictal changes except in a case of absence status or prolonged discharges. Absence seizures may not necessarily be accompanied by classic 3-Hz spike-and-wave activity; and the spike-and-wave discharge could be "atypical" in its frequency, wave form, and topography. In a small number of patients, clinical spells are accompanied by generalized, high-amplitude, rhythmic, 3-Hz activity. Rarely, the clinical absence may be accompanied by 8- to 20-Hz rhythmic waves, or a superimposition of the two rhythms may occur, forming a sawtooth pattern on the EEG (Blume 1982). In some cases, generalized rhythmic fast activity may be followed by spike-and-wave discharges; in others, it may occur following very brief spike-and-wave activity (Figure 3-6).

The spike-and-wave discharges are activated by hyperventilation in a high percentage of patients with absence seizures and are frequently accompanied by clinical attacks (Dalby 1969). In some patients, the activation may occur after only a few deep breaths, whereas, in others, prolonged or repeated hyperventilation is required. Therefore, if an initial 3 minutes of hyperventilation fails to produce spike-

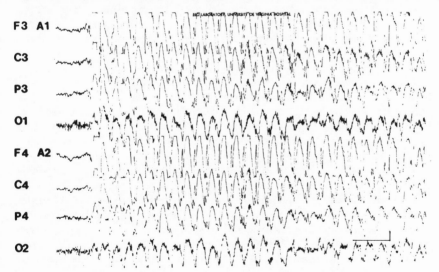

Figure 3-4 Classic, generalized, 3-Hz spike-and-wave activity in an 8-year-old boy with absence seizures. From Dreifuss and Lee (1981). Reproduced with permission from Medical Examination Publishing Co.

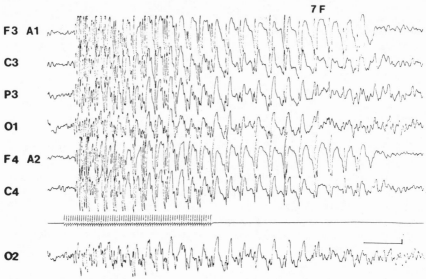

Figure 3-5 Photoparoxysmal response overlasting photic stimulus in a 7-year-old girl with absence seizure. Seventh channel: stimulation marker.

and-wave activity, repeated hyperventilation of 3 to 5 minutes needs to be attempted. Adams and Lueders (1981) reported that 5 minutes of controlled hyperventilation was more reliable than a 6-hour recording as a predictor of clinical seizure frequency in seven patients with poorly controlled absence seizures.

The photoparoxysmal responses to photic stimulation are most commonly observed in absence seizures. According to Reilly and Peters' (1973) study of 132 persons, three types of abnormal responses were recorded. 1) Prolonged: Epileptiform complexes or paroxysmal slow-wave activity, which overlast the stimulus (Figure 3-5) in 54 patients (among whom 50 had a history of convulsive disorder). In seven patients, EEGs were otherwise normal, and five of these had a history of seizures. 2) Self-limited: A similar response, which ceases during stimulation, occurred in 56 patients. Twenty-nine had a seizure disorder, including 23 with an otherwise normal EEG, and 8 of whom had seizures. 3) Flash dependent: Discharges time-locked to the flash occurred in nine patients. Only one had a history of seizures and four of the nine had an otherwise normal EEG with no history of seizures. Doose et al (1969) reported generalized spike-and-wave activity induced by photic stimulation in 3.4% of normal subjects and 19% of siblings of patients with photoparoxysmal responses. Only 10% of the latter subjects had clinical seizures. These data indicate that photoparoxysmal responses are supportive but not diagnostic evidence of seizure disorder.

The spike-and-wave discharges are reactive to different stages of sleep (Ross et al 1966, Sato et al 1973). The discharge rate of spike-and-wave activity progressively increases with deep stages of NREM sleep and is highest during the first sleep cycle. The discharge duration and discharge interval shortens as sleep deepens. During stages I and II of sleep, regular or irregular spike-and-wave complexes occur singly or in bursts of more than two; in stage II, spike-and-wave complexes occur with some periodicity in the discharge pattern. In stages III and IV, polyspike and irregular slow-wave patterns become prominent and are less than 3 Hz in frequency;

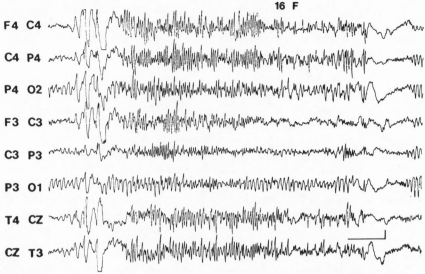

16 F

F4 C4

C4 P4

P4 O2

F3 C3

C3 P3

P3 O1

T4 CZ

CZ T3

Figure 3-6 Clinical absence attack in a 16-year-old girl with generalized fast rhythm preceded by spike-and-wave burst. She spontaneously opened her eyes and remained unresponsive during this discharge.

the spike component increases in number and the wave component becomes longer in duration and distorted in configuration. In stage IV, a preponderance of high-voltage slow waves are interspersed with numerous spikes or multiple spikes. In REM sleep, the morphology of spike-and-wave discharges is similar to that of the waking state, but discharge duration becomes shorter. The spike-and-wave discharges are reactive to eye opening and closure in some cases. Eye opening frequently attenuates or inhibits the discharge, and eye closure may activate it, although the reverse can be observed in rare instances. Alerting or concentration-seeking procedures tend to decrease the spike-and-wave discharges. The discharge rate of spike-and-wave activity, as with clinical absence spells, may change depending on the time of day; it is preferable to record an EEG at the time when the patient is supposed to have more frequent clinical spells.

During absence status, the EEG reveals generalized spike-and-wave activity that may be continuous or intermittent. The activity may be rhythmic, with a frequency of 3 Hz; but it is more commonly irregular at a frequency of 2 to 3 Hz. Multiple spikes are common, and rhythmic slow waves are occasionally found. External stimuli, such as calling the patient's name, making a loud noise, or forcibly opening the patient's eyes may cause momentary cessation of the discharges. Spontaneous changes in the frequency or wave forms of the discharges may be accompanied by clinical changes, such as more obvious myoclonus or interruption or mistakes in counting (Andermann and Robb 1972).

The presence of generalized spike-and-wave activity in the resting record or generalized spike-and-wave activity induced by hyperventilation is strong evidence for the presence of generalized seizure disorder; 97% to 98% of such cases are proved to have generalized seizures (Blume 1982). Eeg-Olofsson et al (1971) found no spike-and-wave activity in the resting record of 743 normal children; and only two of these children demonstrated spike-and-wave discharges during hyperventilation. On the other hand, spike-and-wave activity, even classic, is not found exclusively in patients with absence seizures. The incidence of clinically apparent absence seizures in different series ranges from 26% (Silverman 1954) to 70% (Clark and Knott 1955). However, detailed study of auditory reaction time demonstrated that any spike-wave paroxysm, regardless of duration, can impair consciousness (Browne et al 1974). Penry et al (1975) carefully studied clinical manifestations of absence seizures by using simultaneous recording of video tape and EEG. Only 9.4% of the seizures were simple absence; others most often contained, in order of prevalence, either automatisms, mild clonic components, or decreased postural tone, or a combination of two or more of these features. There was significant correlation between length of seizures and occurrence of automatisms, the latter being seen in almost one-half of seizures lasting more than 6 seconds and in 90% of seizures lasting more than 12 seconds. According to Browne et al (1974), auditory reaction time was normal at the onset of generalized spike-wave paroxysms in only 43% of the tests, and was normal at 0.5 second after onset of the discharge in only 20% of the tests. After 4 seconds of paroxysms, reaction time was normal in 52% of the tests, and responsiveness quickly returned after paroxysms. The degree of impairment markedly decreased when the spike-wave discharge was fully generalized. Typical spike-and-wave activity with normal EEG background is more commonly seen in the cryptogenic variety of absence seizures and is usually accompanied by a favorable prognosis; this is particularly true in cases of early onset absence seizures (Greer and Andriola 1978).

Genetic factors in "centrencephalic" seizures with 3-Hz spike-and-wave discharges were studied by Metrakos and Metrakos (1966, 1974). They observed that siblings of probands with centrencephalic seizure had 4.5 times as high an incidence (45%) of epileptiform dysrhythmia as siblings of normal control subjects (10%). The difference was mainly due to higher incidence (37%) of centrencephalic EEGs in siblings of epileptic probands than in the control group (6%). Similarly high incidence (35%) of centrencephalic EEG changes were found in the offspring of the probands. The penetrance or clinical manifestation of the EEG trait was found to be age dependent, with a high risk period between the ages of 4.5 and 16.5 years. From these studies, they concluded that the inheritance of contrencephalic seizure or 3-Hz spike-and-wave activity is due to an irregular dominant gene with age-dependent penetrance.

ELECTROENCEPHALOGRAM IN OTHER GENERALIZED SEIZURES

Electroencephalograms of other generalized seizures are not unique for children. In grand mal seizures, the ictal recording is characterized by commencement of generalized, low-amplitude, fast activity of rapidly increasing amplitude and decreasing frequency, which becomes generalized, high-amplitude continuous, polyspike activity accompanied by the tonic phase. The subsequent generalized, high-amplitude, bisynchronous, spike-and-wave activity corresponds with clinical clonic seizure and is followed by postictal diffuse slowing and suppression of normal activity. The postictal changes last for various periods depending on the severity of the attacks. As in the partial seizures, it is not unusual to see brief electrodecremental activity at the commencement of generalized electrographic seizure discharge.

Interictal EEG manifestations of grand mal seizures are variable and may include brief paroxysms of generalized, rhythmic, 3-Hz spike-and-wave discharges, irregular spike-and-wave paroxysms (Figure 3-7), generalized multiple spike-and-wave

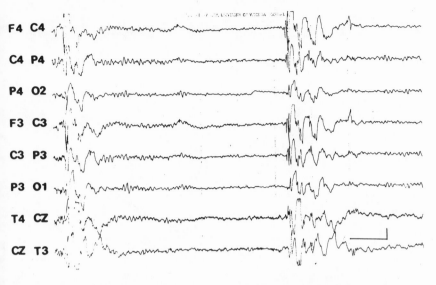

Figure 3-7 Intermittent brief episodes of generalized multiple spike-and-wave discharges in a 23-year-old female with absence and grand mal seizures. From Dreifuss and Lee (1981). Reproduced with permission from Medical Examination Publishing Co.

discharges, or generalized spike, sharp-wave, or multiple-spike discharges or even high-amplitude, paroxysmal, slow-wave activity. The patients with certain focal or multifocal interictal spikes or sharp waves may preferentially manifest generalized or grand mal seizures, presumably by secondary generalization. This phenomenon is often observed in patients with nocturnal seizures and in those who have bilateral foci or epileptic activity.

In generalized myoclonic seizures, brief paroxysms of generalized multiple spike or multiple spike-and-wave discharges are most common (Figure 3-8), frequently accompanied by clinical myoclonic jerks.

In atonic or akinetic seizures, generalized spike-and wave, multiple spike-and-wave, slow spike-and-wave, and electrodecremental activities can be seen.

SLOW SPIKE-AND-WAVE AND LENNOX-GASTAUT SYNDROME

Gibbs and co-workers (1939) noted that some patients with seizure disorder demonstrated spike-and-wave discharges that were different from those of classic petit mal or 3-Hz spike-and-wave activity. They called the pattern "petit mal variant." Gibbs and Gibbs (1952) asserted that the differences were a frequency of 1.5 to 2.5 Hz instead of 3 Hz, a slanting down-slope of the slow waves of the spike-and-wave discharges instead of a round, dome shape, and irregularity of the discharges. Lennox and Davis (1950) reemphasized different clinical seizure patterns accompanying the petit mal variant compared to those with classic spike-and-wave paroxysms, with high incidence of intellectual impairment and intractable seizures. Gastaut et al (1966) reviewed 100 cases of slow spike-and-wave activity or petit mal variant EEG. They found that a large number of the patients did have mixed forms of seizures and demonstrable organic cerebral changes. They found that these pa-

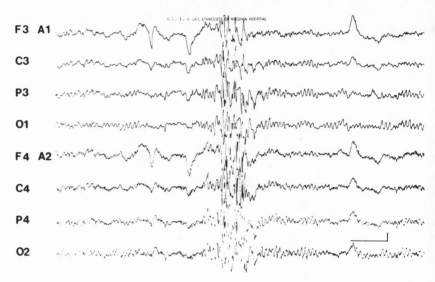

Figure 3-8 Brief discharges of generalized, multiple spikes in a 15-year-old girl with myoclonic seizure. From Dreifuss and Lee (1981). Reproduced with permission from Medical Examination Publishing Co.

tients were suffering from a severe form of childhood epilepsy that is refractory to treatment and is characterized by 1) frequent tonic seizures and a variant of petit mal absences; 2) pronounced mental retardation; 3) interictal EEG records showing pseudorhythmical (1.5–2.5 Hz) diffuse slow spike-and-wave activity. They proposed the term "childhood epileptic encephalopathy with diffuse slow spike-waves" or "Lennox syndrome." Since then, this EEG and clinical entity has been variously known as Lennox syndrome, Lennox-Gastaut syndrome, childhood epileptic encephalopathy, and centrencephalic myoclonic-astatic petit mal.

The EEG in this condition (Gastaut et al 1966, Blume et al 1973, Markand 1977) is characterized by generalized or diffuse 1.5- to 2.5-Hz, irregular, spike-and-wave or sharp-and-slow-wave complexes, which occur as frequent or even almost constant discharges. Both spike and slow-wave components are of longer duration, the former being 100–200 msec and the latter being approximately 350 msec, in comparison with the classic 3-Hz spike-and-wave activity of absence seizures (Figure 3-9). Hence, the terms *slow spike-and-wave* and *sharp-and-slow-wave complexes* were used for their description in addition to *petit mal variant*. The background activity is generally slow, and the degree of slowing has some correlation with mental retardation. It is not uncommon to see focal or multifocal sharp waves and slow waves in addition. The slow spike-and-wave discharges are accentuated during sleep, particularly in REM stage, while their activation by hyperventilation and photic stimulation is less significant than that of typical 3-Hz spike-and-wave discharges. The ictal EEG changes are hard to recognize at times. According to Markand (1977), two main types of EEG changes were observed with the seizures: 1) ictal hypersynchronous EEG activity that was associated with high-amplitude, 1- to 2.5-Hz, bisynchronous, slow spike-and-wave activity lasting 10 to 30 seconds and

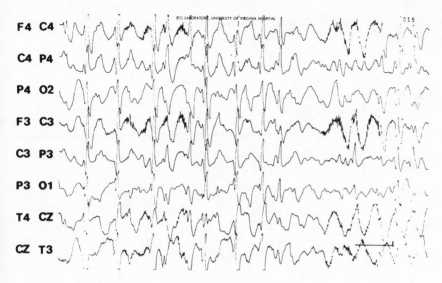

EEG LABORATORY, UNIVERSITY OF VIRGINIA HOSPITAL

Figure 3-9 Slow spike-and-wave activity in a 6-year-old boy with Lennox-Gastaut syndrome. From Dreifuss and Lee (1981). Reproduced with permission from Medical Examination Publishing Co.

that was typically seen during absence attacks; 2) ictal desynchronization of EEG activity that was the most common EEG change associated with clinical seizures, occurring predominantly with myoclonic and tonic seizures and also probably with atonic seizures. During myoclonic seizures, electrodecremental activity or flattening of the EEG activity occurred either with or just following the jerk and lasted 1–2 seconds, but the association was inconsistent. During tonic seizures and some myoclonic seizures, desynchronization of longer duration was observed. The EEG showed sudden disappearance of spike-wave activity with a short period of flattening lasting 1 to 2 seconds; then generalized or focal rhythmic activity appeared and was followed by gradual resumption of spike-wave activity.

The incidence of this pattern is greatest between 2 and 6 years of age, rarely being seen after age 15. Some (5–25%) of the patients with this disorder may have had hypsarrhythmia when they were younger (Daly 1979), and some demonstrated hypsarrhythmia during sleep. Some patients showed multifocal spike activity before development of slow spike-wave activity, and others demonstrated multifocal epileptic activity on follow-up EEGs (Markand 1977). These findings suggest a close relationship among the EEG patterns of hypsarrhythmia, slow spike-and-wave discharges, and independent, multifocal, spike discharges.

There is some disagreement on the incidence of seizure types in slow spike-and-wave activity, but tonic, absence, and major motor seizures seem to be the most common ones, followed by myoclonic, atonic, and focal or multifocal seizures. Most studies confirmed the earlier assertion of Lennox and his co-workers that the slow spike-and-wave pattern carries a poor prognosis for seizure control, intellectual development (85% to 90% mental retardation), and survival rate (88% after 12 years) (Daly 1979).

MULTIPLE INDEPENDENT SPIKE FOCI, SEIZURES, AND INTELLECTUAL IMPAIRMENT

The multiple independent spike foci are defined as "epileptiform discharges (spikes, sharp waves, or both) which, on any single recording, arise from at least three noncontiguous electrode positions with at least one focus in each hemisphere" (Blume 1978). The pattern can occur at any age but is more commonly observed in children, with peak incidence between the ages of 4 and 7 years (Noriega-Sanchez and Markand 1976). The EEG is characterized by abnormally slow and disorganized background activity in 97% of the patients. The spike-and-sharp-wave discharges occur from both hemispheres and are most common (83%) at the temporal areas, followed by (in order of decreasing frequency) occurrence at the occipital, central, frontal, and parietal areas (Figure 3-10). Sleep recording significantly accentuated the epileptic discharges and elucidated new foci. Normal sleep activity, including sleep spindles, was absent, poorly developed, or asymmetric. Hyperventilation and photic stimulation seldom activated any additional abnormality. Previous EEG studies show hypsarrhythmia in 15.9% of the patients and slow spike-and-wave activity in 11.3% (Noriega-Sanchez and Markand 1976).

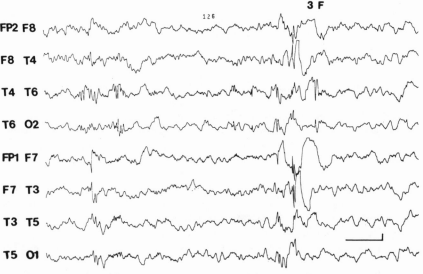

Figure 3-10 Multiple, bilateral, independent spike foci in a 3-year-old girl with staring spells.

The clinical findings were quite similar in the two studies by Noriega-Sanchez and Markand (1976) and Blume (1978). Seizure disorder was present in 84% to 94.4% of the patients, and the most common type of seizure was generalized tonic-clonic seizure, with or without other types of seizures, in 63% to 92%. Other types of seizures consisted of absence, myoclonic, focal motor, and partial complex seizures. Approximately one-half of the patients had more than one type of seizures. The frequency of seizures varied considerably from patient to patient, but 84% had two or more seizures per week in one series and one-half of the cases had daily seizures in another. Intellectual impairment was observed in 68% to 82.3% of the patients.

Subnormal intelligence was correlated with age of seizure onset, neurologic findings, incidence of spikes in the recording, number of spike foci, and presence of excessive delta activity. Seizure onset before the age of 2, abnormal neurologic findings, more than one spike per 10 seconds, ten or more epileptic foci, and excessive amounts of background delta activity were almost invariably accompanied by intellectual impairment.

Probable etiological factors included various prenatal, perinatal, and postnatal insults, including infections, hydrocephalus, and trauma. Noriega-Sanchez and Markand (1976) felt that "independent multiple spike discharges constitute a distinct electrographic entity with a definable clinical correlation." However, it has to be emphasized that the pattern is caused by a wide variety of static and progressive encephalopathies and is not specific to any particular pathological entity.

Hypsarrhythmia, slow spike-and-wave activity, and multiple independent spike foci patterns of EEG could be age-dependent, variable, electrographic expressions of the same static or progressive neurologic disorders. This statement is based on the facts that successive transition from multiple spike foci to hypsarrhythmia, then to slow spike-and-waves and to multiple independent spike discharge in a same patient has been observed and that clinical expression of all three patterns are similar in that they are commonly accompanied by intractable forms of mixed seizure disorders, intellectual impairment in a high percentage of patients, and abnormal neurologic findings suggesting diffuse cerebral affections.

CENTROTEMPORAL SPIKES AND BENIGN FOCAL EPILEPSY OF CHILDHOOD (ROLANDIC SPIKES AND SYLVIAN SEIZURES)

Clinical correlations of rolandic spike discharges were initially and simultaneously described by Bancaud et al (1958) and Nayrac and Beaussart (1958). The correlations have been confirmed and further clarified by many subsequent studies. The syndrome is a common form of childhood epilepsy; it is characterized by temporocentral spike foci, mostly nocturnal generalized seizures of probable focal onset and diurnal partial seizures referable to the lower rolandic area, lack of intellectual impairment or neurologic findings, and benign prognosis.

The EEG pattern has been variously called "rolandic spikes" (Bancaud et al 1958), "midtemporal spikes" (Gibbs and Gibbs 1960, Lambroso (1967), and "centrotemporal spike foci" (Lerman and Kivity 1975). The pattern typically consists of high-amplitude, biphasic, slow spikes that are followed by single slow waves. It is localized at the centrotemporal areas and is synchronous at the central and temporal regions (Figure 3-11). At the temporal area, the potential field is maximal at the midtemporal region, in contrast to the anterior temporal location of psychomotor seizures. At the central area, the spikes occur more at the inferior central rather than at the superior central area. The spikes occur unilaterally in approximately two-thirds of the patients and bilaterally in the remainder. In the latter cases, the spikes are asynchronous, with different amplitude and frequency of discharges. In unilateral discharges of the interictal EEG, the clinical partial seizures may not necessarily be on the contralateral side because the laterality of spikes shifts between EEG recordings. The discharges are usually frequent and may occur in clusters, although clinical seizures are rare. No correlation was found between the intensity of the spike discharges in the EEG and the frequency, length, and duration of the seizures. In a small number of patients (5–7%), in addition to the centrotemporal

50

spikes, generalized spike-and-wave discharges may occur, usually during hyperventilation, photic stimulation, and sleep. During sleep, the spike discharges are augmented and may become bisynchronous. In REM sleep, they remain abundant and tend to be unilateral. The ictal discharges are not well studied because clinical seizures commonly occur in the night. Dalla Bernardina and Tassinari (1975) reported a case in which nocturnal seizure commenced as 20- to 30-μV, 12-Hz activity at the left temporocentroparietal area. The background activity of wake and sleep recordings are characteristically normal. The EEGs normalized within a period ranging from 6 months to 6 years (Lerman and Kivity 1975).

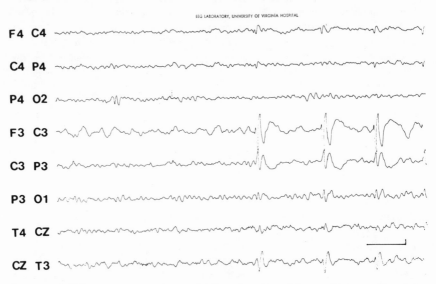

Figure 3-11 Right centrotemporal or rolandic spikes in a 4.5-year-old boy with sylvian seizures. From Dreifuss and Lee (1981). Reproduced with permission from Medical Examination Publishing Co.

The clinical seizures occur exclusively during sleep in 76% of patients, during both wake and sleep in 17%, and only during wakefulness in 7% (Lerman and Kivity 1975). The nocturnal seizures are reported as generalized tonic-clonic seizures with or without facial twitching. They may be of focal onset but may not be noticed by others until they become generalized. They also may be associated with drooling or excessive salivation and vomiting. The seizures during the waking state are mostly partial seizures, with twitching at the corner of the mouth, drooling, and inability to speak; full consciousness is retained. In a small number of patients, paresthesias of the cheek, chin, gums, and tongue were reported.

The syndrome occurred in 14.4% of childhood epileptics, with age of onset at 3 to 13 years (mean, 9.9 years) (Lerman and Kivity 1975). The seizures are easily controlled with anticonvulsant medications and disappear by puberty, being hardly seen after age 15. Beaussart and Faou (1978) studied evolution of epilepsy with rolandic paroxysmal foci in 324 cases and found that there was no significant difference between treated and untreated patients with extremely favorable prognosis. They even proposed the possibility of avoiding all medications. Neurologic examinations and other diagnostic procedures are usually normal, and intellectual impairment is not observed. Genetic studies (Heijbel et al 1975) demonstrated that the centrotemporal spike foci are inherited as an autosomal dominant trait with age-dependent penetrance, similar to findings in 3-Hz or "centrencephalic" spike-and-wave discharges.

OTHER FOCAL EPILEPTIC DISCHARGES AND PARTIAL SEIZURES

Interictal focal epileptic discharges consist of spikes, sharp waves, spikes and waves, or paroxysmal slow waves. Spikes are sharp, transient, and stand out from the background activity; they have a duration of 20 to 70 msec. Sharp waves have the same characteristics, except that their duration is 70 to 200 msec (Chatrian et al 1974). Focal ictal discharges or electrographic seizure activity usually commence as low-amplitude rhythmic activity, most commonly having a frequency range of 13 to 30 Hz and less commonly of 4 to 12 Hz; the low-amplitude rhythmic activity progressively increases its amplitude and decreases its frequency (Figure 3-12). The activity may spread to adjacent areas or become widely distributed (Figure 3-13). The discharges then change into spike-wave or slow-wave activity, which gradually decreases in frequency and gives way to postictal suppression or slowing. Quite often, interictal spikes or sharp-wave discharges decrease or abruptly cease just before the onset of rhythmic fast activity and may be replaced by focal or generalized flattening of the ongoing activity (Geiger and Harner 1978). The ictal activity may be of low amplitude and may become barely recordable from the scalp electrodes in some partial simple seizures.

Scarpa and Carassini (1982) studied 261 patients aged 1 to 13 years with partial seizures. Most of them (73%) had single foci, and 19% had multiple foci. General-

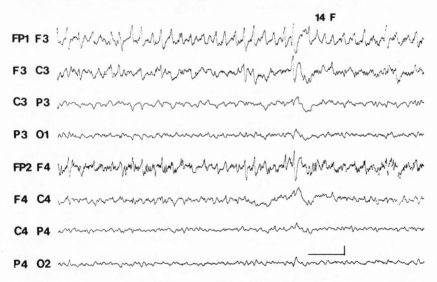

Figure 3-12 Focal electrographic seizure at the left frontopolar region with spread to the right side in a 14-year-old girl. Seizure consists of blank stare, eye deviation to the right, twitching of right face or upper extremities, and fearful expression with jitteriness.

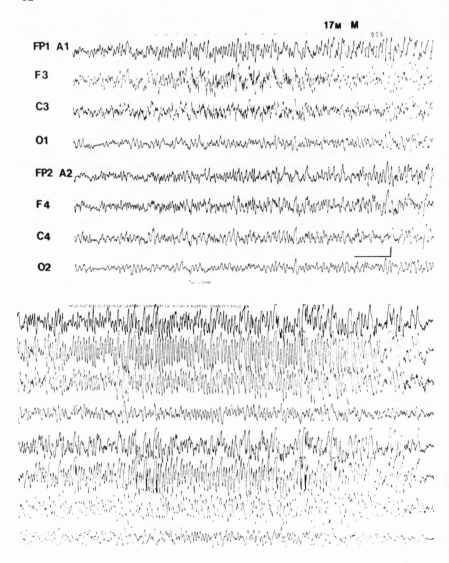

Figure 3-13 Left frontal seizure activity rapidly becoming generalized in a 17-year-old boy.

ized abnormality was found in 27% and a normal EEG in 4%. Temporal foci were most frequent (44%), followed by rolandic foci (32%) and occipital foci (30%). They observed migration of EEG foci and modification of EEG findings in 73% of their follow-up studies. Focal seizures in children generally had favorable prognosis, particularly so in patients with nonfocal EEG findings. In longitudinal studies of 242 children with spike foci, Trojaborg (1968) demonstrated pronounced variations of spike foci with respect to their localization and number of involved areas. Localization changes were observed in 85%, and a change from one focus into two or multiple foci on repeat EEG was observed in more than two-thirds of the children. He cautioned that spike discharges in children are of limited value as an indicator of focal cortical damage unless serial EEGs over many years show consistent focal abnormality. Location of the epileptic focus in EEG generally corresponds with type of clinical seizures. However, interictal spike focus does not necessarily correspond with originating site of seizures (Gloor 1975). Daly (1979) summarized the significance of focal spikes in children as a) having high association with clinical seizures; b) probably associated with structural disease of the brain in patients without clinical seizures; and c) having rare occurrence in normal children.

Focal epileptic EEG discharges in children may not necessarily be accompanied by clinical seizure disorders. Most of the spikes not associated with seizures in children are localized at the centrotemporal areas and, in smaller numbers, at the occipital region. These children have been referred with a variety of nonrelated complaints, such as headaches, bed-wetting, syncope, behavioral problems, and learning difficulties. In contrast to an earlier belief that these syndromes represented masked seizures or seizure equivalents (Green 1961, Kellaway et al 1965), more recent studies (Fois et al 1968, Cavazzuti et al 1980, Lerman and Kivity-Ephraim 1981) indicate that "these children are not to be considered as epileptic and should not be treated with anticonvulsant drugs." The latter opinions are based on benign prognosis demonstrated in longitudinal studies of these children and on the generally accepted benign nature of centrotemporal or rolandic spikes in children (see section on centrotemporal spikes).

OCCIPITAL SPIKES

Occipital spike foci are most commonly observed in children younger than 3 to 4 years of age; occipital spike foci gradually decrease as the children become older (Gibbs et al 1954, Smith and Kellaway 1964). The spikes may involve unilateral or bilateral occipital areas with or without involvement of the adjacent temporal and parietal regions (Figure 3-14). Rapid spread of occipital lobe seizure to the temporal lobe was documented in man and experimental animals (Babb et al 1981). The occipital spike discharges are more frequent when the patient's eyes are closed, and central vision seems to have an inhibitory effect on occipital lobe seizures (Panayiotopoulos 1981). The finding is interesting because of the fact that 19% of children with occipital spike foci have visual or ocular abnormalities, as reported by Smith and Kellaway (1964). Intermittent photic stimulation significantly activates interictal occipital discharges in 13% of patients, resulting in widespread paroxysmal activity and clinical seizure in some of them. Consistent asymmetry of photic driving was observed in 26% (Ludwig and Ajmone Marsan 1975).

A comprehensive study of 452 children with occipital spikes by Smith and Kellaway (1964) demonstrated protean clinical seizure patterns. Seizure occurred in 54% of the children with spike focus and 60% of the children with slow-wave focus. The most common seizure type was generalized tonic-clonic (40%); pure focal seizures were observed in 34%; generalized seizures with focal onset or focal features in 14%. There was an aura of flashing light in 24% and transient loss of vision in 9%. Nineteen percent of the patients with occipital spikes had ocular abnormalities, such as strabismus and congenital cataract. Only 34% of these children had seizures in contrast to the high incidence of seizures in the whole group. The study of clinical ictal pattern in epileptic patients with occipital spikes by Ludwig and Ajmone

54

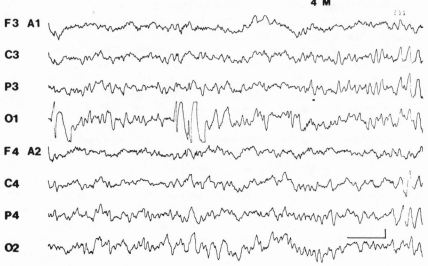

4 M

F3 A1

C3

P3

O1

F4 A2

C4

P4

O2

Figure 3-14 Left occipital spike focus in a 4-year-old boy.

Marsan (1975) again emphasized clinical pleomorphism. Even though motor manifestation was most common (53%) and visual symptoms were observed in 47%, epigastric, psychic, somatic, and other sensory phenomena were not infrequently observed. Focal motor seizures and partial complex seizures were frequent. They felt that synchronous bioccipital discharges may relfect a different type of seizure disorder because of different clinical manifestations, including lack of visual symptoms in all. However, they found no significant difference in clinical or ictal manifestations between patients with purely focal occipital involvement and those with temporal or temporoparietal spread (Figure 3-15).

TEMPORAL SPIKE FOCI

There has been increasing awareness that significant numbers of cases of temporal lobe epilepsy have their onset in childhood. The study of Ounsted et al (1966) of temporal lobe epilepsy in 100 patients less than 15 years of age demonstrated that the median age of onset was 5 years 4 months. Twenty-six percent of the patients studied by Currie et al (1971) had onset of their temporal lobe seizures before age 15, and 46% of Falconer's (1971) subjects developed their seizures during the first decade. Hughes and Olson (1981) demonstrated that peak incidence of posterior temporal and midtemporal epileptic discharges occurred between 6 and 10 years of age and that of anterior temporal and anterior/midtemporal epileptic discharges between the ages of 16 and 20 years. Both groups had a second peak at middle age.

The interictal temporal lobe spikes or sharp waves may occur unilaterally or bilaterally—in the latter case, either independently or bisynchronously (Figure 3-16). The bisynchronous discharges often are of mesiobasal temporal origin. The bilateral discharges occur more frequently in older patients (Hughes and Olson 1981). It is important to differentiate anterior temporal spikes from centrotemporal or rolandic spikes because of marked differences in their clinical manifestations and prognostic significance. The anterior temporal spikes seldom extend beyond the Sylvian fissure,

9 F

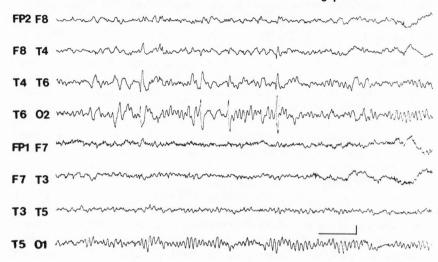

Figure 3-15 Right posterior temporal spike focus in a 9-year-old girl. The seizures consist of loss of vision, followed by loss of consciousness, shaking of all extremities, and postictal confusion.

being of maximum potential field at the anterior temporal or mesiobasal temporal region. Rolandic spikes are localized at the centrotemporal region with apparent originating focus at the lower rolandic area, and their potential field in the temporal lobe is maximal at the midtemporal region. Small sharp spikes and 14- and 6-Hz positive spikes also need to be differentiated from the anterior temporal spikes as they

13 F

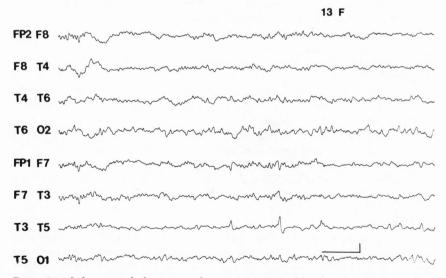

Figure 3-16 Left temporal sharp wave focus in a 13-year-old girl with partial complex, generalized, tonic-clonic, and absence seizures.

do not have specific correlation with seizure disorders (Klass 1975, Blume 1977).

The temporal spikes are best activated by sleep or sleep deprivation, and sleep recording following sleep deprivation seems to be even more effective. The activation occurs during NREM sleep, particularly the first through third stage, and occurs at different stages in different patients. Hyperventilation may also activate temporal lobe spikes even though it is not as effective as in patients with generalized spike-and-wave discharges. Photic stimulation may activate posterior temporal and occipital spike foci at lower frequency of stimuli as well as generalized discharges. The nasopharyngeal or sphenoidal electrodes are useful to record the spikes or sharp waves originating from the mesiobasal temporal or orbital frontal areas, which may or may not be recorded from the scalp electrodes and may be equivocal even when recorded.

The anterior temporal spikes are most commonly associated with clinical partial complex seizures. In a series of 666 patients of all ages having temporal lobe epilepsy, 92% of the patients showed temporal spike foci (Currie et al 1971). On the other hand, automatisms or partial complex symptoms occur most commonly in patients with temporal or frontal foci (60% to 80%), followed by occipital foci (40%) and centroparietal foci (25%) (Ajmone Marsan and Goldhammer 1973, Ludwig and Ajmone Marsan 1975).

In patients with persistent temporal spike foci and partial complex seizures, the underlying cause is frequently a statis one, such as mesial temporal sclerosis or hamartoma (Daly 1979). Blume (1982) emphasized that the possibility of a temporal spike representing a tumor must be considered if the patient is devoid of history for trauma, febrile convulsions, anoxia, and central nervous system infection and has refractory seizures.

MIDLINE PARASAGITTAL SPIKE FOCI

Tukel and Jasper (1952) reported the case of a man who showed generalized seizures and generalized spike-and-wave activity in his EEG and who was found to have a paramedian lesion. They first proposed the idea of secondary bilateral synchrony in the same paper. However, little attention has been paid to the midline parasagittal spike foci. According to the recent studies of Pedley et al (1981) and Ehle et al (1981), the midline parasagittal spikes appear to be predominantly indicative of childhood EEG abnormality. Among the 14 subjects of the first paper, 11 were 15 years old or younger, and all of the patients of the second paper were 3- to 12-year-old patients of a children's medical center.

The spikes were most commonly localized at the central vertex, followed by, in decreasing order, parietal vertex and frontal vertex. They may be confined at the midline or may spread to the adjacent parasagittal areas of one hemisphere. In approximately one-third of the EEGs, the midline spikes occurred exclusively during sleep. The background activity was diffusely or focally slow in approximately two-thirds of the patients. On follow-up studies, the longest persistence of midline spikes was 3 years.

Seizures were the most common clinical manifestation (71%; 91%). The remaining patients had migraine or headache, mental retardation of unknown cause, and premature birth with subsequent normal development. The most common seizure type was generalized tonic-clonic (50%; 63%), but seizure manifestations were diverse in the remainder and consisted of partial motor, generalized myoclonic, atypical absence, partial complex, atonic, and mixed. Neurologic abnormalities were not uncommon (36%; 25%).

PERIODIC DISCHARGES

Periodic lateralized epileptiform discharges (PLEDs) [a term coined by Chatrian et al (1964)] are characterized by recurrent discharges with intervals of 1 to 2 seconds of spikes, sharp waves, spike-waves, sharp-and-slow-waves, or multiple spike-waves, which are lateralized to one hemisphere. They may be reflected synchronously but with lower amplitude on the contralateral hemisphere. The discharges are self-limited, usually disappearing in a few days to a few weeks. They are accompanied with a high incidence of decreased level of consciousness, focal seizures, and focal neurologic deficits. They are caused by a variety of acute or progressive focal organic lesions—most commonly cerebral infarct, but also rapidly growing brain tumors, herpes encephalitis, chronic seizure disorder, and subdural hematoma. A large number of patients also have systemic metabolic disturbances. The bilateral, independent PLEDs are most often EEG manifestations of anoxic encephalopathy, CNS infections such as herpes encephalitis or meningitis, and multiple vascular lesions due to sickle cell disease; they are accompanied with a high incidence of coma (de la Paz and Brenner 1981, Daly 1979). Cases with Jakob-Creutzfeldt disease with EEG finding of PLEDs or bilateral PLEDs have been reported (Au et al 1980). The PLEDs can occur in all ages but are less frequent in children. PeBenito and Cracco (1979) studied seven infants and children, 2 months to 16 years old, who had PlEDs. The wave form, periodicity, and transitory nature of the discharges were similar to those in adults and so was an accompaniment of structural abnormalities and metabolic changes. However, they were accompanied by little or no alteration in consciousness and often were accompanied by chronic, nonprogressive lesions of the central nervous system.

In *herpes encephalitis*, the periodic discharges often occur focally at the temporal or temporofrontal regions and consist of monophasic or biphasic sharp slow waves that recur every 2 to 4 seconds (Ch'ien et al 1977). As mentioned earlier, PLEDs and bilateral periodic discharges are also observed. The focal EEG periodic discharges may occur earlier than changes in isotope or CT scan of the brain and may lead to early diagnosis of herpes encephalitis. This fact has become critically important with recent availability of antiviral medications because the earlier the treatment, the better the prognosis.

Generalized periodic discharges in childhood are most often EEG manifestations of subacute sclerosing panencephalitis (Figure 3-17). Periodic discharges in SSPE are initially described by Radermecker (1949), and the periodic complexes are characteristically 1) bilateral, usually bisynchronous, and symmetric; 2) stereotyped in their wave form; 3) usually composed of two or more delta waves: diphasic, triphasic, or multiphasic; 4) of amplitude of approximately 500 μV; 5) repeat with a fair regularity every 4 to 5 seconds; and 6) correlate with myoclonic jerks if present (Markand and Panszi 1975). They may be activated solely during sleep in some cases (Westmoreland et al 1977). Cobb (1966) remarked that spikes and true sharp waves did not occur; but Markand and Panszi (1975) observed bisynchronous spike-wave activity, random frontal spikes, and focal spike-and-slow-wave foci in addition to periodic slow-wave discharges. A child with SSPE had clinical and electrographic epilepsia partialis continua without development of periodic discharges (Lombroso

12 M

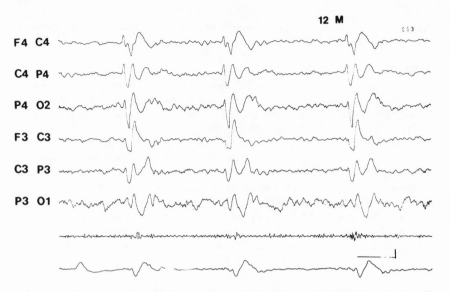

F4 C4

C4 P4

P4 O2

F3 C3

C3 P3

P3 O1

Figure 3-17 Generalized periodic discharges in a 12-year-old boy with SSPE. Seventh channel: movement monitor of the left arm. Eighth channel: eye movement monitor, recording between bilateral epicanthal electrodes.

1968). Another 10-year-old girl had atypical absence attacks and EEG patterns of diffuse 2.5-Hz spike-wave complexes with desynchronization during absence attacks and recruiting rhythm during the tonic seizure (Ishikawa et al 1981). Periodic complexes resembling those of SSPE have been reported in other forms of encephalitis (Ibrahim and Jeavons 1974), during the postictal state in a child with orbitofrontal seizure (Tharp 1972) and during phencyclidine (PCP) intoxication (Fariello and Black 1978).

FEBRILE SEIZURES

The usefulness of electroencephalography in febrile seizures is controversial as reflected in the statement of the NIH Consensus Development Conference Summary on Febrile Seizures (Nelson and Ellenberg 1981) that "the role of the EEG in the workup of febrile seizures remains controversial. Abnormal EEGs do not reliably predict the development of epilepsy in patients with febrile convulsions."

The EEGs taken during the first week following febrile seizures demonstrates excessive posterior slowing in approximately one-third or more of the children (Frantzen et al 1968, Lennox-Buchthal 1973, Yamamura 1977). However, paroxysmal activity is rarely recorded in the immediate postseizure period, and another cause must be considered if such occurs.

The longitudinal follow-up studies (Doose et al 1966, Frantzen et al 1968, Thorn 1981) demonstrated increasing incidence of abnormal EEGs as the children with febrile seizures become older, showing generalized spike-and-wave discharges in 35% to 45% of cases by age 5, and focal spikes mostly at the temporal and occipital areas in 10%. Siblings of patients with febrile seizures also have an increased incidence of generalized spike-wave discharges (Metrakos and Metrakos 1970). These studies also revealed that the paroxysmal discharges in EEG are of little predictive value about recurrence of febrile seizures or subsequent development of nonfebrile seizures. The findings are contradictory with the earlier statement, "the value of the electroencephalogram in assessment of prognosis [in febrile seizures] is established" (Millichap 1968). The results are contradictory to those associated with nonfebrile seizures, where overall recurrence rate in 2.5 years is approximately 30% and development of second nonfebrile seizures approaches 65% to 70% in the presence of spike-wave discharges in their EEG (Hauser 1981). The controversy in the role of EEG here could be due to "lack of double-blind controlled study done by experienced pediatric electroencephalographers" (Nealis 1981) and/or the variety of criteria or definitions of febrile seizures being used in the studies.

With the information available at present, it seems that the EEG is of little value in evaluation of diagnosed cases of febrile seizures. However, the EEG may be used in febrile patients with seizures to identify or confirm structural or organic abnormalities of the brain.

BIBLIOGRAPHY

Adams DJ, Lueders H: Hyperventilation and 6-hour EEG recording in evaluation of absence seizures. *Neurology* 1981;31:1175-1177.

Aicardi J, Chevrie JJ, Rousselie F: Le syndrome spasmies en flexion, agénésie calleuse, anomalies chriorétiniennes. *Arch Fr Pediatr* 1969;26:1103-1120.

Ajmone Marsan C, Goldhammer L: Clinical ictal patterns and electrographic data in cases of partial seizures of frontal-central-parietal origin, in Brazier MAB (ed): *Epilepsy: Its Phenomena in Man*. New York, Academic Press, 1973, pp 236-260.

Ajmone Marsan C, Zivin LS: Factors related to the occurrence of typical paroxysmal abnormalities in the EEG records of epileptic patients. *Epilepsia* 1970;11:361-381.

Andermann F, Robb JP: Absence status: A reappraisal following review of 38 patients. *Epilepsia* 1972;13:177-187.

Au WJ, Gabor AJ, Vijayan N, et al: Periodic lateralized epileptiform complexes (PLEDs) in Creutzfeldt-Jakob disease. *Neurology* 1980;30:611-617.

Babb TL, Halgren E, Wilson C, et al: Neuronal firing patterns during the spread of an occipital lobe seizure to the temporal lobes in man. *Electroencephalogr Clin Neurophysiol* 1981; 51:104-107.

Bancaud J, Colomb D, Dell MB: Les pointes rolandiques "un symptôme E.E.G. propre à l'enfant." *Rev Neurol (Paris)* 1958;99:206-209.

Beaussart M, Faou R: Evolution of epilepsy with rolandic paroxysmal foci: A study of 324 cases. *Epilepsia* 1978;19:337-342.

Bickford RG, Klass DW: Electroencephalography in children having seizures, in Keith HM (ed): *Convulsive Disorders in Children*. Boston, Little Brown and Co, 1963, pp 117-145.

Blume WT: Temporal lobe seizures in childhood: Medical aspect, in Blaw MS, Rapin I, Kinsbourne M (eds): *Topics in Child Neurology*. New York and London, Spectrum Publications, 1977, pp 105-125.

Blume WT: Clinical and electroencephalographic correlates of the multiple independent spike foci pattern in children. *Ann Neurol* 1978;4:541-547.

Blume WT: *Atlas of Pediatric Electroencephalography*. New York, Raven Press, 1982, pp 139-148.

Blume WT, David R, Gomez M: Generalized sharp and slow wave complexes. *Brain* 1973;96: 289-306.

Browne TR, Penry JK, Porter RJ, et al: Responsiveness before, during and after spike-wave paroxysms. *Neurology* 1974;24:659-665.

60

Cavazzuti GB, Cappella L, Nalin A: Longitudinal study of epileptiform EEG patterns in normal children. *Epilepsia* 1980;21:43–55.

Chatrian GE, Bergamini L, Dondey M, et al: A glossary of terms most commonly used by clinical electroencephalographers. *Electroencephalogr Clin Neurophysiol* 1974;37:538–548.

Chatrian GE, Shaw CM, Leffman H: The significance of periodic lateralized epileptiform discharges in EEG: An electrographic, clinical and pathological study. *Electroencephalogr Clin Neurophysiol* 1964;17:177–193.

Ch'ien L, Boehm R, Robinson H, et al: Characteristic early electroencephalographic changes in herpes simplex encephalitis. *Arch Neurol* 1977;34:361–364.

Clark EC, Knott JR: Paroxysmal wave and spike activity and diagnostic subclassification. *Electroencephalogr Clin Neurophysiol* 1955;7:161–164.

Cobb W: The periodic events of subacute sclerosing leukoencephalitis. *Electroencephalogr Clin Neurophysiol* 1966;21:278–294.

Cukier F, Andre M, Monod N, et al: Apport de l'EEG au diagnostic des hémorrhagies intraventriculaires du prématuré. *Rev Electroencephalogr Neurophysiol Clin* 1972;2:318–322.

Currie S, Heathfield RW, Henson RA, et al: Clinical course and prognosis of temporal lobe epilepsy. A survey of 666 patients. *Brain* 1971;94:173–190.

Dalby MA: Epilepsy and 3 per second spike and wave rhythms. *Acta Neurol Scand* [Suppl] 1969;40:1–183.

Dalla Bernardina B, Tassinari CA: EEG of a nocturnal seizure in a patient with "benign epilepsy of childhood with rolandic spikes." *Epilepsia* 1975;16:497–501.

Daly DD: Use of the EEG for diagnosis and evaluation of epileptic seizures and nonepileptic episodic disorders, in Klass DW, Daly DD (eds): *Current Practice of Clinical Electroencephalography*. New York, Raven Press, 1979, pp 221–268.

de la Paz D, Brenner RP: Bilateral independent periodic lateralized epileptiform discharges: Clinical significance. *Arch Neurol* 1981;38:713–715.

Doose H, Gerken H, Kien-Volpel KF, et al: Genetics of photosensitive epilepsy. *Neuropaediatrie* 1969;1:56–73.

Doose H, Voelzke E, Petersen CE, et al: Fieberkraempfe und Epilepsie. II. Elektrencephalographische Verlaufsuntersuchungen bei sogenanten Fieberoder Infektkraempfen. *Neurologie* 1966;208:413–432.

Dreifuss FE, Lee SI: *Epilepsy Case Studies*. New York, Medical Examination Publishing Co, 1981.

Eeg-Olofsson O, Petersen I, Selldén U: The development of the electroencephalogram in normal children from the age of 1 through 15 years. Paroxysmal activity. *Neuropaediatrie* 1971;2:375–404.

Ehle A, Co S, Jones MG: Clinical correlates of midline spikes: An analysis of 21 patients. *Arch Neurol* 1981;38:355–357.

Ellingson RJ: EEGs of premature and full-term newborns, in Klass DW, Daly DD (eds): *Current Practice of Clinical Electroencephalography*. New York, Raven Press, 1979, pp 149–178.

Engel RCH: *Abnormal Electroencephalograms in the Neonatal Period*. Springfield, IL, Charles C Thomas, 1975.

Falconer MA: Genetic and related aetiological factors in temporal lobe epilepsy. A review. *Epilepsia* 1971;12:13–31.

Fariello RG, Black JA: Pseudoperiodic bilateral EEG paroxysms in a case of phencyclidine intoxication. *J Clin Psychiatry* 1978;39:579–581.

Fariello RG, Chun RWM, Doro JM, et al: EEG recognition of Aicardi's syndrome. *Arch Neurol* 1977;34:563–566.

Fois A, Borgheresi S, Luti E: Clinical correlate of focal epileptic discharges in children without seizures. A study of 110 cases. *Helv Paediatr Acta* 1968;3:257–265.

Frantzen E, Lennox-Buchthal M, Nygaard A: Londitudinal EEG and clinical study of children with febrile convulsions. *Electroencephalogr Clin Neurophysiol* 1968;24:197–212.

Friedman E, Pampiglione G: Prognostic implications of electroencephalographic findings of hypsarrhythmia in first year of life. *Br Med J* 1971;4:323-325.

Gastaut H, Roger J, Soulayrol R, et al: Childhood epileptic encephalopathy with diffuse slow spike-waves (otherwise known as "petit mal variant") or Lennox syndrome. *Epilepsia* 1966;7:139-179.

Geiger LR, Harner RN: EEG patterns at the time of focal seizure onset. *Arch Neurol* 1978;35: 276-286.

Gibbs FA, Davis H, Lennox WG: The electroencephalogram in epilepsy and in conditions of impaired consciousness. *Arch Neurol Psychiatr* 1935;34:1134-1148.

Gibbs FA, Gibbs EL, Lennox WG: Influence of the blood sugar level on the wave and spike formation in petit mal epilepsy. *Arch Neurol Psychiatr* 1939;41:1111-1116.

Gibbs FA, Gibbs EL: *Atlas of Electroencephalography.* Cambridge, MA, Addison-Wesley Publishing Co, 1952, vol 2.

Gibbs FA, Gibbs EL: Good prognosis of midtemporal epilepsy. *Epilepsia* 1960;1:448-453.

Gibbs EL, Gillen HW, Gibbs FA: Disappearance and migration of epileptic foci in childhood. *Am J Dis Child* 1954;88:596-603.

Gloor P: Contributions of electroencephalography and electrocorticography to the neurosurgical treatment of the epilepsies, in Purpura DP, Penry JK, Walter RD (eds): *Advances in Neurology.* New York, Raven Press, 1975, vol 8, pp 59-105.

Green JB: Association of behaviour disorder with an electroencephalographic focus in children without seizures. *Neurology* 1961;11:337-344.

Greer M, Andriola MR: Convulsive disorders of childhood, in Thompson RA, Green JR (eds): *Pediatric Neurology and Neurosurgery.* New York and London, SP Medical and Scientific Books, 1978, pp 241-281.

Hauser WA: The natural history of febrile seizures, in Nelson KB, Ellenberg JH (eds): *Febrile Seizures.* New York, Raven Press, 1981, pp 5-17.

Heijbel J, Blom S, Rassmuson M: Benign epilepsy of childhood with centrotemporal EEG foci: A genetic study. *Epilepsia* 1975;16:285-293.

Hrachovy RA, Frost JD, Kellaway P: Sleep characteristics in infantile spasms. *Neurology* 1981;31:688-694.

Hughes JR, Olson SF: An investigation of eight different types of temporal lobe discharges. *Epilepsia* 1981;22:421-435.

Ibrahim MM, Jeavons PM: The value of electroencephalography in the diagnosis of subacute sclerosing panencephalitis. *Dev Med Child Neurol* 1974;16:295-307.

Ishikawa A, Murayama T, Sakuma N, et al: Subacute sclerosing panencephalitis: Atypical absence attacks as first symptom. *Neurology* 1981;31:311-315.

Jeavons PM, Bower B, Dimitrakoudi M: Long-term prognosis of 150 cases of "West syndrome." *Epilepsia* 1973;14:153-164.

Jeavons PM, Bower BD: Infantile spasms, in Magnus O, de Haas L (eds): *Handbook of Clinical Neurology.* Amsterdam, North-Holland Publishing Co, 1974, vol 15, pp 219-234.

Kellaway P, Crawley J, Maulsby R: The electroencephalogram in psychiatric disorders in childhood, in Wilson WP (ed): *Applications of Electroencephalography in Psychiatry.* Durham, NC, Duke University Press, 1965, pp 30-53.

Klass DW: Electroencephalographic manifestations of complex partial seizures, in Penry JK, Daly DD (eds): *Advances in Neurology.* New York, Raven Press, 1975, vol 11, pp 113-141.

Kurokawa T, Goya N, Fukuyama Y, et al: West syndrome and Lennox-Gastaut syndrome: A survey of natural history. *Pediatrics* 1980;65:81-88.

Lacy J, Penry JK: *Infantile spasms.* New York, Raven Press, 1976.

Lennox WG, Davis JP: Clinical correlates of the fast and slow spike-wave electroencephalogram. *Pediatrics* 1950;5:626-644.

Lennox-Buchthal MA: Febrile convulsions. A reappraisal. *Electroencephalogr Clin Neuro-*

physiol 1973;suppl 32:1–132.

Lerman P, Kivity S: Benign focal epilepsy of childhood. A follow-up study of 100 recovered patients. *Arch Neurol* 1975;32:261–264.

Lerman P, Kivity-Ephraim S: Focal epileptic EEG discharges in children not suffering from clinical epilepsy: Etiology, clinical significance, and management. *Epilepsia* 1981;22: 551–558.

Lombroso CT: Sylvian seizures and midtemporal spike foci in children. *Arch Neurol* 1967; 17:52–59.

Lombroso CT: Remarks on the EEG and movement disorder in SSPE. *Neurology* 1968;18(part 2):60–75.

Lombroso CT: Convulsive disorders in newborns, in Thompson RA, Green JR (eds): *Pediatric Neurology and Neurosurgery*. New York, SP Medical and Scientific Books, 1978, pp 205–239.

Lombroso CT, Fejerman N: Benign myoclonus of early infancy. *Ann Neurol* 1977;1:138–143.

Ludwig BI, Ajmone Marsan C: Clinical ictal patterns in epileptic patients with occipital electro-encephalographic foci. *Neurology* 1975;25:463–471.

Markand ON: Slow spike-wave activity in EEG and associated clinical features: Often called 'Lennox' or 'Lennox-Gastaut' syndrome. *Neurology* 1977;27:746–757.

Markand ON, Panszi JG: The electroencephalogram in subacute sclerosing panencephalitis. *Arch Neurol* 1975;32:719–726.

Metrakos JD, Metrakos K: Childhood epilepsy of subcortical ("centrencephalic") origin. *Clin Pediatr* 1966;5:536–542.

Metrakos JD, Metrakos K: Genetic factors in epilepsy, in Niedermeyer E (ed): *Modern Problems in Pharmacopsychiatry*, vol 4, *Epilepsy*. Basel, Karger, 1970, pp 71–86.

Metrakos K, Metrakos JD: Genetics of epilepsy, in Magnus O, de Haas L (eds): *Handbook of Clinical Neurology*. Amsterdam, North-Holland Publishing Co, 1974, vol 15, pp 429–439.

Millichap JG: *Febrile Convulsions*. New York, Macmillan Inc, 1968, pp 37–53.

Nonod N, Dreyfus-Brisac C: Prognostic value of the neonatal EEG in full-term newborns, in *Handbook of Electroencephalography and Clinical Neurophysiology*. Amsterdam, Elsevier, 1972, vol 15B, pp 89–112.

Nayrac P, Beaussart M: Les pointes-ondes pre-rolandiques. Expression E.E.G. trés particuliére de 21 cas. *Rev Neurol* 1958;99:201–206.

Nealis JG: Management of febrile seizures by pediatricians in the United States, in Nelson KB, Ellenberg JH (eds): *Febrile Seizures*. New York, Raven Press, 1981, pp 81–86.

Nelson KB, Ellenberg JH: *Febrile Seizures*. New York, Raven Press, 1981, pp 297–306.

Noriega-Sanchez A, Markand ON: Clinical and electroencephalographic correlation of independent multifocal spike discharges. *Neurology* 1976;26:667–672.

Ounsted C, Lindsay J, Norman R: Biological factors in temporal lobe epilepsy. London, William Heinemann Medical Books, 1966.

Pampiglione G, Moynahan EJ: The tuberous sclerosis syndrome: Clinical and EEG studies in 100 children. *J Neurol Neurosurg Psychiatry* 1976;39:666–673.

Panayiotopoulos CP: Inhibitory effect of central vision on occipital lobe seizures. *Neurology* 1981;31:1331–1333.

PeBenito R, Cracco JB: Periodic lateralized epileptiform discharges in infants and children. *Ann Neurol* 1979;6:47–50.

Pedley TA, Tharp BR, Herman K: Clinical and electroencephalographic characteristics of midline parasagittal foci. *Ann Neurol* 1981;9:142–149.

Penry JK, Porter RJ, Dreifuss FE: Simultaneous recording of absence seizures with videotape and electroencephalography: A study of 374 seizures in 48 patients. *Brain* 1975;98: 427–440.

Radermecker J: Aspects électroéncephalographiques dans cas d'encéphalite subaigue. *Acts Neurol Psychiatr Belg* 1949;49:222–232.

Reilly EL, Peters JF: Relationship of some varieties of electroencephalographic photosensitivity to clinical convulsive disorders. *Neurology* 1973;23:1050-1057.

Rose AL, Lombroso CT: Neonatal seizure states. A study of clinical, pathological, and electroencephalographic features in 137 full-term babies with a long-term follow-up. *Pediatrics* 1970;45:404-425.

Ross JJ, Johnson LC, Walter RD: Spike and wave discharges during stages of sleep. *Arch Neurol* 1966;14:399-407.

Sato S, Dreifuss FE, Penry JK: The effect of sleep on spike-wave discharges in absence seizures. *Neurology* 1973;23:1335-1345.

Saunders MG, Westmoreland BF: The EEG in evaluation of disorders affecting brain diffusely, in Klass DW, Daly DD (eds): *Current Practice of Clinical Electroencephalography*. New York, Raven Press, 1979, pp 343-379.

Scarpa P, Carassini B: Partial epilepsy in childhood: Clinical and EEG study of 261 cases. *Epilepsia* 1982;23:333-341.

Silverman D: Clinical correlates of spike-wave complex. *Electroencephalogr Clin Neurophysiol* 1954;6:663-669.

Smith JMB, Kellaway P: The natural history and clinical correlates of occipital foci in children, in Kellaway P, Petersen I (eds): *Neurological and Electroencephalographic Correlative Studies in Infancy*. New York, Grune & Stratton Inc, 1964, pp 230-249.

Tharp BR: Orbital frontal seizures. An unique electroencephalographic and clinical syndrome. *Epilepsia* 1972;13:627-642.

Tharp BR: Neonatal and pediatric electroencephalography, in Aminoff MJ (ed): *Electrodiagnosis in Clinical Neurology*. New York, Churchill Livingstone, 1980, pp 67-117.

Thorn I: Prevention of recurrent febrile seizures: Intermittent prophylaxis with diazepam compared with continuous treatment with phenobarbital, in Nelson KB, Ellenberg JH (eds): *Febrile Seizures*. New York, Raven Press, 1981, pp 119-126.

Tjiam A, Stefanko S, Schen KV, et al: Infantile spasms associated with hemihypsarrhythmia and hemimegalencephaly. *Dev Med Child Neurol* 1978;20:779-798.

Trojaborg W: Changes in spike foci in children, Kellaway P, Petersen I (eds): *Clinical Electroencephalography in Children*. New York, Grune & Stratton Inc, 1968; pp 213-226.

Tukel K, Jasper H: The electroencephalogram in parasagittal lesions. *Electroencephalogr Clin Neurophysiol* 1952;4:481-494.

Volpe J: Neonatal seizures. *N Engl J Med* 1973;289:413-416.

Watanabe K, Iwase K, Hara K: The evolution of EEG features in infantile spasms: A prospective study. *Dev Med Child Neurol* 1973;15:584-596.

Weir B: The morphology of the spike-wave complex. *Electroencephalogr Clin Neurophysiol* 1965;19:284-290.

Werner SS, Stockard JE, Bickford RG: *An Atlas of Neonatal Electroencephaloggraphy*. New York, Raven Press, 1977.

Westmoreland BF, Gomex MR, Blume WT: Activation of periodic complexes of subacute sclerosing panencephalitis by sleep. *Ann Neurol* 1977;1:185-187.

Yamamura H: A follow-up study of febrile convulsions. *Epilepsia* 1977;18:129.

CHAPTER 4

Generalized Seizures: Absence

Susumu Sato

The "absence seizure" is characterized by interruption of activity, a blank stare, and unresponsiveness. The first description of such an episode was given by Poupart in 1705 (Temkin 1971). Since then, a variety of terminologies have been introduced to describe such events.

Daly in 1968 offered an excellent, brief, historical review of the definition of the event associated with electrographic discharges. Although Tissot was often credited with introducing the term *petit mal* in 1769, Esquirol used this term to describe all minor epileptic seizures, including absences in 1815 (Temkin 1971). In 1824, Calmeil introduced the term *epileptic absence* to describe a passing mental confusion without any definite physical symptoms but to comprise the great variety of attacks that did not have the character of generalized tonic-clonic seizures (Temkin 1971). Since Jackson's era, the term *petit mal* gradually came to refer to a particular type of seizure occurring perdominantly in children (Daly 1968). The first description of absence seizure in English literature was given under the name *pyknolepsy* by Adie in 1924 and first in the United States by Jelliffe and Notkin in 1934.

In 1935, Gibbs and co-workers reported that EEGs from patients with characteristic petit mal epilepsy showed bursts of 3-per-second spike-wave discharges during attacks. In 1954, Penfield and Jasper introduced the concept of a centrencephalic integrating system to explain the generalization of spike-wave discharges. Although this system has never been demonstrated in an anatomical sense, the term *centrencephalic seizure* has been used since then to describe primarily generalized seizures.

Lennox and Lennox (1960) described the petit mal triad: pure petit mal, myoclonic attacks, and akinetic or atonic attack; they also added the fourth member: petit mal variant or petit mal with psychomotor components. In recent years, the term *absence* has been used widely and has been thought to give a better description of the attack.

CLASSIFICATION

In the *Dictionary of Epilepsy* (Gastaut 1973), petit mal epilepsy is defined as the epilepsy of subjects who have only petit mal seizures and, especially, typical absences. The typical absence is further defined as a type of simple or complex absence associated with bilateral, synchronous and symmetrical EEG discharges of 3-per-second spike-and-wave complexes. The simple absence is characterized mainly or exclusively by clouding or loss of consciousness. The complex absence is an

66

absence in which the impairment of consciousness is accompanied by other symptoms; and it includes many clinical manifestations.

According to the International Classification of Epilepsy (Merlis 1970), petit mal epilepsy is one of the primarily generalized epilepsies, the characteristic of which is that epileptic seizures are generalized from the onset. Likewise, the International Classification of Epileptic Seizures (Gastaut 1970, Dreifuss 1981) categorizes the petit mal seizure or absence seizure in the generalized epileptic seizures and classified the absence seizures, as shown in Table 4-1.

Table 4-1
Classification of Absence Seizures (Dreifuss 1981)

---

a. Absence seizures with impairment of consciousness only
b. Absence seizures with mild clonic components
c. Absence seizures with atonic component
d. Absence seizures with tonic component
e. Absence seizures with automatisms
f. Absence seizures with autonomic components

The hallmarks of the absence attack are sudden onset, interruption of ongoing activities, a blank stare, and possibly a brief upward rotation of the eyes. The ictal EEG abnormality usually consists of regular and symmetrical 2- to 4-Hz spike-wave complexes or multiple spike-slow-wave complexes of bilateral distribution. The EEG background activity usually is normal.

INCIDENCE

Petit mal epilepsy is a relatively uncommon type of epileptic disorder (Livingston 1972, Currier et al 1963, Lennox 1960). Among various seizure types, reported incidences of petit mal seizures range between 2-5% (median, 3%) (Commission Report 1978) and 8-11% (Cavazzuti 1980, Blom et al 1978); reported prevalences of petit mal seizures with other types of seizures range from 5% to 20% (median, 11%) in adults (Commission report 1978) and from 6% to 12% in children with seizures.

The variation in these figures probably represents differences in classification, as well as in the different populations studied (Commission Report 1978). In a Swedish county, the prevalence of simple and complex absences was estimated as 10 per 100,000 in the age group of 0-15 years (Blom et al 1978). In Rochester, Minnesota, the prevalence of petit mal seizures was 3.3 per 100,000. If this rate is applied to the United States population, the number of new cases each year would be approximately 6000 (Kurland 1959/1960). The prevalence of absence (petit mal) seizures was highest in the first ten years of life and then fell to a negligible level (Hauser and Kurland 1975).

GENETICS

Genetic aspects of absence seizures have been extensively reviewed by Newmark and Penry in 1980. Matthes and Weber in 1968 reported that a significant number (13.3%) of probands with absence attacks had a family history of epilepsy involving either the siblings or parents: 3.7% of the siblings had epilepsy and another 6.3%

experienced occasional childhood convulsion (mainly febrile convulsions before the age of 5 years), whereas 3.1% of the patients had epilepsy and another 2.3% had occasional childhood convulsions. An even higher prevalence of epileptic seizures in relatives was reported by Doose et al in 1973. Thirty percent of 239 patients with absence epilepsy had relatives with seizures of various types, and convulsions occurred in 7% of the siblings and in 6% of the parents.

Metrakos and Metrakos (1961) found a centrencephalic type of electroencephalogram in approximately 37% of the siblings of the probands with centrencephalic epilepsy, up to 50% between the ages of 4.5 and 7.5 years. However, only 7.69% of the parents had a centrencephalic EEG abnormality. They proposed that the major gene in centrencephalic epilepsy is an irregular, autosomal, dominant gene with age-dependent expression. On the other hand, Matthes (1968) found the 3-per-second spike-wave discharges in only 9.2% of the siblings and in 2.5% of the parents.

In monozygotic twins, there was 84% concordance for 3-per-second spike-wave discharges and 75% concordance for petit mal seizures. No dizygotic twins were concordant for petit mal seizures (Lennox and Lennox 1960). Although the increased prevalence of epilepsy and epileptiform discharges in the probands' relatives was amply shown, investigators other than Metrakos and Metrakos (1961) concluded that the 3-per-second spike-wave discharges are not controlled by an autosomal dominant gene; rather, they suggested that several genetic factors are responsible, some mutually independent and some either reinforcing or inhibiting the others (Doose et al 1973).

ETIOLOGY

In 1969, Dalby reviewed the etiology of generalized spike-wave discharges. Evidence of brain damage was found in 40% of patients with 3-per-second spike-wave rhythm, although only 14% had a known causative factor that could be related to the presence of epilepsy and the presence of spike-wave activity in the EEG: birth trauma, 5.8%; cranial traumas, 2.0%; encephalitis, 2.0%; and developmental abnormalities, brain tumor, and endocrinopathies, 4.2%. Thus, the author concluded that brain damage is not an important pathogenic factor in the causation of spike-wave epilepsy, although it may act as a trigger mechanism when other factors of heredity, age, and sex are present. No cases with a probable organic cause were found among 24 patients with classic spike-wave paroxysms (Silverman 1954). Patients with petit mal epilepsy were not found among patients with epilepsy following birth trauma, congenital brain lesions, encephalitis, or cranial trauma (Livingston 1954).

Generalized spike-wave patterns were noted in children with precocious puberty (Scherman and Abraham 1963) and in a 40-year-old man with an astrocytoma of very long standing in the left frontal mesial cortex (Loiseau et al 1971). Autopsy showed no major neuropathologic lesion in a 13.5-year-old female with absence, who died of aplastic anemia (Cohn 1968).

Focal and diffuse abnormalities were seen in 35 of 100 patients with petit mal seizures, but possible causative factors were found in the history of only six patients in spite of extensive diagnostic workup (O'Brien et al 1959).

Ajmone Marsan and Lewis reported two patients with brain tumors who also had "centrencephalic" electroencephalographic patterns. On the basis of a statistical analysis on reported cases of brain tumors and 3-per-second spike-wave discharges, they concluded that brain tumor and a centrencephalic EEG pattern are related.

PATHOPHYSIOLOGY

In 1977, Sarnat presented a compact but thorough review of pathogenesis of absence seizures. Currently, there are three models of the neurophysiological mechanism of absence seizures, although they are not necessarily mutually exclusive. In 1952, Penfield defined the "centrencephalic" system as the central system within the brain stem that is responsible for integration of the function of the two cerebral hemispheres (see Penfield and Jasper 1954). This proposal was preceded by Morison and Dempsey's work (1942) in which two thalamocortical projection systems in cats were described, namely, a specific projection system and a nonspecific diffuse projection system. The stimulation of the nonspecific system produced recruiting responses diffusely over the cortex of both hemispheres. Rhythmical electrical stimulation to a small area in the medical intralaminal region of the thalamus (Jasper and Droogleever-Fortuyn 1946) and the mesencephalic reticular formation (Weir 1964) elicited the bilaterally synchronous 3-per-second wave-and-spike discharges. In unanesthetized cats or in cats with chronically implanted electrodes, electrical stimulation of the thalamic reticular system (Hunter and Jasper 1949) and the mesencephalic reticular formation (Weir 1964) produced a spike-wave response concurrently with an arrest reaction, head nodding, and facial twitching. In kittens ranging in age from 21 to 30 days, implantation of alumina into the intralaminar nuclei of the thalamus and mesencephalic reticular formation produced the EEG patterns of 3-per-second spike-wave discharges associated with behavior absences (Guerrero-Figueroa et al 1963). Cats similarly prepared with alumina when 30 days old or older did not develop these EEG or behavior patterns. Small coagulations around the medial part of the lamina medularis interna at the level of the commissura media reduced the frequency of petit mal attacks in patients with grand mal and petit mal. The authors concluded that this observation supports the assumption that there exists a group of petit mal cases caused by foci in the diencephalon (Spiegel and Wyeis 1950).

On the basis of the clinical similarity of attacks elicited from the gyrus cinguli in cats, Lennos and Robinson (1951) questioned the model of hemispherical focus for petit mal seizures. The centrencephalic EEG pattern was observed in patients with epileptic lesions in the anterior parasagittal regions and in the medial aspect of the brain (Tückel and Jasper 1952). In 1964, Pollen and his colleagues (Pollen 1964, Pollen and Sie 1964, Pollen et al 1964) did a series of experiments in which extracellular and intracellular recordings of cortical unit activity were made during the surface wave-and-spike response elicited by 3-per-second intralamina stimulation of the thalamus. Their results suggest that the thalamic-induced wave-spike response originates within the cortex. The spike component corresponds to a recruiting response associated with excitatory postsynaptic potentials generalized in the superficial layer of the cortex, and the long-duration, surface, negative wave was believed to be produced by the apical dendrites acting as passive sinks for active sources of current in the deeper cortical layers.

In adult cats or monkeys with intact thalamus and brain stem, it is possible to reproduce both the bilateral spike-slow wave discharge (2.5–4 cycles/second) and the absence seizures by introducing lesions limited to cerebral cortex in a bilateral manner. This capacity for bilateral discharges was retained following extensive ablation of diencephalic and mesencephalic structures. This model does not rule out a role for diencephalic and brain stem structures or other subcortical structures, although section of the corpus callosum disrupted the synchrony of discharge of bilateral foci (Marcus and Watson 1966, 1968).

Stewart and Dreifuss (1967) reported "centrencephalic seizure discharges" in five patients with focal hemispherical lesions; they stated that there is no constant and reliable way to distinguish primary bilateral synchrony from secondary bilateral synchrony or an EEG. Thus, they thought it reasonable to postulate that most cases of presumed primary brain stem epilepsy are in fact examples of secondary bilateral synchrony.

Depth recording in epileptic patients with generalized spike-wave discharges failed to show any evidence of a primary thalamic focus; however, in two patients, primary focal discharges in the frontal lobe were observed (Niedermeyer et al 1969). Similarly, Rossi et al (1968) observed that thalamic participation was not essential for the occurrence of an otherwise generalized discharge.

In 1974, Bancaud et al demonstrated that electrical stimulation of the human frontal cortex, particularly mesial cortex, is capable of producing generalized spike-wave burst and clinical absences, both of which are indistinguishable from spontaneous spike-wave burst and absences. The effective areas were distributed in the two frontal areas in most cases and were practically symmetrical.

Microelectrode recording of unit firing and of local slow wave activity from the precentral motor cortex of monkey showed the focal events of 3-per-second spike-and-wave discharges and associated tonic eye movements during drowsiness that occurred spontaneously or was specifically thalamic-induced. The EEG components of focal spike-and-wave discharges were closely associated with the epileptic firing of interneurons. The spike is regarded as reflecting extracellularly the synchronous and powerful depolarization of excitatory interneurons, which set in motion inhibitory Golgi II elements that are responsible for the subsequent, long-lasting wave (Steriade 1974).

Gloor et al (1967) have shown that a small amount of penicillin applied to the reticular formation of the mesencephalon is capable of producing self-sustained seizure discharge at a rhythm of 3 per second which, however, did not show any cortical projection. Penicillin injection into other subcortical structures, such as the thalamus, never produced any epileptic discharges unless there was some escape of the penicillin into CFS-containing spaces or some diffusion toward the cerebral cortex. Lange and Julien (1978) made a similar observation in cats which failed to produce spike-wave discharges after thalamic injection of estrogens.

In 1968 and 1969, Gloor described two patients with generalized epilepsy who received intracarotid injections of amytal and metrazol and two patients who received intravertebral injection of metrazol. Unilateral intracarotid injection of metrazol on either side precipitated the clinical and electrographic features of centrencephalic epilepsy. A bilateral arresting effect of unilateral intracarotid injection of amytal was noted. Intravertebral injection of metrazol failed to activate the bilateral spike-wave paroxysms but, instead, decreased their number and amplitude. He proposed the term *generalized corticoreticular epilepsies* to emphasize the role of a cortical mechanism as the origin of epileptiform discharges although suggesting involvement of the diffuse projection system of the brain stem and thalamus. The term meant that centrencephalic epilepsy results from an abnormal interaction of cortical and subcortical gray matter. Diminution of the desynchronizing effect upon the cerebral cortical activity exerted by the ascending reticular formation may be a factor for the occurrence and spread of bilaterally synchronous spike-and-wave discharges of cortical or thalamocortical origin in cats (Gloor et al 1973, Testa and Gloor 1974).

Intramuscular injection of penicillin (large amount) in cats produced clinical and EEG features resembling human myoclonic petit mal (Gloor and Testa 1974). Unilateral intracarotid injections of pentylenetetrazol produced a bilateral activation of the generalized epileptiform discharges. Intravertebral injection of pentylenetetrazol diminished and, in chronic animals, invariably eliminated spontaneous generalized epileptiform activity. Unilateral intracarotid injection of amobarbital produced either an ipsilateral or bilateral diminution of paroxysmal discharges or an ipsilateral activation. Responses to intravertebral injections of amobarbital were variable: with EEG desynchronization induced by intravertebral injection of amobarbital, generalized epileptiform discharges were diminished or arrested; with EEG synchronization, they were increased. Gloor and Testa (1974) concluded that the origin of the convulsive discharges in this animal model is most likely cortical. Brain stem structures, however, exert a powerful influence upon these discharges; increased desynchronizing drive of brain stem reticular origin markedly reduced or even eliminates them. Conversely, a reduction in ascending reticular drive markedly promotes their occurrence. Gloor and Testa (1974) proposed similar mechanisms are at work in human generalized corticoreticular epilepsy.

An observation that was made in an 8-year-old girl with petit mal suggested a similar mechanism, namely, that seizures evoked by various stimuli were best developed during light drowsiness and clearly potentiated by the use of partial sensory restriction (Cleeland and Booker 1967).

In cats with penicillin-induced, generalized, spike-wave activity, diffuse cortical hyperexcitability is shown by increased amplitude of both visual- and auditory-evoked potentials during spike-and-wave activity. However, intact brain stem, auditory-evoked potentials during spike-wave activity suggested that a deficit in sensory processing occurs rostral to the brain stem (Burchiel et al 1976).

In 1972 and 1980, Fromm and his colleagues postulated that petit mal spells represent paroxysmal activity in cortical inhibitory pathways, because anti-absence drugs had a depressant effect on cortical as well as subcortical inhibitory pathways.

Interesting observations have been provided by blood flow studies (Sakai et al 1978) and position emission tomography studies (Engel et al 1981), both of which showed diffuse cortical involvement in the form of increased gray matter blood flow and cortical fluorodeoxyglucose uptake during typical absence seizures.

CLINICAL MANIFESTATIONS

Clinical manifestations of absence seizures were detailed by Penry et al (1975) as a result of video-EEG analysis of 374 seizures in 48 patients with absence seizures.

Specific Clinical Manifestations

A. *Simple Absences.* This type of absence is characterized by sudden cessation of ongoing activities: interruption of speech, walking, eating, and so forth. The patient will remain stock-still and normal breathing continues. Hyperventilation will stop at the onset of the seizure and normal respiration supervenes. The eyes become vacant;

occasionally the lids droop slightly; the eyes may rotate upward, but usually stare straight ahead as if in a trance. There is no other manifestation in the motor or behavior spheres. During the attack, the patient is usually unresponsive, but the postictal recovery is immediate. The patient will usually resume his preictal activities as if nothing had happened, or he may resume speaking where he left off. The patient is frequently unaware of the fact that he has had an attack, but he spontaneously recommences hyperventilation if it had been interrupted by an attack (Figure 4-1).

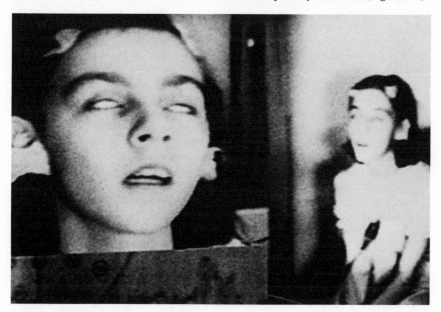

Figure 4-1 Brief absence seizure with interruption of speech and upward rotation of the eyes.

B. *Complex Absences.* This type of absence has other symptoms in addition to those seen in simple absence.

1. *Absences with mild clonic components.* During the attack, clonic movements may involve the eyelids (blinking), the mouth corner, fingers, arms, or shoulders. The eyes may go upward, with blinking of the eyelids. Blinking is the most common type and tends to occur early in the seizure. The severity varies considerably up to a series of generalized myoclonic jerks (Lance 1970). Clonic movements are often bilaterally symmetrical and do not become severe enough to impair the patient's posture. However, if the patient holds something in his hands at the onset of the attack, the attack may cause him to lose his grip; if a spoon is full, the contents may spill.

2. *Absence with increase in postural tone.* During the attack, tonic muscular contraction may occur and cause an increase in muscle tone; the extensor or flexor muscles may be affected symmetrically or asymmetrically. If the patient is standing, the patient may be drawn backward and the trunk may arch; this condition leads to retropulsion. If the contraction oc-

curs asymmetrically, the patient's head or trunk will be pulled to one side.

3. *Absence with diminution in postural tone.* During the attack, there may be diminished tone in the muscle subserving posture as well as the limb musculature, leading to drooping of the head, occasionally slumping of the trunk, dropping of the arms, and relaxation of grip. During these attacks, the patient may drop what he is holding in his hands. If the patient is standing, the knees may buckle. Rarely, tone is sufficiently diminished to cause the patient to fall.

4. *Absence with automatisms.* Purposeful or quasi-purposeful movements occur without awareness during the absence attack. The patient may lick his lips, chew, swallow, yawn, grimace, stick out his tongue, rub his face, fumble with his clothes or with a necklace, or he may even perform such complex activities as putting objects in his hand into his pocket. Penry and Dreifuss (1969) studied 93 absence seizures from 12 patients with video-telemetry and analyzed in detail automatisms occurring during absence attacks and generalized spike-wave abnormalities in the electroencephalogram. They noted that simple and complex automatisms occur in patients with absence seizures and that automatisms were easily induced and influenced by environmental stimuli; they proposed a classification of automatisms. However, these automatisms have no characteristics that would distinguish them from those seen in temporal lobe epilepsy. The automatisms are divided into two major categories: ictal and postictal automatisms. Ictal automatisms are further divided into two groups: perseverative and de novo automatisms. The ictal automatism is the one that is characteristic of absence seizures. In the perseverative automatisms, the patient continued an activity initiated before the seizure, such as persistence of the bimanual transfer, manual forearm rubbing, walking, and raising the outstretched arms. Changes in rhythm may be seen: slowing down or speeding up, sometimes preceded by a pause. Hyperventilation ceases at the onset of an absence attack and usually does not recur until the attack is over. De novo automatism is one that occurs after the beginning or during absence seizures. The mechanism of de novo automatism is thought to be mainly of reactive type: either externally or internally (spontaneous, occult stimulation). Spontaneous automatisms such as scratching, rubbing, or picking at the clothes or pulling at the microphone around the neck are postulated as responses to occult stimuli. De novo automatisms may be triggered by various external stimulations: reacting to stimulation, the patient may withdraw the stimulated extremity, beat at the stimulus, or vocalize. The patient may scratch or chew. Released automatisms are rare but, for instance, the patient initiates a prohibited behavior such as scratching genitalia in public during an absence attack. Humming has been known, but formed speech does not occur. If spoken to, the patient may turn towards the sound of the voice. When touched or tickled, he may rub the site. These manifestations indicate that the nature of the automatism may sometimes by determined by reaction to environmental stimuli (Penry and Dreifuss 1969, Klass and Daly 1961). Automatisms are frequently quite complex and may consist of combinations of the above described movements, or they may be so simple and fleeting as to be missed by casual

observation. Automatisms are related to the duration of seizures and rarely occur as the initial clinical event. More than 50% of the seizures longer than 7 seconds have automatisms.

5. *Absence with autonomic phenomena.* Pupil dilatation, pallor, flushing, piloerection, tachycardia, salivation, and urinary incontinence occasionally occur in association with absence seizures. The most frequently observed phenomena are circumoral pallor and pupil dilatation.

6. *Mixed form.* Seizures may be classified as a combination of two or more of the previous categories, except simple absence.

The 374 seizures ranged in duration from 1 to 45 seconds (mean, 10.5 seconds; median, 9.0 seconds). Of 374 absence seizures analyzed, simple absence (35 seizures) constituted only 9.4% and complex absence seizures 90.6% with 39.8% of the seizures comprising the mixed category with multiple components. Automatisms were observed in 63.1% and mild clonic components were observed in 45.5% of the seizures. Decreased postural tone occurred in 22.5% of the seizures; increased tone occurred in only 4.5% of the seizures. Although the occurrence of two components in the same seizure was not uncommon (34.8%), the occurrence of three or more components in the same seizures was infrequent (5.1%). Individual patients tended to have seizures of the same kind on different occasions (Penry et al 1975). However, some patients may have different types of seizures at different times (Klass and Daly 1961).

Frequent seizures interfere with school performance. Such children are often thought to be daydreaming, lazy, or depressed or to have a learning disability, which is the complaint that may lead the parents to medical help (Grossman 1969, Lawall 1976). A polygraphic study showed that in almost every case of absence, the apnea was the only respiratory phenomenon and no changes in EEG were noted (Bogacz and Yanicelli 1962).

Sex

The ratio of males to females in populations of patients with absence seizures is reported as 36% to 64% by Gibberd (1966) and as 48% to 52% by Sato et al (1976a).

Onset

Onset occurred between the ages of 5 and 15 years in 68.3% of patients, in 24% below the age of 5 years, and in 7.9% above the age of 15 years (Gibberd 1966). In the study by Sato et al (1976a), 22.9% had a seizure before the age of 5 years, 60.4% had their first seizure between the ages of 5 and 9 years, and 16.7% experienced their first seizure between the ages of 10 and 13.2 years. Onset of seizures occurs most commonly between 4 and 8 years of age and rarely occurs much before the age of 3 or after 15 years of age.

Family History of Seizure Disorder

A family history of seizure disorder was noted in 39.6% (Sato et al 1976a) and in 19% (Gibberd 1966).

Neurologic Findings

Mild, nonprogressive, neurologic abnormalities such as corticospinal tract signs and mental retardation were noted in 18.8% (Sato et al 1976a). The reported prevalences of abnormal neurologic findings are 5.1% (Livingston et al 1965), 24% (Holowach et al 1962), 21% (Dreifuss 1972).

Intelligence Quotient

Lennox and Lennox (1960) and Livingston (1954) stated that the patient with petit mal is of average or above average intelligence. However, prevalence of low IQ (< 90) was noted in 20-24% of patients (Holowach et al 1962, Hertoft 1963); IQ scores of less than 80 were noted in 35 of 116 patients with petit mal epilepsy (Charlton and Yahr 1967). Twenty-five of 48 patients with absence seizures had IQ scores of less than 89 (Sato et al 1976a). Although the mean IQ scores of the patients with epilepsy were within or near the "average" ranges, they scored lower than the average (median IQ) of their close, nonepileptic relatives. Investigators felt it unlikely that anticonvulsant therapy truly reduces intellectual function in many patients (Needham et al 1969).

Generalized Tonic-Clonic Seizures

The occurrence of generalized tonic-clonic seizures was noted in 38% to 59% of patients with petit mal epilepsy (Currier et al 1963, Charlton and Yahr 1967, Gibberd 1966, Sato et al 1976a). Generalized tonic-clonic seizures may precede or follow the onset of absence seizures. The patient may stop having absence seizures but may continue to have generalized tonic-clonic seizures (Currier et al 1963, Hertoft 1963, Gordon 1965, Sato et al 1976a). Lennox and Lennox (1960) stated that petit mal epilepsy of late onset is more likely to be complicated by grand mal seizures; Charlton and Yahr (1967) stated that the earlier the age of onset of petit mal, the less likely the development of grand mal.

Psychological Aspects

Patients with petit mal epilepsy were found to have impairment in sustaining attention (continuous performance test) but to have a better memory as compared to those with focal epilepsy (Mirksy et al 1960, Fedio and Mirsky 1969).

Social Adjustment

The patient should be treated as a normal subject and encouraged to participate in various sports activities. Contrary to popular belief, physical activity favorably affects an epileptic disorder in most cases. Restricted activities are horseback riding, climbing to heights, swimming alone, and driving a car; these activities should not be undertaken until seizures are judged to have ceased (Livingston 1978).

Precipitating Factors

Various stimuli (tactile, auditory, olfactory, and photic stimulation; simple mental tasks; and behavioral responses) evoked absence seizures best during light drowsiness with partial sensory restriction (Cleeland and Booker 1967). Reflex or voluntary closing of the eyes precipitated absence seizures (Dobrzynska and Mierzejewska 1974). Environmental influences, seizure frequency, and emotional stress triggered clinical seizures (Sato et al 1976b). The petit mal EEG paroxysms occurred more often during the patient's silence and school exercises than during the patient's speech, indicating that more focused attention or activity during speech tends to reduce these paroxysms (Luborsky et al 1975, Guey et al 1969). Sleep deprivation is also noted to be a triggering factor (Sibley 1974).

DIAGNOSIS

Diagnosis of absence seizures can be made without difficulty in most cases. A good history describing sudden onset and sudden cessation of the ictus usually is diagnostic, but witnessing actual seizures during neurologic examination is confirmatory. Further confirmation can be obtained with an EEG examination documenting bursts of generalized 3-Hz spike-wave discharges with ictal manifestation. When the patients or relatives are poor historians, the EEG recording with simultaneous clinical observation is confirmatory.

Other testings such as CT scans, brain scan, hematology, blood chemistry, or urinalysis are not helpful in establishing the diagnosis of absence seizures. No abnormality of skull x-ray films were noted (Sato et al 1976a), but some abnormalities were reported in neuroradiographic examination (Hertoft 1963).

CT Scan Findings

Gastaut described abnormal CT findings of atrophic lesions in 7% of patients with simple absences, in 17% of patients with complex absences, and in 24% of patients with both generalized tonic-clonic and absence seizures (Gastaut and Gastaut 1977). Sato et al (1982) observed abnormal CT findings of nonprogressive types in 9 (11%) of 83 patients with absence seizures. However, a rather high prevalence (41%) of abnormal CT findings (atrophic) has also been reported (Langenstein et al 1979).

EEG Findings

In 1935, Gibbs et al gave the first description of EEG findings in patients with absence seizures. During the seizure, a burst of 3-per-second waves of 100 to 300 μV was noted, with a constant wave component and a variable spike component.

A thorough description of EEG characteristics of the petit mal discharge in man was given by Jasper and Droogleever-Fortuyn in 1946.

The petit mal discharge is generalized; it appears suddenly and disappears suddenly. The onset of the discharges appears as a phase reversal in the midfrontal area, where the maximal voltage occurs in most patients with true petit mal. In exceptional cases, the discharges may appear first in the parietooccipital regions and spread with extreme rapidity to involve frontal regions. The most constant component is the regular series of rounded waves, but the spike component is highly variable and may in fact disappear for a time during the course of a seizure. The spikes appear between the slow waves or on the descending or ascending limbs of the slow waves. The discharge seldom varies more than 0.2 cycles per second above or below 3 cycles per second, slowing down a bit toward the end of a long series of waves.

The background activity is usually normal for the patient's age. The spike-wave discharges may also be associated with generalized tonic-clonic seizures. In children, the 3-cycle-per-second spike-wave is well associated with absence seizures (Nuffield 1961).

The bursts of generalized spikes and waves were divided into three categories: 1) 3-per-second spike-and-wave bursts exclusive of absence seizures; 2) 4- to 6-per-second spike-and-wave bursts almost always associated with generalized tonic-clonic seizures; 3) 2- to 2.5-per-second spike-and-wave bursts associated with Lennox-Gastaut syndrome (Gastaut 1968).

Runs of bilateral slow waves without spike components are often seen in the records from patients with absence seizures and predominate in the posterior head regions. Focal spikes or spike-wave components are occasionally seen in the frontal polar position, unilaterally or bilaterally (O'Brien et al 1959). The interictal occurrence of focal or lateralized epileptic transients is thought to be consistent with centrencephalic epilepsy (Gianturco et al 1968). Four elements (namely, spike 1, positive transient, spike 2, and wave) were described to be characteristic of the complex, though spike 1, spike 2, or the wave might be absent (Weir 1965). The EEG is thought not only to be prognostic but also actually to pinpoint the degree of organicity (Paty and Boucebci 1972). During sleep, the spike-wave discharges undergo changes in frequency and morphology (Niedermeyer 1965, Sato et al 1973).

Activation

Hyperventilation may induce a burst of spike-wave discharges in nearly every patient with absence seizures. Photic stimulation may induce absence seizures in 20–35% of patients who are photosensitive (Newmark and Penry 1979). Sleep and sleep deprivation are effective methods of activating EEG discharges (Sato et al 1973, Pratt et al 1967). Methohexital (Brevital), an ultra short-acting agent, injected intravenously in small doses, activates 3-per-second spike-and-wave discharges in the majority of patients with absence seizures (Wilder et al 1971).

SPECIAL TESTING

After unilateral intracarotid injection of amobarbital into patients with primary bilateral synchrony, three types of EEG responses may be seen: 1) no changes in the rate of bilateral spike-wave discharges, though some reduction of amplitude may occur on the injected side; 2) arrest or diminution of bilateral spike-and-wave discharges for several minutes; 3) temporary activation of bilateral or unilateral spike-and-wave discharges immediately after injection. Intracarotid injection of pentylenetetrazol on either side produced identical responses of bilaterally synchronous spike-and-wave activity and clinical seizures (Gloor et al 1976). Fractional intravenous injections of Na-thiopentone (Pentothal) in 19 patients with petit mal produced a prolonged stage of symmetrically induced beta rhythms, suppression of bilateral spike-waves, and no activation of focal elements. The same test in patients with lateralized neurological signs showed good beta rhythms (except for some areas varying in extent), suppression of the spike-wave activity, and emergence or reinforcement of focal elements, usually within the area of beta suppression (Lombroso and Erba 1969).

Flash stimulation in photosensitive patients produced a large visual-evoked potential in the occipital area (Green 1969, Lücking et al 1970).

Prolonged EEG monitoring with telemetry showed a waxing and waning of spike-wave activity both day and night (Stevens et al 1972).

DIFFERENTIAL DIAGNOSIS

From a behavioral point of view, absence seizures are most often confused with complex partial seizures (Daly 1968), especially those characterized by an impairment of consciousness only or by automatisms (Penry et al 1975, Daly 1977). However, it should be possible to correctly identify nearly all of the seizures on the basis of 1) seizure duration, 2) presence or absence of an aura, 3) rate of mental clearing following the seizure (Penry et al 1975). Escueta et al (1982) has added another differential sign, namely, 4) presence or absence of de novo ambulatory automatism and complex bilateral motor symptoms. They are more common in complex partial seizures. In those rare instances when differentiation by clinical criteria fails, the EEG characteristics should help differentiate complex partial seizures from absence seizures. The important differentiating features are summarized in Table 4-2.

Table 4-2
Characteristics of Absence Seizures and Complex Partial Seizures

Characteristics	Absence Seizures	Complex Partial Seizures
Age	Childhood	Any age, though rare in childhood
Predisposition	None	Febrile convulsion
Aura	None	In the majority
Onset	Instantaneous	Commonly preceded by aura
Automatisms	Seen in longer seizures, somewhat simpler	Almost always, more complex
Duration	Majority ten seconds or less	Almost always longer than ten seconds, often longer than 30 seconds
Postictal recovery	Immediately with resumption of partial activity	Slowly (many seconds to minutes), confused
Hyperventilation	A great precipitant	Occasional precipitant
Photic	Frequent precipitant	Almost nil
EEG	Generalized spike-wave	Focal spikes

In the so-called Lennox-Gastaut syndrome, the age at onset is generally between 1 and 6 years and clinical manifestation is characterized by periodic bursts of frequent severe seizures such as tonic, atypical absence, or atonic seizures, usually in combination. These patients may show a pronounced mental retardation with a generally low IQ and their interictal EEG records show 1.5- to 2.5-cycle-per-second diffuse slow spike-wave discharges, often in generalized bursts and not very susceptible to activation procedures (Gastaut et al 1966). Other differential diagnoses include hypoglycemia, fainting, micturition syncope, cataplexy, transient global amnesia, transient cerebral ischemia, cardiac causes of syncope, and psychological causes. They are not necessarily easy to differentiate from absence seizures but have other clues not characteristic of absence seizures (Burns 1976).

CONSCIOUSNESS AND RESPONSIVENESS DURING ABSENCE SEIZURE

In some cases, consciousness is never lost or amnesia does not occur (Howell 1955). In others, it is always lost. In some, it is lost during some of the attacks and preserved in others. Consciousness during an absence seizure was initially tested by responsiveness to visual stimulation, auditory stimulation (Schwab 1939, 1941), and various verbal stimulations (Shimazono et al 1953). During a given petit mal seizure, the degree of disturbance of consciousness is not constant but is altered from almost no loss of consciousness to complete lapse of consciousness (Shimazono et al 1953).

It was found that response time slowed significantly even for discharges of 0.5 to 1.5 seconds, even though there was no increase in errors of omission during the short discharges (Tizard and Margerison 1963). Behavioral alterations become manifest before the burst itself is evident in the EEG and they dissipate somewhat earlier than EEG abnormalities (Mirsky and Van Buren 1965). The spike-wave discharge has a differential effect: performance on the continuous performance test with random critical stimuli and a response of key pressing was significantly more impaired by the generalized spike-wave discharges than performance on either a delayed identification test (the letters are presented visually and orally before and during the seizure and are identified after the seizure end) or a simple motor response test (continuous key pressing). Thus, the motor task performance is less affected by burst activity than is performance on the sensory task (Mirsky and Orren 1977).

There is a strong relationship between the duration of spike-wave activity and incidence of errors in performance. The longer the spike-wave burst, the higher the incidence of errors during the paroxysm. Three seconds was a critical duration in that the percentage of spike-wave episodes associated with errors was much greater than paroxysms lasting longer than 3 seconds. Spike-wave paroxysms that lasted longer than 3 seconds nearly always produced clearly observable errors in tracking the target and were associated with phenomena such as arrest of movement, picking up the pointer, or staring ahead with no attention to the test (Goode et al 1970). In pursuit rotor performance, the erorrs begin well after the onset of generalized spike-wave discharge and end well before the end of EEG abnormality; during the error period, the "broken" or fluctuating level of consciousness was noted (Goode et al 1970).

With a paroxysm-triggered technique, reaction time was delayed at the exact onset of spike-wave discharges in more than half of the paroxysms (Porter et al 1973). Nearly half of the patients had normal reaction times at the onset of spike-wave discharges regardless of the length of paroxysmal bursts (Porter et al 1973). It was postulated that normal reaction time at the onset was due to incomplete generalization of spike-wave discharges at the onset of the paroxysm (Penry 1973).

All reaction times during the 1 second before a paroxysm were within normal limits, but only 43% of the reaction times at the onset of a paroxysmal were normal, and after a delay of 0.5 seconds into a paroxysm, only 20% were normal. Responsiveness was recovered quickly after a paroxysm. The degree of maximal impairment of auditory responsiveness was the same in paroxysms of both long and short duration. Thus, any spike-wave paroxysm, regardless of duration, can impair consciousness, and therapy for absence seizure should aim at controlling all spike-wave paroxysms, not just the longer bursts (Browne et al 1974).

The average visual-evoked potential was altered 0.5 seconds or less before the onset of generalized spike-wave discharges, suggesting that behavioral unresponsiveness starts well before the discharges (Orren 1978). A blocking effect of sensory arousal and of activated attentiveness-nociceptive and acoustic fear stimuli were noted (Jung 1962).

Freeman et al (1973), with simultaneous video and telemetered EEG recording, studied environmental interaction and memory during petit mal seizures and concluded that a patient retains some degree of visual-motor coordination during a petit mal seizure. The patient may be totally amnestic for complex environmental interactions or may have detailed memory for environmental events.

ABSENCE STATUS

Since Lennox named this condition "petit mal status," this status has received a variety of names: "petit mal epilepsy occurring in status," "status epilepticus in petit mal," "petit mal status epilepticus," and "spike-wave stupor." In 1973, Penry reviewed the subject extensively. Behavior during absence status may be stuporous, confused, dazed, groggy; the patient may show slow or incomplete responses, wandering, and automatisms or may be in a catatonic state (Thompson and Greenhouse 1968). The duration of such behavior may vary from hours to several days. The electroencephalographic recording during such episodes reveals almost continuous spike-and-wave activity with only occasional episodes of very brief duration of relative normality (Kellaway and Chao 1955). However, the morphology of spike-wave discharges may not be as regular as those seen in absence seizures. A strong or repeated stimulus will elicit a response during paroxysmal discharges when none result from a weaker or single stimulus. These stimuli often alter or temporarily normalize the EEG (Jung 1962). During absence status, the patient may have a period of confusion or stupor but can follow a simple command, which often has to be repeated. All movements are slow. Speech consists of simple responses such as "yes" or "no" (Penry and Dreifuss 1969).

Absence status is considered important as a cause of psychotic manifestations in children (Asperger et al 1974, Groh and Rosenmayr 1974). The 3-Hz spike-wave discharges in adults may be associated with depression characterized by withdrawal, hostility and suicidal thoughts (Wells 1973), and confusional psychosis (Flor-Henry 1972).

During the status, the impairment of higher cortical function is selective rather than global, because intact or partially preserved contact, time and space orientation though diminution of praxic function, or motor and speech slackening occurred (Geier 1978). Absence status may terminate in generalized tonic-clonic seizures (Hess et al 1971). Petit mal status without impairment of consciousness was recorded in a 17-year-old girl (Assael 1969). Physical examination during the ictus may show dull facies with twitching around the eyes or mouth and local or generalized myoclonic jerks.

Absence status must be differentiated from the status of complex partial seizures, although it may be difficult to distinguish the two conditions on clinical grounds. An EEG makes it possible to differentiate them (Lugaresi et al 1971). In a status of complex partial seizures, EEG shows bilateral diffuse slowing interrupted by intermittent temporal 4- to 12-Hz discharges (Belafsky et al 1978). The diagnosis of spike-wave stupor is not difficult when both the clinical picture and the EEG are taken into consideration (Niedermeyer and Khalifeh 1965). However, absence status clinically is often misdiagnosed as a functional disorder or psychotic disease. The frequency of absence status is greater in the female than in the male, and petit mal status occurs most frequently in the fourth decade of life (Shev 1968, Rennick et al 1969) and is common in adults who have had petit mal since childhood (Thompson and Greenhouse 1968). However, absence status in children may be different from similar episodes in adults without prior history of absences or seizure disorders, because the latter responded well to antiepileptic drugs such as phenobarbital or phenytoin (Ellis and Lee 1978).

Petit mal status does not produce sufficiently typical mental changes to enable diagnosis; therefore, it is imperative to perform EEG examination in all cases of episodic mental disturbances (Domyslawski and Kość 1971).

Petit mal status also has to be differentiated from postictal twilight states, organic brain syndrome, interictal psychosis, and drug intoxication (Weissberg 1975, Mor 1971).

Diazepam is the drug of choice and should be given intravenously. Its initial maximal dose is 10 mg; the most serious complication is respiratory arrest and is due to excessive doses. Respiratory arrest is particularly likely to occur when diazepam is used immediately after intravenous administration of phenobarbital (Forman 1974). Ethosuximide and nitrazepam also are effective, though the onset of effectiveness may be delayed (Schwartz and Scott 1971, Celesia 1976). Clonazepam IV also is noted to be effective for terminating the status (Rosenmayr and Groh 1975).

COURSE AND PROGNOSIS

Petit mal is not transformed into psychomotor seizures (Currier et al 1963, Sato et al 1976a). The prognosis is good for patients with absence seizures only but is less favorable for patients with supervening grand mal seizures (Hertoft 1963, Dalby 1969, Currier et al 1963, Gordon 1965, Barnhart et al 1969, Sato et al 1976a). Petit mal epilepsy of late onset is more likely to be complicated by grand mal seizures (Lennox and Lennox 1960, Currier et al 1963, Dalby 1969, Livingston et al 1965), ie, the prognosis is regarded as slightly better for those patients whose petit mal commenced before the age of 10 years (Gibberd 1966). The earlier the age of onset of petit mal, the less likely the patient is to develop grand mal (Charlton and Yahr 1967).

The prognostic importance of immediate, energetic treatment has been emphasized (Rodin 1972). It is said that petit mal epilepsy seldom continues into adult life (Lennox and Lennox 1960, Livingston et al 1965). However, in adult patients with petit mal persisting after the age of 20 years, the chance of cessation of petit mal was 50% at the age of 20 years and 30% by the age of 40 years (Gibberd 1972). In a study of 39 adult patients (30–74 years) with spike-and-wave discharges, petit mal uncomplicated by the appearance of grand mal tends to subside by the age of 30; however, persisting spike-wave abnormalities are usually associated with grand mal seizures (Crews and Sidell 1973). Early cessation of seizures was noted to be more frequent in males than in females (Dalby 1969); however, there is no prognostic difference between sexes (Hertoft 1963, Gibberd 1966). A normal neurologic examination and normal EEG background activity favor a better outcome (Sato et al 1976a).

A prospective follow-up study in 48 patients with absence seizures showed that significant prognostic factors for cessation of any seizure type were a negative history of generalized tonic-clonic seizures, normal or above-normal intelligence, and a negative family history of seizure disorders. Nearly 90% of the patients with all three significant factors ceased having seizures (Sato et al 1976a). Overall remission rate ranges between 37.5% and 57.8% (Currier et al 1963, Dalby 1969, Hertoft 1963, Gordon 1965, Lees and Liversedge 1962, Kuhlo 1965, Sato et al 1976a).

TREATMENT

The goal of therapy is complete seizure control from psychological, social, and economic points of view (Sibley 1974). Early and adequate treatment is recommended (Bergamini 1969). Treatment should begin with the administration of only one medication, the dosage being adjusted until effective blood concentrations are achieved and maintained. If there is no improvement, the patient should be crossed over to another drug. If there is partial improvement, a second drug should be added and the effect on seizures observed while effective serum concentrations of both compounds are maintained (Penry and Newmark 1979). The two major groups of compounds used in the treatment of absence seizures are the oxazolidine dione derivatives (trimethadione and paramethadion) and the succinimides (phensuximide, methsuximide, and ethosuximide). The oxazolidines have been effective agents but have produced serious side effects; therefore, they are now rarely used.

As early as 1964, ethosuximide was the drug of first choice for the treatment of petit mal in children (O'Donohoe 1964); this is still true even though valproate has been introduced as an agent for treatment of absence seizures and has been found to be as effective as ethosuximide (Sato et al 1982). Treatment with ethosuximide may be initiated at the maintenance level of the drug, whereas the dosage of valproic acid should be gradually increased. Livingston and co-workers advocated a combined therapy of antiabsence agents and other antiepileptic agents because of the high prevalence of generalized tonic-clonic seizures in patients with absence seizures (Livingston et al 1965). However, this has not been routinely adopted by most neurologists (Singer and Freeman 1975) and may be contraindicated.

There is no clear rule for deciding when to stop treatment. Some investigators have recommended a minimal seizure-free period of two years before discontinuation of medication (Hamilton 1972, Forman 1974); some have recommended a longer period (Gibberd 1975). A minimum period of three years free of seizures with a further year to withdraw anticonvulsants has also been recommended (Barry 1978).

Ethosuximide

Ethosuximide (2-ethyl-2-methylsuccinimide; Zarontin) is a heterocyclic compound with one nitrogen. Ethosuximide is well absorbed and reaches a peak level 1 to 4 hours after oral administration. Protein binding is not significant. The rate of metabolism and the half-life of ethosuximide vary with the age of patient: the average half-life is only 30 hours in children and is 60 hours in adults. Microsomal enzyme induction in man has not been documented. Serum concentrations of 40 to 100 $\mu g/mL$ have been reported to be effective (Browne et al 1975), though higher levels are occasionally needed. The usual dosage ranges from 20 to 40 mg/kg/day (Penry et al 1972); this dosage may be started at the beginning of therapy. Response to ethosuximide is rapid, within 48 hours. Dose-related toxic effects include nausea, vomiting, anorexia, headache, fatigue, lethargy, dizziness, and hiccups. Toxic effects may diminish after a slight reduction in the dosage; withdrawal of the drug is rarely required (Browne et al 1975). Toxic effects unrelated to the dosage include skin rash, blood dyscrasias, allergic reactions, and systemic lupus erythematosis. Frequent blood counts are recommended (Weinstein and Allen 1966). Gastrointestinal side effects are relatively common but may be lessened by giving the drug with food. The mechanism of action is not known. Seventy percent of patients with petit mal attacks obtained approximately 90% or better seizure control with ethosuximide treatment (Weinstein and Allen 1966). Improvement was observed in 17 of 21 patients who were previously refractory to trimethadione: complete control in 8 and partial control in 9 (Livingston et al 1962).

Valproic Acid

Use of sodium valproate as an antiepileptic drug was extensively reviewed by Simon and Penry (1975). In the United States, valproic acid in capsules and sodium valproate in syrup are available. Valproic acid (2-propylpentanoic acid; Depakene) is a simple, eight-carbon, branched-chain carboxylic acid; it is rapidly absorbed, reaching its peak blood level in less than 4 hours. Valproic acid is extensively bound by protein and interacts with other agents. The half-life of valproic acid, which may be more variable in children than in adults, ranges between 8 and 15 hours. Valproic acid appears to have no enzyme-inducing properties, may increase phenobarbital levels, and may reduce total serum phenytoin while increasing free phenytoin. Phenytoin, phenobarbital, or primidone may decrease the half-life of valproic acid. The starting dosage is below 15 mg/kg/day, with weekly increase of 5 mg/kg/day. A daily maintenance dosage of 20 to 60 mg/kg may be needed to achieve optimal control of seizures. A reported therapeutic blood plasma level ranged between 50 and 100 μg/mL. Valproic acid is usually given three to four times a day because of its relatively short half-life, but schedules with less frequent administration have also been effective.

The most common side effects of valproic acid are nausea, vomiting, and cramps; these symptoms appear early in treatment and usually respond to reduction of the dosage or administration with some food. Sedation and ataxia are rarely noted with valproic acid alone, though interaction with phenobarbital may be responsible. Increased weight gain and transient hair loss have been noted. Inhibition of platelet aggregation has been noted, but no bleeding disorders secondary to its use have been reported. A total of 43 fatal cases of hepatoxicity of valproic acid have been reported in the FDA Drug Bulletin (July 1981;11[2]). When abnormal liver function test findings occur, particularly elevation of SGOT and SGPT, volproic acid should be reduced or stopped. The mechanism of action has been postulated as inhibition of discharge spread, increased γ-aminobutyric acid activity through a reduction of GABA degrading enzyme, decrease of cyclic GMP concentration in the cerebellum, and increase in potassium conductance.

Clonazepam

Clonazepam, a chlorinated derivative of nitrazepam, is a potent antiepileptic drug for controlling absence seizures. Clonazepam was found to be as effective as ethosuximide (Sato et al 1977). Clonazepam appears to be well absorbed, and the peak plasma level occurs in 1 to 4 hours after oral administration. Distribution is rapid because of its high lipid solubility. Clonazepam is 47% protein-bound. It has a half-life between 22 and 33 hours in children with absence seizures (Dreifuss et al 1975). A starting dosage is 0.5 mg/day; this dosage is slowly increased to a maximum of 8 mg/day. Gradual increment is essential to avoid excessive drowsiness. Reduction in the frequency of absence seizures was seen with serum levels of 13 to 72 μg/mL (Dreifuss et al 1975). A high rate of side effects limits its extensive use (Dreifuss and Sato, 1982). The common side effects include drowsiness, ataxia, and behavior and personality changes such as hyperactivity, restlessness, short attention span, irritability, disruptiveness, and aggressiveness. Nystagmus, dizziness, dysarthria, hypotonia, and slight weight gain also are fairly common. Increased frequency of various seizure types have been noted. Hypersecretion and hypersalivation may be troublesome in infants and children. Hematological and dermatological complications have been occasionally reported, but hepatic or renal complications have not been seen. The preceding side effects often result in withdrawal of clonazepam; however, withdrawal has to be done very gradually in order to avoid a withdrawal effect. The mechanism of action is not known.

Other agents that are occasionally used for the treatment of absence seizures include methsuximide (Celontin) (Scholl et al 1959, Trolle and Kiørboe 1959/60), phensuximide (Milontin), and acetazolamide (Lombroso and Frosythe 1959/60).

BIBLIOGRAPHY

Adie WJ: Pyknolepsy: A form of epilepsy occurring in children with a good prognosis. *Brain* 1924;47:96–102.

Ajmone Marsan C: A newly proposed classification of epileptic seizures. Neurophysiological basis. *Epilepsia* 1965;6:275–296.

Ajmone Marsan C, Lewis WR: Pathologic findings in patients with "centrencephalic" electroencephalographic patterns. *Neurology* 1960;10:922–930.

Arushaian EB, Avalian RM: Metrazol-induced petit mal: The role played by monoaminergic mechanisms and striatum. *Pharmacol Biochem Behav* 1978;8:113–117.

Asperger H, Groh Ch, Rosenmayr FM: Psychotische Manifestationen bei Kindern II bei Epilepsien. *Paediatr Paedol* 1974;9:226–236.

Assael MI: Petit mal status without impairment of consciousness. *Electroencephalogr Clin Neurophysiol* 1969;27:218.

Bancaud J, Talairach P, Morel M, et al: "Generalized" epileptic seizures elicited by electrical stimulation of the frontal lobe in man. *Electroencephalogr Clin Neurophysiol* 1974;37: 275–282.

Barnhart DA, Newsom TD, Crawley JW, et al: Long-term prognosis of petit mal epilepsy. *Electroencephalogr Clin Neurophysiol* 1969;27:549–550.

Barry JE: Epilepsy in childhood. *N Engl J Med* 1978;88:412–415.

Belafksy MA, Carwille S, Miller P, et al: Prolonged epileptic twilight states: Continuous recordings with nasopharyngeal electrodes and videotape analysis. *Neurology* 1978;28: 239–245.

Bergamini von L: Zur Therapie des echten Petit Mal. *MMW* 1969;36:1807–1809.

Bickford RG: The application of depth electroencephalography in some varieties of epilepsy. *Electroencephalogr Clin Neurophysiol* 1956;8:526–527.

Blom S, Heijbel J, Bergfous PG: Incidence of epilepsy in children: A follow-up study three years after the first seizure. *Epilepsia* 1978;19:343–350.

Bogacz J, Yanicelli E: Vegetative phenomena in petit mal epilepsy. *World Neurol* 1962;3: 195–208.

Böhm M: Status epilepticus petit mal: Further observation of an adult case. *Electroencephalogr Clin Neurophysiol* 1969;26:229.

Browne TR, Dreifuss FE, Dyken PR, et al: Ethosuximide in the treatment of absence (petit mal) seizures. *Neurology (Minneap)* 1975;25:515–524.

Browne TR, Penry JK, Porter RJ, et al: Responsiveness before, during, and after spike-wave paroxysms. *Neurology* 1974;24:659–665.

Burchiel KJ, Myers RR, Bickford RC: Visual and auditory evoked responses during penicillin-induced generalized spike-and-wave activity in cats. *Epilepsia* 1976;17:293–311.

Burns R: Transient disturbances of consciousness. *Aust Fam Physician* 1976;5:935–938.

Cavazzuti GB: Epidemiology of different types of epilepsy in school age children of Modena, Italy. *Epilepsia* 1980;21:57–62.

Celesia GG: Modern concepts of status epilepticus. *JAMA* 1976;235:1571–1574.

Charlton MH, Yahr MD: Long-term follow-up of patients with petit mal. *Arch Neurol* 1967;16:595–598.

Cleeland CS, Booker HE: Petit mal evoked by arousal during sensory restriction. *Arch Neurol* 1967;17:324–330.

Cohn R: A neuropathological study of a case of petit mal epilepsy. *Electroencephalogr Clin Neurophysiol* 1968;24:282.

Crews RD, Sidell AD: The clinical significance of spike and wave abnormalities in the adult. *Bull Los Angeles Neurol Soc* 1973;38:60–68.

Currier RD, Kooi KA, Saidman LJ: Prognosis of "pure" petit mal. A follow-up study. *Neurology (Minneap)* 1963;13:959–967.

Commission for the Control of Epilepsy and Its Consequences: *Plan for Nationwide Action on Epilepsy,* vol 1. DHEW Publication No. (NIH) 78-276, 1978.

Dalby MA: Epilepsy and 3 per second spike and wave rhythms. A clinical electroencephalographic and prognostic analysis of 346 patients. *Acta Neurol Scand* 1969;(supp 40):45.

Daly DD: Reflections on the concept of petit mal. *Epilepsia* 1968;9:175–178.

Daly DD: Differentiation of automatisms of focal or general origin. *Folia Psychiatr Neurol Jpn* 1977;31:539–542.

Degen R: Die Atiologie der Kindlichen Epilepsien aufgrand anamnestischer Erhebungen im Vergleich mit einer Kontrollgruppe. *Fortschr Neurol Psychiatr* 1977;46:43–60.

DeMarco P: Petit mal epilepsy during early infancy. *Clin Electroencephalogr* 1980;11:38–40.

Dobrzynska L, Mierzejewska E: Activation of epileptic discharges by closing of eyes. *Neurol Neurochir Pol* 1974;6:713–716.

Domyslawski M, Kość B: Petit mal status. *Psychiatr Pol Rok* 1971;1040:27–32.

Doose H, Gerken T, Horstmann T, et al: Genetic factors in spike-wave absences. *Epilepsia* 1973;14:57–75.

Dorazco VJ: Cuantas clases de'pequeno mal'existen. *Cubana Med* 1979;18:449–453.

Dreifuss FE: The prognosis of petit mal, in Alter M (ed): *Epidemiology of Epilepsy.* Washington, DC, NINDS Monographs, 1972.

Dreifuss FE: The differential diagnosis of partial seizures with complex symptomatology, in Penry JK, Daly DD (eds): *Advances in Neurology.* New York, Raven Press, 1975, vol 2, pp 187–199.

Dreifuss FE, Penry JK, Rose SW, et al: Serum clonazepam concentrations in children with absence seizures. *Neurology* 1975;25:255–258.

Dreifuss FE: Proposal for revised clinical and electroencephalographic classification of epileptic seizures. *Epilepsia* 1981;22:489–501.

Dreifuss FE, Sato S: Clonazepam, in Woodbury DM, Penry JK, Pippenger CE (eds): *Antiepileptic Drugs.* New York, Raven Press, 1982.

Ellis JM, Lee SI: Acute prolonged confusion in later life as an ictal state. *Epilepsia.* 1978;19:119–128.

Engel J Jr, Kuhl DE, Phelps ME, et al: Metabolic correlates of 3 per second spike-and-wave absences. 35th American EEG Society Annual Meeting, Chicago, June 11–13, 1981.

Englander RN, Johnson RN, Brickley JJ, et al: Effects of antiepileptic drugs on thalamocortical excitability. *Neurology* 1977;27:1134–1139.

Escueta AVD, Bacsal FE, Treiman DM: Complex partial seizures on closed circuit television and EEG. A study of 691 attacks in 79 patients. *Ann Neurol* 1982;11:292–300.

Fedio P, Mirsky AF: Selective intellectual deficits in children with temporal lobe or centrencephalic epilepsy. *Neuropsychologia* 1969;7:287–300.

Flor-Henry P: Ictal and interictal psychiatric manifestations in epilepsy: Specific or nonspecific? A critical review of some of the evidence. *Epilepsia* 1972;13:773–783.

Forman PM: Therapy of seizures in children. *Am Fam Physician* 1974;10:144–148.

Freeman FR, Douglas EFO, Penry JK: Environmental interaction and memory during petit mal (absence) seizures. *Pediatrics* 1973;51:911–918.

Fromm GH, Kohli CM: The role of inhibitory pathways in petit mal epilepsy. *Neurology (Minneap)* 1972;22:1012–1020.

Fromm GH, Glass JD, Chattha AS, et al: Antiabsence drugs and inhibitory pathways. *Neurology* 1980;30:126–131.

Gastaut H, Roger J, Soulayrol R, et al: Childhood epileptic encephalopathy and diffuse slow spike-waves (otherwise known as "petit mal variant") or Lennox syndrome. *Epilepsia* 1966;7:139–179.

Gastaut H: Clinical and electroencephalographic correlates of generalized spike and wave bursts occurring spontaneously in man. *Epilepsia* 1968;9:179–184.

Gastaut H: Clinical electroencephalographical classification of epileptic seizures. *Epilepsia* 1970;11:102–113.

Gastaut H: *Dictionary of Epilepsy. Part 1: Definitions.* Geneva, World Health Organization, 1973.

Gastaut H, Gastaut J: Computerized axial tomography in epilepsy, in Penry JK (ed): *Epilepsy, The Eighth International Symposium.* New York, Raven Press, 1973, pp 5–15.

Geier S: Prolonged psychic epileptic seizures: A study of the absence status. *Epilepsia* 1978; 19:431–445.

Gianturco DT, Wilson WP, Harris BS: Interictal focal or lateralized discharges occurring in the electroencephalograms of patients suffering from centrencephalic epilepsy. *Confin Neurol* 1968;30:368–374.

Gibberd FB: The clinical features of petit mal. *Acta Neurol Scand* 1966;42:176–190.

Gibberd FB: The prognosis of petit mal in adults. *Epilepsia* 1972;13:171–175.

Gibberd FB: Diseases of the central nervous system: Epilepsy. *Br Med J* 1975;365/75:270–272.

Gibbs FA, Davis H, Lennox WG: The electro-encephalogram in epilepsy and in conditions of impaired consciousness. *Arch Neurol Psychiatr* 1935;34:1133–1148.

Gibbs FA: Petit mal variant revisited. *Epilepsia* 1971;12:89–96.

Gloor P, Hall G, Coceani F: Differential epileptogenic action of penicillin on cortical and subcortical brain structures. *Electroencephalogr Clin Neurophysiol* 1967;23:491.

Gloor P: Generalized cortico-reticular epilepsies: Some considerations on the pathophysiology of generalized bilaterally synchronous spike and wave discharge. *Epilepsia* 1968;9: 249–263.

Gloor P: Neurophysiological bases of generalized seizures termed centrencephalic, in Gastaut H, et al (eds): *The Physiopathogenesis of the Epilepsies.* Springfield, IL, Charles C Thomas Publisher, 1969, pp 209–248.

Gloor P, Testa G, Guberman A: Brain-stem and cortical mechanisms in an animal model of generalized corticoreticular epilepsy. *Trans Am Neurol Assoc* 1973;98:203–205.

Gloor P, Testa G: Generalized penicillin epilepsy in the cat: Effects of intracarotid and inervertebral pentylenetetrazol and amobarbital injections. *Electroencephalogr Clin Neurophysiol* 1974;36:499–515.

Gloor P, Rasmussen T, Altuzarra X, et al: Role of the intracarotid amobarbital pentylentetrazol EEG test in the diagnosis and surgical treatment of patients with complex seizure problems. *Epilepsia* 1976;17:15–31.

Godschalk M, Dzoljic MR, Bonta IL: Slow wave sleep and a state resembling absence epilepsy induced in the rat by α-hydroxybutyrate. *Eur J Pharmacol* 1977;44:105–111.

Goode DJ, Penry JK, Dreifuss FE: Effects of paroxysmal spike-wave on continuous visual-motor performance. *Epilepsia* 1970;11:241–254.

Gordon N: The natural history of petit mal epilepsy. *Dev Med Child Neurol* 1965;7:537–542.

Green JB: Cerebral evoked responses in epilepsy. *Electroencephalogr Clin Neurophysiol* 1969; 21:666–667.

Groh C, Rosenmayr FW: Isolierter Petit Mal Status. *Dtsch Med Wochenschr* 1974;99:379–385.

Grossman HJ: Convulsive disorders in infants and children. *J Med J* 1969;135:260–267.

Guerrero-Figueroa R, Barros A, de Balbian VM, et al: Experimental "petit mal" in kittens. *Arch Neurol* 1963;9:297–306.

Guey J, Bureau M, Dravet C, et al: A study of the rhythm of petit mal absences in children in relation to prevailing situations. The use of EEG telemetry during psychological examinations, school exercises, and periods of inactivity. *Epilepsia* 1969;10:441-451.

Hamilton DG: Epilepsy in childhood. *Med J Aust* 1972;1:587-591.

Hauser WA, Kurland LT: The epidemiology of epilepsy in Rochester, Minnesota, 1935 through 1967. *Epilepsia* 1975;16:1-66.

Hertoft P: The clinical, electroencephalographic and social prognosis in petit mal epilepsy. *Epilepsia* 1963;4:298-314.

Hess R, Scollo-Lavizzari G, Wyss FE: Borderline cases of petit mal status. *Eur Neurol* 1971; 5:137-154.

Holowach J, Thurston DL, O'Leary L: Petit mal epilepsy. *Pediatrics* 1962;30:893-901.

Howell DA: Unusual centrencephalic seizure patterns. *Brain* 1955;78:199-208.

Hunter J, Jasper HH: Effects of thalamic stimulation in unanesthetized animals: Arrest reaction and petit mal-like seizures, activation patterns, and generalized convulsions. *Electrocephalogr Clin Neurophysiol* 1949;1:305.

Jasper HH, Droogleever-Fortuyn J: Experimental studies on the functional anatomy of petit mal epilepsy. *Res Publ Assoc Res Nerv Ment Dis* 1946;26:272-298.

Jung R: Blocking of petit mal attacks by sensory arousal and inhibition of attacks by an active change in attention during the epileptic aura. *Epilepsia* 1962;3:407-434.

Jelliffe ES, Notkin J: The pyknolepsies. *Am J Psychiatry* 1934;91:679.

Kawai I, Fujii S, Shinzu K, et al: Uncontrollable cases of absence. *Folia Psychiatr Neurol Jpn* 1980;34:97-105.

Kellaway P, Chao D: Prolonged status epilepticus in petit mal. *Electroencephalogr Clin Neurophysiol* 1955;7:145.

Klass D, Daly DD: Petit mal seizures. *Electroencephalogr Clin Neurophysiol* 1961;13:824.

Kogeargos J, Henson RA, Scott DF: Pattern sensitive epilepsy: A case report. *J Neurol Neurosurg Psychiatry* 1979;42:635-639.

Kuhlo W: Katammestische Untersuchungen zur pyknolepsie. *Arch Psychiatr Nervenkr* 1965; 207:254-268.

Kurland LT: The incidence and prevalence of convulsive disorders in a small urban community. *Epilepsia* 1959/60;1:143-161.

Lagenstein I, Kühne D, Sternowsky HJ, et al: Computerized cranial transverse axial tomography (CTAT) in 145 patients with primary and secondary generalized epilepsies, West syndrome, myoclonic-astatic petit mal, absence epilepsy. *Neuropaediatrie* 1979;10:15-28.

Lange SC, Julien RM: Reevaluation of estrogen-induced cortical and thalamic paroxysmal EEG activity in the cat. *Electroencephalogr Clin Neurophysiol* 1978;44:94-103.

Lance JW: Classification and treatment of myoclonus. *Proc Aust Assoc Neurol* 1970;133: 61-64.

Lawall J: Psychiatric presentations of seizure disorders. *Am J Psychiatry* 1976;3:321-323.

Lees F, Liversedge LA: The prognosis of "petit mal" and minor epilepsy. *Lancet* 1962;2:797-799.

Legg NJ, Swash M: Clinical note: Seizures and EEG activation after trimipramine. *Epilepsia* 1974;15:131-135.

Lennox WG, Robinson F: Cingulate-cerebellar mechanisms in the physiological pathogenesis of epilepsy. *Electroencephalogr Clin Neurophysiol* 1951;3:197-205.

Lennox WG, Lennox MA: *Epilepsy and Related Disorders.* Boston, Little Brown & Co, 1960.

Lima JGC, Longo RH, Di Migueli HB: Anomalidades focals no pequeno mal epilépeptico. *Arq Neuropsiquiatr* 1972;30:331-334.

Livingston S: *The Diagnosis and Treatment of Convulsive Disorders in Children.* Springfield, IL, Charles C Thomas Publisher, 1954.

Livingston S, Pauli L, Najmatadi A: Ethosuximide in the treatment of epilepsy. *JAMA* 1962; 180:822-825.

Livingston S, Torres I, Pauli LL, et al: Petit mal epilepsy. Results of a prolonged follow-up study of 117 patients. *JAMA* 1965;194:113-118.

Livingston S: *Comprehensive Management of Epilepsy in Infancy, Childhood, and Adolescence.* Springfield, IL, Charles C Thomas Publisher, 1972.

Livingston S, Berman W: Participation of epileptic patients in sports. *JAMA* 1973;224: 236–238.

Livingston S: Guest editorial: Epilepsy and sports. *Am Fam Physician* 1978;17:67, 69.

Loiseau P, Cohadon F, Cohadon S: Recording of absences of petit mal type in a man of 40, with epileptic attacks since the age of 3, who had a frontal glioma. *Electroencephalogr Clin Neurophysiol* 1971;30:251.

Lombroso CT, Forsythe I: A long-term follow-up of acetazolamide (Diamox) in the treatment of epilepsy. *Epilepsia* 1959/60;1:493–500.

Lombroso CT, Erba G: A test for separating secondary from primary bilateral synchrony in epileptic subjects. *Epilepsia* 1969;10:415–420.

Lorentz de Haas AM, Kuilman M: Ethosuximide (α-ethyl-α-methylsuccinimide) and grand mal. *Epilepsia* 1964;5:90–96.

Luborsky L, Dockerty P, Todd C, et al: A context analysis of psychological states prior to petit mal EEG paraoxysms. *J Nerv Ment Dis* 1975;160:282–298.

Lücking CH, Creutzfeldt OD, Heinenmann U: Visual evoked potentials of patients with epilepsy and of a control group. *Electroencephalogr Clin Neurophysiol* 1970;30:557–566.

Lugaresi E, Pazzaglia P, Tassinari CA: Differentiation of absence status and temporal lobe status. *Epilepsia* 1971;12:77–87.

Marcus EM, Watson CW: Bilateral synchronous spike wave electrographic patterns in the cat: Interaction of bilateral cortical foci in the intact, the bilateral cortical callosal, and adiencephalic preparation. *Arch Neurol* 1966;14:601–610.

Marcus EM, Watcon CW: Symmetrical epileptogenic foci in monkey cerebral cortex: Mechanisms of interaction and regional variations in capacity for synchronous discharges. *Arch Neurol* 1968;19:99–116.

Marcus EM, Watson CW, Simon SA: An experimental model of some varieties of petit mal epilepsy: Electrical-behavior correlations of acute bilateral epileptogenic foci in cerebral cortex. *Epilepsia* 1968;9:233–248.

Marcus EM, Jacobson S, Watson CW, et al: An experimental model of "petit mal epilepsy" in the monkey: Additional studies of the anterior premotor area. *Trans Am Neurol Assoc* 1970;95:279–281.

Matthes A, Weber H: Klinische und elektroencephalographische Familienuntersuchungen bei Pykuolepsien. *Dtsch Med Wschr* 1968;93:429–435.

Merlis JK: Proposal for an international classification of the epilepsies. *Epilepsia* 1970;11: 114–119.

Metrakos JD, Metrakos K: Genetics of convulsive disorders. Part 1: Introduction, problems, methods, and base lines. *Neurology (Minneap)* 1960;10:228–240.

Metrakos K, Metrakos JD: Genetics of convulsive disorders. Part 2: Genetic and electroencephalographic studies in centrencephalic epilepsy. *Neurology (Minneap)* 1961;11:464–483.

Metrakos JD, Metrakos K: Genetic factors in epilepsy, in Niedermeyer E (ed): *Modern Problems of Pharmacopsychiatry,* vol 4, *Epilepsy.* Basil, Karger, 1970, pp 71–86.

Mirsky AF, Primac DW, Ajmone Marsan C, et al: A comparison of the psychological test performance of patients with focal and nonfocal epilepsy. *Exp Neurol* 1960;2:75–89.

Mirsky AF, Van Buren JM: On the nature of the "absence" in centrencephalic epilepsy: A study of some behavioral, electroencephalographic and autonomic factors. *Electroencephalogr Clin Neurophysiol* 1965;18:334–348.

Mirsky AF, Orren MM: Attention, in Miller LH, Sandman CA, Kastin AJ (eds): *Neuropeptide Influences on the Brain and Behavior.* New York, Raven Press, 1977, pp 233–267.

Mirsky AF: Epilepsy, attentiveness, and consciousness. Recent contributions from behavioral and physiological investigations. A summary and commentary, in Cobb WA, Van Dujin H (eds): *Contemporary Clinical Neurophysiology.* Amsterdam, Elsevier, 1978, (EEG

Suppl No 34), pp 269–275.

Mor PG: Spike-wave stupor. *Am J Dis Child* 1971;12:307–313.

Morillo A, Baylor D: A brief report on the experimental production of electroclinical patterns of petit mal type. *Electroencephalogr Clin Neurophysiol* 1964;16:519–521.

Morison RS, Dempsey EW: A study of thalamo-cortical relations. *Am J Physiol* 1942;135: 281–292.

Needham WE, Bray PE, Wiser WC, et al: Intelligence and EEG studies in families with idiopathic epilepsy. *JAMA* 1969;207:1497–1501.

Newmark ME, Penry JK: *Photosensitivity and Epilepsy: A Review.* New York, Raven Press, 1979.

Newmark ME, Penry JK: *Genetics of Epilepsy: A Review.* New York, Raven Press, 1980.

Niedermeyer E: Sleep electroencephalograms in petit mal. *Arch Neurol* 1965;12:625–630.

Niedermeyer E, Khalifeh R: Petit mal status ("spike-wave stupor"). An electro-clinical appraisal. *Epilepsia* 1965;6:250–262.

Niedermeyer E: Generalized seizure discharges and possible precipitating mechanisms. *Epilepsia* 1966;7:23–29.

Niedermeyer E, Laws ER Jr, Walker AE: Depth EEG findings in epileptics with generalized spike-wave complexes. *Arch Neurol* 1969;21:51–58.

Niedermeyer E, Walker AE, Burton C: The slow spike-wave complex as a correlate of frontal and fronto-temporal post-traumatic epilepsy. *Eur Neurol* 1970;3:330–346.

Nuffield EJ: Electro-clinical correlations in childhood epilepsy. *Epilepsia* 1961;2:178–196.

O'Brien JL, Goldensohn ES, Hoefer PF: Electroencephalographic abnormalities in addition to 3 per sec spike and wave activity in petit mal. *Electroencephalogr Clin Neurophysiol* 1959; 11:747–761.

O'Donohoe NV: Treatment of petit mal with ethosuximide. *Dev Med Child Neurol* 1964; 6:498–501.

Okama T, Kumashiro H: Natural history and prognosis of epilepsy: Report of a multi-institutional study in Japan. *Epilepsia* 1981;22:35–53.

Orren MM: Evoked potential studies in petit mal epilepsy, in Cobb WA, Van Dujin H (eds): *Contemporary Clinical Neurophysiology.* Amsterdam, Elsevier, 1978, EEG Suppl No 234, pp 251–257.

Ottino CA, Meglio M, Rossi GF, et al: An experimental study of the structures mediating bilateral synchrony of epileptic discharges of cortical origin. *Epilepsia* 1971;12:299–311.

Paty J, Boucebci M: Étude de 192 absences du type petit mal considérations sur les critéres d'organicité. *Bord Med* 1972;5:2593–2608.

Penfield W, Jasper H: *Epilepsy and the Functional Anatomy of the Human Brain.* Boston, Little Brown & Co, 1954.

Penry JK, Dreifuss FE: Automatisms associated with the absence of petit mal epilepsy. *Arch Neurol* 1969;21:142–149.

Penry JK, Porter RJ, Dreifuss FE: Ethosuximide: Relation of plasma levels to clinical control, in Woodbury DM, Penry JK, Schmidt RP (eds): *Antiepileptic Drugs.* New York, Raven Press, 1972, pp 431–441.

Penry JK: Behavioral correlates of generalized spike-wave discharge in the electroencephalograph, in *Epilepsy. Its Phenomena in Man.* UCLA Forum in Medical Sciences, no. 17. New York, Academic Press Inc, 1973, pp 171–188.

Penry JK, Porter RJ, Dreifuss FE: Simultaneous recording of absence seizures with video tape and electroencephalography. A study of 374 seizures in 48 patients. *Brain* 1975;98:427–440.

Penry JK, Newmark ME: The use of antiepileptic drugs. *Ann Intern Med* 1979;90:207–218.

Pollen DA, Perot P, Reid KH: Experimental bilateral wave and spike from thalamic stimulation in relation to level of arousal. *Electroencephalogr Clin Neurophysiol* 1963;15:1017–1028.

Pollen DA, Reid KH, Perot P: Microelectrode studies of experimental 3/sec wave and spike in the cat. *Electroencephalogr Clin Neurophysiol* 1964;17:57–67.

Pollen DA, Sie PG: Analysis of thalamic induced wave and spike by modifications in cortical excitability. *Electroencephalogr Clin Neurophysiol* 1964;17:154–163.

Pollen DA: Intracellular studies of cortical neurons during thalamic induced wave and spike. *Electroencephalogr Clin Neurophysiol* 1964;17:398–404.

Pollen DA: Experimental spike and wave responses and petit mal epilepsy. *Epilepsia* 1968; 9:221–232.

Porter RJ, Penry JK, Dreifuss FE: Responsiveness at the onset of spike-wave bursts. *Electroencephalogr Clin Neurophysiol* 1973;34:239–245.

Pradham SN, Ajmone Marsan C: Chlorambucil toxicity and EEG "centrencephalic" patterns. *Epilepsia* 1963;4:1–14.

Pratt KL, Mattson RH, Weikers NJ, et al: EEG activation of epileptics following sleep deprivation: A prospective study of 114 cases. *Electroencephalogr Clin Neurophysiol* 1968;24: 11–15.

Rabending G, Klepel H: Fotokonvilsiv Reaktion und Fotomyoklonus: Altersabhängige Genetisch Determinierte Varianten der Gesteigerten Fotosensibilitate. *Neuropaediatrie* 1970; 2:164–172.

Rennick PM, Perez-Borja C, Rodin EA: Transient mental deficits associated with recurrent prolonged epileptic clouded state. *Epilepsia* 1969;10:397–405.

Rodin E, Gonzalez S, Caldwell D, et al: Photic evoked responses during induced epileptic seizures. *Epilepsia* 1966;7:202–214.

Rodin EA: Medical and social prognosis in epilepsy. *Epilepsia* 1972;13:121–131.

Rosenmayr F, Groh CH: Petit mal status initiated by photic stimulation. *Acta Univ Carol* 1975;23:193.

Rossi GF, Walter RD, Crandall PH: Generalized spike and wave discharges and nonspecific thalamic muclei. *Arch Neurol* 1968;19:174–183.

Sakai F, Myer JS, Hsu M-C, et al: EEG correlation with noninvasive measurement of cerebral blood flow in epilepsy and narcolepsy. *Trans Am Neurol Assoc* 1977;102:73–76.

Sarnat HB: Changing concepts of the absence seizure: A review of the pathogenesis of petit mal epilepsy. *Aust Paediatr J* 1977;13:158–162.

Sato S, Dreifuss FE, Penry JK: The effect of sleep on spike-wave discharges in absence seizures. *Neurology (Minneap)* 1973;23:1335–1345.

Sato S, Dreifuss FE, Penry JK: Prognosis factors in absence seizures. *Neurology (Minneap)* 1976a;26:788–796.

Sato S, Penry JK, Dreifuss FE: Electroencephalographic monitoring of generalized spike-wave paroxysms in the hospital and at home, in Kellaway P, Petersen I (eds): *Quantitative Analysis Studies in Epilepsy*. New York, Raven Press, 1976b, pp 237–251.

Sato S, Dreifuss FE, Penry JK, et al: Long-term follow-up study of absence seizures, in Akimoto H, Hazamatsuri H, Seizro M, et al (eds): *Advances in Epileptology*. New York, Raven Press, 1982, pp 41–42.

Sato S, White BG, Penry JK, et al: Valproic acid versus ethosuximide in the treatment of absence seizures. *Neurology (Minneap)* 1982;32:157–163.

Scherman RG, Abraham K: "Centrencephalic" electroencephalographic patterns in precocious puberty. *Electroencephalogr Clin Neurophysiol* 1963;15:559–567.

Scholl ML, Abbott JA, Schwab RS: Celontin—A new anticonvulsant. *Epilepsia* 1959;1: 105–109.

Schwab RS: Method of measuring consciousness in attacks of petit mal epilepsy. *Arch Neurol Psychiatr* 1939;41:215–217.

Schwab RS: The influence of visual and auditory stimuli on the electrographic tracing of petit mal. *Am J Psychiatry* 1941;97:1301–1312.

Schwartz MS, Scott DF: Isolated petit-mal status presenting de novo in middle age. *Lancet*

1971;2:1399-1401.

Seki T, Yamawaki H, Suzuki N, et al: Prognosis of typical absence with special reference to relationship with EEG findings. *Brain Dev* 1980;12:273-280.

Shev EE: Adult petit mal with special reference to petit mal status. *Electroencephalogr Clin Neurophysiol* 1968;24:393-398.

Shimazono Y, Hirai T, Okuma T, et al: Disturbance of consciousness in petit mal epilepsy. *Epilepsia* 1953;2:49-55.

Sibley WA: Diagnosis and treatment of epilepsy: Overview and general principles. *Pediatrics* 1974;53:531-535.

Silverman D: Clinical correlates of the spike and wave complex. *Electroencephalogr Clin Neurophysiol* 1954;6:663.

Simon D, Penry JK: Sodium di-n-propylacetate (DPA) in the treatment of epilepsy: A review. *Epilepsia* 1975;16:549-573.

Singer HS, Freeman JM: Seizures in adolescents. *Med Clin North Am* 1975;59:1461-1472.

Snead CO: Gamma hydroxybutyrate in the monkey. I. Electroencephalographic, behavioral, and pharmacokinetic studies. *Neurology* 1978a;28:636-642.

Snead CO: Gamma hydroxybutyrate in the monkey. II. Effect of chronic oral anticonvulsant drugs. *Neurology* 1978b;28:643-648.

Spiegel EA, Wyeis HT: Thalamic recordings in man with special reference to seizure discharges. *Electroencephalogr Clin Neurophysiol* 1950;2:23-27.

Steriade M: Interneuronal epileptic discharges related to spike-and-wave cortical seizures in behaving monkeys. *Electroencephalogr Clin Neurophysiol* 1974;37:247-263.

Stevens JR, Lonsbury BL, Goel SL: Seizure occurrence and interspike interval: Telemetered electroencephalographic studies. *Arch Neurol* 1972;26:409-419.

Stewart LF, Dreifuss FE: Centrencephalic seizure discharges in focal hemispheric lesions. *Arch Neurol* 1967;17:60.

Swaiman KF: Petit mal seizures. *Postgrad Med* 1969;46:93-96.

Swaiman KF: Brief lapses of consciousness in children. *Postgrad Med* 1971;50:107-109.

Temkin O: *The Falling Sickness. A History of Epilepsy from the Greeks to the Beginnings of Modern Neurology*, ed 2. Baltimore, Johns Hopkins Press, 1971.

Testa G, Gloor P: Generalized penicillin epilepsy in the cat: Effect of midbrain cooling. *Electroencephalogr Clin Neurophysiol* 1974;36:517-524.

Thompson SW, Greenhouse AH: Petit mal status in adults. *Ann Intern Med* 1968;68:1271-1279.

Tizard B, Margerison JH: The relationship between generalized paroxysmal EEG discharges and various test situations in two epileptic patients. *J Neurol Neurosurg Psychiatry* 1963;26:308-313.

Trolle E, Kiørboe E: Treatment of petit mal epilepsy with the new succinimides: PM 680 and Celontin. *Epilepsia* 1959/60;1:587-591.

Tucker JS, Solitare GB: Infantile myoclonic spasms. Clinical, electrographic and neuropathologic observations. *Epilepsia* 1963;4:45-59.

Tückel K, Jasper H: The electroencephalogram in parasagittal lesions. *Electroencephalogr Clin Neurophysiol* 1952;4:481-494.

Van Gelder NM, Janjua NA, Metrakos K, et al: Plasma amino acids in 3/sec spike-wave epilepsy. *Neurochem Res* 1980;5/6:659-671.

Weinstein AW, Allen RJ: Ethosuximide treatment of petit mal seizures. *Am J Dis Child* 1966;111:63-67.

Weir B: Spike-wave from stimulation of reticular core. *Arch Neurol* 1964;11: 209-218.

Weir B: The morphology of the spike-wave complex. *Electroencephalogr Clin Neurophysiol* 1965;19:284-290.

Weissberg MP: A case of petit mal status: A diagnostic dilemma. *Am J Psychiatry* 1975;132:1200-1201.

Wells C: Petit mal status presenting as a psychosis. *Trans Am Neurol Assoc* 1973;98:321–323.

Whitehouse D: Psychological and neurological correlates of seizure disorders. *Johns Hopkins Med J* 1971;129:36–42.

Wilder BJ, Musella L, Van Horn G, et al: Activation of spike and wave discharge in patients with generalized seizures. *Neurology* 1971;21:517–527.

Zegans LS, Kooi KA, Waggoner RW, et al: Effects of psychiatric interview upon paraoxysmal cerebral activity and autonomic measures in a disturbed child with petit mal epilepsy. *Psychosom Med* 1964;26:151–161.

CHAPTER 5

Generalized Tonic-Clonic Seizures

Fritz E. Dreifuss

Generalized tonic-clonic seizures are often known as major seizures or grand mal. It is difficult to define where the seizure begins and where it ends. The incontestable nucleus of the seizure consists of loss of consciousness and a sharp tonic contraction of muscles; there is often a cry and the patient falls to the ground in a tonic state (usually rigid and opisthotonic, but sometimes flexed), occasionally injuring himself in falling. The patient lies rigid; during this stage, tonic contraction inhibits respiration and cyanosis may occur. The tonic stage gives way to clonic convulsive movements, which last for a variable period of time; during this stage, small gusts of grunting respiration may occur between the convulsive movements. The patient may remain cyanotic; saliva may froth from the mouth; and if the tongue has been bitten, saliva may be blood-tinged. At the end of this stage, deep respiration occurs and all the muscles relax. After relaxation, the patient remains unconscious for variable periods of time and often awakes feeling stiff and sore all over.

Occasionally, there is an aura prior to the attack. The aura is a short ill-defined warning, which may consist of an epigastric sensation, a prodrome or foreboding, and sometimes a series of myoclonic jerks or an exacerbation of absence attacks. Usually, the attack begins abruptly, and consciousness is lost at the beginning. Occasionally, the patient may remember the initial cry as the last memory prior to loss of consciousness (Janz 1969). The cry is the result of forced expiratory muscle contraction, which forces air through a partially closed glottis, although it may occur during forced inspiration. Usually, the tonic phase, which may be asymmetrical, lasts approximately a minute and then gives way to the jerking movements of the clonic phase. The jerks gradually diminish in frequency, although the amplitude remains unchanged. After the last jerk the patient lies completely exhausted, perspiring, and gradually regaining normal color. The breathing in the postconvulsive period is stertorous. During the seizure, there is frequently involuntary passage of urine and infrequently involuntary passage of feces. The tongue is frequently bitten, and the mucosa of the cheek may be lacerated. Occasionally, the convulsion may be sufficiently severe to lead to bony injury, particularly spinal compression fractures. The seizure may be followed by vomiting, sleep, and a variable period of confusion with gradual regaining of consciousness over a period of minutes to hours.

Attacks can occur at any time of the day or night. If they occur during sleep, the first indication may be the noise of the bed shaking. The frequency of attacks may be greater on first going to sleep or on awakening in the morning. Attacks may be precipitated by lack of sleep or fatigue, by fever, by failure to take anticonvulsants, and sometimes by reflex sensory stimuli, such as flashing lights. The classic generalized tonic-clonic seizure is not difficult to diagnose by history, especially the history obtained from an observer or by observation of a seizure. Secondary generalized seizures, beginning as partial seizures and rapidly projecting to subcortical structures and becoming generalized, may be clinically indistinguishable, especially if the aura is short or if an amnesia for the aura takes place as a result of a seizure. In partial seizures, secondarily generalized, the aura imparts a focal signature. The focal signature may be a focal motor phenomenon with or without march; a somatosensory symptom, or a special sensory symptom; autonomic symptomatology such as vomiting, flushing, sweating, or piloerection; or gustatory or olfactory symptoms. Psychic symptomatology, including dynmnesic symptoms, cognitive disturbances, affective symptoms, illusions, hallucinations, or dreamy states may constitute the focal element prior to generalization of the seizure (Commission on Classification and Terminology 1981). Apart from the clinical description, the electroencephalogram may be helpful in distinguishing paroxysmal instability of the corticoreticular system that is manifested as primary generalized tonic-clonic seizures from the asymmetries and focal discharges in those attacks that arise focally and become secondarily generalized tonic-clonic seizures. This distinction is of more than theoretical importance, both from the point of view of etiological significance and that of approach to treatment.

Generalized tonic-clonic seizures may occasionally be seen as a consequence of syncope on a vasovagal or a cardiac basis. Here the prodrome is different. The patient is usually quite pale, the seizure is short, and consciousness is usually rapidly regained when the patient become recumbent. There is frequently a clear precipitating factor associated with convulsive syncope, particularly in children, and this is often an injury or a frightening spectacle.

From the point of view of management, reflex-induced seizures should be distinguished from other forms of generalized tonic-clonic seizures. Precipitating factors may include flashing lights, visual patterns, and certain sounds, including music. Photically induced seizures are nearly always generalized (Bickford and Klass 1969, Newmark and Penry 1979). It is not known what sets the seizures off and what causes the discharges to persist after cessation of the stimulus. Startle epilepsy may be set off by touch or by movement as well as by sudden noise. Movement-induced seizures may be localized or generalized.

The physiological basis of generalized seizures associated with bilaterally synchronous spike-and-wave discharges has long been of interest. Experimentally, there is evidence that stimulation of subcortical structures can induce bilateral symmetrical spike-wave discharges over both hemispheres (Jasper and Drooglever-Fortuyn 1946). Later, Penfield and Jasper (1954) induced similar EEG changes and clinical evidence of absence-like seizures in cats and monkeys, using 10- and 20-cycles-per-second stimuli through implanted electrodes. Young animals responded better than older animals to this type of stimulation. These findings led to the theory that an area of the central nervous system, later termed the centrencephalon, was responsible for mediating or forming the substratum of consciousness. Subsequently this concept engendered much controversy, particularly as to whether the centrencephalon represented the "fons et origo" of the epileptic discharge or whether this region represented a mediating pathway for centrencaphalic integration of seizure discharge to both hemispheres. This then represents the crux of the argument as to whether bilateral synchrony is truly primary or whether it is frequently secondary and occurs in response to a focal cortical discharge as proposed by Howell. There have been many examples of what appears to be a "centrencephalic" EEG pattern in patients who in fact had focal hemispheric diseases (Bray and Wiser 1965, Madsen and Bray 1966, Stewart and Dreifuss 1964, Tückel and Jasper 1952). Williams (1965) stated that "generalized epilepsy does not arise in brain stem structures, though it involves brain stem structures in its development." Bancaud et al (1965) on the basis of painstaking stereoelectroencephalographic studies suggested that the mesial orbital frontal cortex was a frequent initiating site for discharge ultimately involving brain stem structure and concluded that the scalp EEG could not resolve the question of what constituted primary and what constituted secondary bilateral synchrony if rapid provocation of the seizure discharge to contralateral homologous areas occurred. They emphasized that provocation of seizure discharge is altogether too rapid to be amenable to clinical analysis and that in the face of a generalized tonic-clonic motor convulsion a focal onset might well be missed. Marcus and Watson (1966) reproduced what appeared to be bilaterally synchronous spike-and-wave discharges with the appropriate clinical manifestations by means of cerebral lesions following destruction of centrencephalic structures. So long as the corpus callosum remained intact they were able to reproduce the spike-and-wave discharges. Thus evolved the concept of cortical-reticular epilepsy as proposed by Gloor (1968). This model postulates involvement of several levels of the nervous system in the elaboration of the spike-and-wave discharge, including the cerebral cortex in a hyperexcitable state, the thalamus, and the reticular formation of the brain stem.

The generalized spike-and-wave discharge appears to be in some measure an age-related phenomenon and may reflect the stage in the maturation of the nervous system, the nature of which is at present unknown, during which epilepsy developed and as a result of what there is participation by predilection of the brain stem in the elaboration of the epileptic discharge. This age relatedness may account for the fact that, unlike what is seen in adults where partial seizures predominate, over 75% of the seizures of childhood are of the generalized tonic-clonic type.

In the treatment of generalized tonic-clonic seizures, several anticonvulsant drugs are effective (Chapter 15). Under various circumstances, phenytoin, carbamazepine, phenobarbital, or valproate may be the drug of choice. The chance of successful control is good. However, when the seizure is secondarily generalized and when there is evidence of other neurologic dysfunction, such as intellectual impairment or the presence of abnormal neurologic signs and the presence of other seizure types, the prognosis becomes considerably less favorable with respect to cessation of seizures upon cerebral maturation. A theme that recurs repeatedly is that the prognosis for cessation of seizures or for their control depends on factors that indicate that the condition under discussion consists of more than one statistical population. Similar factors obtain in febrile seizures (Nelson and Ellenberg 1976), generalized tonic-clonic seizures that are not febrile, absence seizures, and, to an extent, infantile spasms. These factors include the presence of a history of other seizure types, of abnormal neurologic development, of a family history of epilepsy of a type other than that under discussion, and of seizures that are complex (that is, prolonged, occur in clusters, or possess a focal signature) and interictal EEG slowing, indicating ongoing cerebral abnormalities between seizures.

BIBLIOGRAPHY

Bancaud J, et al: La stéréo-electroéncephalographic dans l'épilepsie. Paris, Masson and Cie, 1965.

Bickford RG, Klass DW: Sensory precipitation and reflex mechanisms, in Jasper HH, Ward AA Jr, Pope A (eds): *Basic Mechanisms of the Epilepsies.* Boston, Little Brown & Co, 1969.

Bray PR, Wiser WC: The relation of focal to diffuse epileptiform EEG discharges in genetic epilepsy. *Arch Neurol* 1965;13:225-237.

Commission on Classification and Terminology, International League against Epilepsy: Proposal for revised clinical and electroencephalographic classification of epileptic seizures. *Epilepsia* 1981;22:489-501.

Gloor P: Generalized cortico-reticular epilepsies. Some considerations on the pathophysiology of generalized bilaterally syncrhonous spike and wave discharge. *Epilepsia* 1968;9:245-263.

Janz D: *Die Epilepsien: Spezielle Pathologie und Therapie.* Stuttgart, Georg Thieme Verlag, 1969.

Jasper HH, Droogleever-Fortuyn J: Experimental studies on the functional anatomy of petit mal epilepsy. *Res Publ Assoc Res Nerv Ment Dis* 1946;26:272-298.

Madsen JA, Bray PF: The coincidence of diffuse electroencephalographic spike-wave paroxysms and brain tumors. *Neurology* 1966;16:546-555.

Marcus EM, Watson CW: Bilateral synchronous spike-wave electrographic patterns in the cat. *Arch Neurol* 1966;14:601-610.

Newmark ME, Penry JK: *Photosensitivity and Epilepsy: A Review.* New York, Raven Press, 1979.

Nelson KB, Ellenberg JH: Predictors of epilepsy in children who have experienced febrile seizures. *N Engl J Med* 1976;295:1029-1033.

Penfield W, Jasper HH: *Epilepsy and the Functional Anatomy of the Human Brain.* Boston, Little Brown & Co, 1954.

Stewart LF, Dreifuss FE: "Centrencephalic" seizure discharges in focal hemispheric lesions. *Arch Neurol* 1964;17:60-68.

Tückel K, Jasper HH: The electroencephalogram in parasaggital lesions. *Electroencephalogr Clin Neurophysiol* 1952;4:481-494.

Williams D: The thalamus and epilepsy. *Brain* 1965;88:539-556.

CHAPTER 6

Infantile Spasms

Fritz E. Dreifuss

This form of epilepsy constitutes a syndrome of early childhood. Although to a large degree it is age specific, it appears to be heterogeneous in etiology and in clinical detail. Since its early description by West—an English pediatrician who described the manifestations in his own child in 1841 as a "peculiar form of infantile convulsions"—many synonyms have appeared to describe the syndrome, including massive spasms (Levin and Pearce 1968), Blitz-Nick und Salaam Krämpfe (Zellweger 1948), infantile spasms (Gibbs et al 1954), jack-knife, maladie des spasmes en flexion (Chevrie and Aicardi 1978), Propulsive-Petit mal (Janz 1969), West syndrome (Pampiglione 1964), and encephalopathie myoclonique infantile avec hypsarrythmie (Gastaut et al 1964).

The cardinal feature of the syndrome is the appearance in infancy of single or repetitive short muscular contractions that usually lead to flexion and occasionally to extension. They may be characterized as tonic contractions lasting for a fraction of a second to several seconds or as myoclonic contractions. When the attacks occur in flexion, they may be fragmentary and consist only of a drop of the head or they may be more complete with a forward flinging of the head and with flexion of the neck and trunk and of the arms at the elbow with abduction of shoulders—movements reminiscent of the Moro reflex. The movement may be so severe that the head ends up between the legs. The head nod is the "Nick," the sudden flexion the "Blitz," and the more prolonged tonic flexion spasm with outflung arms the "Salaam" element. Occasionally an extensor spasm will take place; it is characterized by extension of the neck and trunk with forward extension of the limbs, or abduction of the shoulders and extension of the lower extremities, which has been described by Druckman and Chao (1964) as "cheerleader spasm" (Figure 6-1). It is not clear whether consciousness is impaired during the attacks. Sometimes there appears to be a warning and the child may look startled or begin to cry even before the attack commences. At other times the child may cry at the termination of an episode. Sometimes attacks occur in clusters of up to 30 or 40 spasms; at other times they are more isolated. They may be several days apart or they may occur up to 200 times or more a day. They are more frequent at times of awakening from sleep or when startled, though other precipitating features may include feeding and other forms of stimulation.

In addition to the typical movements that characterize this disorder, there may be autonomic manifestations including pallor, flushing, sweating, pupil dilatation, hiccups, lacrimation, and changes in respiratory pattern, including arrest of respiration. Occasionally laughter may be seen, and this may occur in association with flushing and urination. Fluttering of the eyelids and upward rotation of the eyes is seen usually in those infantile spasms associated with extension (Jeavons and Bower 1964).

In pediatric neurologic practice, infantile spasms are seen quite frequently and have been reported in 7.5% to 15% of childhood seizure disorders. In the infantile age groups, this syndrome represents an even larger proportion of seizures. The incidence is estimated at 1 per 4000 to 6000 live births. There is a preponderance of involvement of males over females to the extent of 1.7 to 1 (Jeavons et al 1973) to 2 to 1. There is occasionally a family history of epilepsy and infantile spasms, the frequency of which varies from 7% to 17% (Gibbs et al 1954, Trojaborg and Plum 1960). In view of the fact that the syndrome is frequently associated with tuberous sclerosis, a family history of epilepsy is to be expected at least in that proportion of cases in which this causative factor is responsible.

THE ETIOLOGY OF INFANTILE SPASMS

Most authors divide etiological factors into idiopathic factors and symptomatic factors. This continues to be an important distinction despite the fact that the idiopathic group is shrinking in relation to the symptomatic group. In patients in whom there is no detectable cause, the condition usually appears later, resolves spontaneously, and is largely unassociated with flagrant neurologic abnormalities; whereas, in the symptomatic group, abnormality of development is seen earlier in life, normal progress is not achieved at any stage of development, and the seizures do not resolve, though they may change in character. Intermediate between these groups is that group in which seizures are associated with tuberous sclerosis, which makes up approximately 6% to 15% of children with infantile spasms. The epileptic course frequently does not begin until the third or fourth month of life; prognosis is not uniformly unfavorable.

The symptomatic factors may be described according to the time of development during which the causative factor is operative.

Prenatal Factors

Predisposing elements include toxemia of pregnancy, pregnancy in older age groups, history of miscarriage, pregnancy complications including first trimester infections such as cytomegalic inclusion disease (Feldman and Schwartz 1968), hemorrhages, and injury. Congenital illnesses include phakomatoses (Charlton and Mellinger 1970, Livingstone et al 1958, Roth and Epstein 1971, Rizzuto and Ferrari 1968) (Figures 6-1 to 6-5), Down's syndrome (Coleman 1971), and Aicardi's syndrome (Aicardi et al 1969, Dennis and Bower 1972) a condition primarily occurring in females and characterized by absence of the corpus callosum, chorioretinitis, and cortical heterotopia. Amino acidurias, including phenylketonuria, may be associated with infantile spasms.

Perinatal Factors

Perinatal factors associated with infantile spasms include traumatic delivery, birth anoxia, and icterus neonatorum. A relatively large proportion of these children had low birth weights (Crichton 1969).

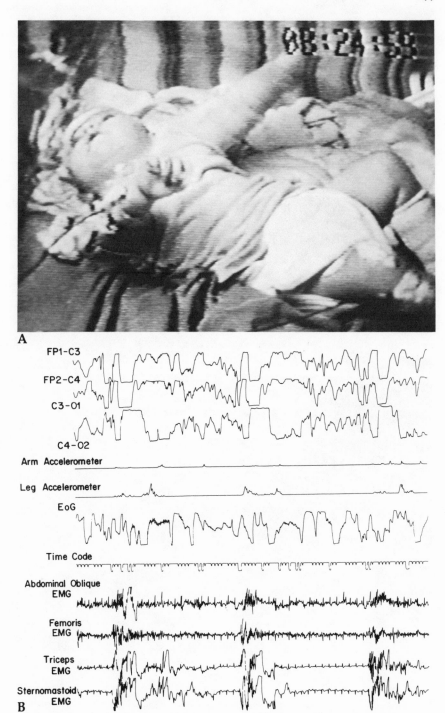

Figure 6-1 A An infantile spasm. B Polygraphic recording of a cluster of three seizures.

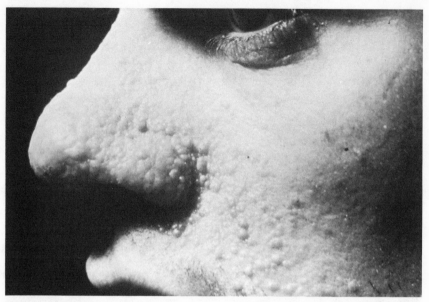

Figure 6-2 Tuberous sclerosis showing the characteristic distribution of adenoma sebaceum.

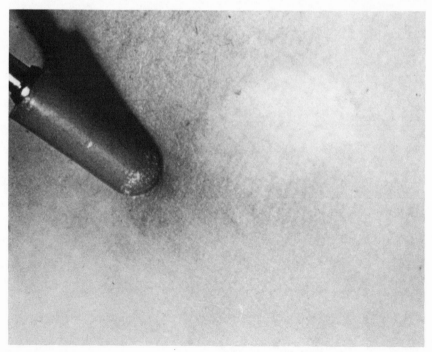

Figure 6-3 Tuberous sclerosis—hypopigmented skin area, the so-called achromatic or ash-leaf patch.

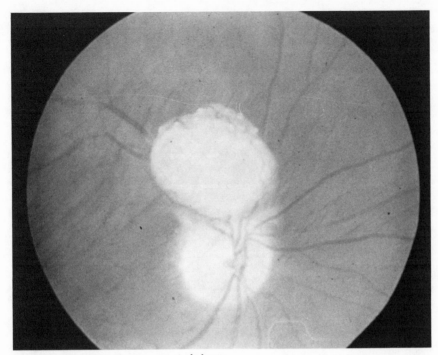

Figure 6-4 Tuberous sclerosis—retinal phakoma.

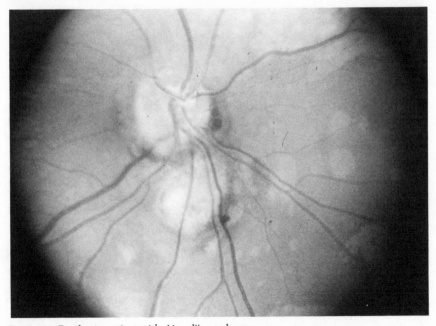

Figure 6-5 Fundus in patient with Aicardi's syndrome.

Postnatal Factors

Postnatal factors include infections such as neonatal meningitis and traumatic brain afflictions including hemorrhages, dehydration with venous thrombosis, and subdural hematoma. Various encephalitides have been reported, and there appears to be a relationship between certain immunizations and the onset of infantile spasms (Jeavons et al 1964). The pertussis component of DPT has been implicated (Low 1955), though this may be coincidental insofar as the time of onset of infantile spasms is very similar to the time of immunization. The question of such a relationship is unresolved.

Hypoglycemia may be a precipitating cause. Hypoglycemia should be considered in children particularly as risk, such as those born to a toxemic mother, children of low birth weight, and the smaller child in twin pairs. Hypoglycemia may be related to leucine sensitivity.

In many cases the cause of seizures appears to be multifactorial. The majority of patients who have evidence of perinatal etiological factors also have evidence of prenatal contributing causes. It is likely that the latter play the predominant role.

Neurologic Abnormalities

Abnormalities evident on examination include the stigmata of prenatal disease such as spasticity, flaccidity, microcephaly or macrocephaly, chorioretinitis, and evidence of Down's syndrome or of tuberous sclerosis. For tuberous sclerosis, hypopigmented patches may be the only evidence early in life, as the other cutaneous manifestations do not appear until somewhat later. In children with the idiopathic variety of infantile spasms and those in whom immunizations are thought to have played a part, neurologic development is usually normal until the onset of the epilepsy and examination does not usually reveal any significant abnormalities. In the symptomatic group, the CT scan is usually quite abnormal, showing as a rule a communicating hydrocephalus or evidence of congenital anomalies such as genesis of the corpus callosum or the presence of a cavum of the velum interpositum.

COURSE AND PROGNOSIS

Onset of infantile spasms usually occur by 6 months and nearly always occur by 1 year (Jeavons et al 1973). Again one has to distinguish between the symptomatic and the idiopathic groups. In the symptomatic group, the age of onset is frequently much earlier. In the idiopathic group, it is characteristically between 3 and 6 months of age. Also, in severely brain-damaged children, infantile spasms supervene on already existing seizures of other types, such as generalized tonic-clonic attacks. In some patients, the onset may be missed, and the movements may be attributed to something such as irritability, startle responses, or colic. Once the spasms begin, they tend to increase in frequency and in severity. With onset of the attacks, normal neurologic development is slowed, may reach a plateau, and may, in fact, regress. The child may no longer be able to raise its head and may not be as attentive to its surroundings; it may become hypotonic. At least some regression is reversible with appropriate intervention and with cessation of the attacks and normalization of the electroencephalogram. The natural course of the seizures is that they frequently spontaneously remit between 3 and 4 years of age; however, they may give rise to other seizure types, particularly drop attacks, absence seizures, and generalized and focal seizures characteristic of the Lennox-Gastaut syndrome, or they may give way to generalized tonic-clonic seizures. With adequate therapy, the natural course can be modified in many instances, particularly in the idiopathic variety where the prognosis for cessation of seizures is favorable with the institution of ACTH therapy. Jeavons and Bower (1964) and Jeavons et al (1973) indicated that most spasms are expected within the first year of life; approximately 50% will cease before 2 years of age and the majority by 5 years of age.

In the days before adequate treatment, mortality rate exceeded 30%. To some extent mortality rate depends on the underlying cause but the mortality rate has been changed by steroid treatment. The average mortality rate in recently reported series has been approximately 20%, and the symptomatic cases predominated. Most of them were severely retarded and had a significant number of neurologic abnormalities. The most common cause of death was aspiration pneumonia.

Morbidity outcome in terms of abnormal neurologic findings and developmental retardation is again strikingly different in the idiopathic and symptomatic groups. Mental retardation is one of the cardinal features of the illness. As mentioned earlier, neurologic abnormality and retarded development are frequently present in the symptomatic group before the onset of spasms; it is therefore not surprising that it is also prominent after cessation of the seizures. However, the patients in the idiopathic group apparently develop normally before the onset of their illness. It is among this group that the majority of the favorable prognoses reside. There are some patients whose infantile spasms are associated with tuberous sclerosis and for whom a reasonably favorable prognosis of intellectual development can be made. Outcome statistics suggest that 15% to 20% of these patients will have normal intelligence, 10% to 20% will be moderately retarded, and 40% to 50% severely retarded (Freidman and Pampiglione 1971, Jeavons et al 1973). Recent data (Charlton and Mellinger 1970, Chevrie and Aicardi 1978, Singer et al 1980) suggest that early adequate intervention with ACTH beneficially influences the ultimate outcome of intellectual development. It would certainly appear that the duration of infantile spasms prior to intervention may well influence the ultimate intellectual outcome and early treatment is therefore indicated. It is of course evident that the patient whose disease is caused by perinatal and postnatal encephalopathies, with the cerebral malformation attendant thereon, will have an unfavorable outcome.

ELECTROENCEPHALOGRAPHIC ABNORMALITIES

The electroencephalographic patterns associated with infantile spasms characteristically are those described as hypsarrhythmia. According to Gibbs et al (1954), hypsarrhythmia is characterized by random high-voltage slow waves and spikes. The spikes are said to vary from moment to moment both in duration and amplitude; they may be focal, multi-focal, or generalized, and the abnormality is almost continuous. During the seizures themselves, Frost et al (1978) noted various features, including 1) a high-voltage, frontal-dominant, generalized, slow-wave transient followed by attenuation, 2) a generalized sharp- and slow-wave complex, 3) a generalized sharp- and slow-wave discharge followed by attenuation, 4) there may be attenuation only, 5) generalized slow-wave transients only, 6) attenuation with superimposed fast activity, 7) a generalized slow-wave discharge followed by attenuation with superimposed fast activity, 8) attenuation and rhythmic slow activity, 9) fact activity only, 10) a sharp- and slow-wave complex followed by attenuation and superimposed fast activity, or 11) attenuation with superimposed fast activity followed by rhythmic slow activity.

The onset of hypsarrhythmia is similar to that of infantile spasms, and like infantile spasms, it appeares to be an age-related and age-limited phenomenon. Although hypsarrhythmia usually ceases as the infantile spasms cease, infantile spasms may continue, with an EEG that may have changed to a multiple polyspike-and-wave abnormality superimposed on a slow background with shifting hemisphere-emphasis or one with focal characteristics. Conversely, this type of EEG pattern may be associated with infantile spasms from the beginning, and no hypsarrhythmia may be seen. This is more frequently the case in the symptomatic group than in the idiopathic group. In the idiopathic group, hypsarrhythmia is nearly always the EEG pattern of record. Hypsarrhythmia may be a relatively transient phenomenon in the natural history of the EEG abnormality. In many cases hypsarrhythmia spontaneously resolves. This is a less common consequence than evolution into other focal or generalized abnormalities. Occasionally hypsarrhythmia may be seen in seizures other than infantile spasms, a finding that indicates that hypsarrhythmia is not pathognomonic for or synonymous with infantile spasms.

TREATMENT OF INFANTILE SPASMS

Prior to the introduction of steroids in the treatment of infantile spasms, this was one of the most frustrating conditions to treat by virtue of its resistance to standard forms of anticonvulsant therapy. Although many anticonvulsant drugs were used, few were used with benefit. The ketogenic diet was occasionally successful in the alleviation of the syndrome (Low 1955). However, the ketogenic diet is a difficult form of treatment in small children, is difficult to prepare, and over the long term is associated with deficiency problems, including those of protein malnutrition. The present era of therapy was ushered in in 1958 when Sorel and Dusaucy-Bauloye (1958) introduced ACTH, with strikingly beneficial results in a number of cases. Since then, many different treatment regimens with either ACTH or corticosteroids have been recommended. Adrenocorticotropic hormone is administered intramuscularly; and in different series the doses have varied from 5 units a day (Trojaborg and Plum 1960) to as much as 240 units a day (Gamstorp 1970). The most widely used range has been 40 to 80 units of ACTH per day. For corticosteroids, the usual recommended dose (Jeavons and Bower 1974) is 2 mg/kg/day of hydrocortisone. The duration of therapy has also varied from 2 to 6 weeks. Response, when it occurs, is usually rapid, with resolution of seizures within 2 weeks and normalization of the electroencephalogram in the majority of cases in which the seizures are controlled. In different series, the controls have varied from 20% to 80%. The most satisfactory results have occurred in the so-called idiopathic or cryptogenic group of cases and the symptomatic group has responded less well. In both groups, the lapses occur on occasion after discontinuation of therapy; this event is, once again, more frequent in those whose infantile spasms have an underlying structural abnormality and an abnormal premorbid neurologic development. Long-term studies also reported a larger relapse rate (Chevrie and Aicardi 1978, Freidman and Pampiglione 1971, Hrachovy et al 1980a, Jeavons et al 1970, Lennox and Davis 1958, Pollack et al 1979). These have all dealt essentially with the outcome following treatment with corticotropins and/or corticosteroids. Several controversies continue concerning the optimal regimen and the ultimate outcome. Much controversy has resulted from insufficient categorization of the patients being studied into definitive prognostic groups. The relative efficacy of corticotropins and corticosteroids is not fully settled, though it would appear that ACTH is more effective than corticosteroids. The reason may well be that ACTH does not exert its total effect through mobilization of corticosteroids; this may also account for the recommendation that large doses rather than small doses be used despite the fact that small doses will usually produce a maximal corticosteroid response. Adrenocorticotropic hormone may contain a peptide neurotransmitter substance that may exert a beneficial effect over and above that of the steroid component. Hrachovy et al (1980a), however, suggests that there is no difference in response between patients receiving 20 units of ACTH per day and those receiving 30 or 40 units per day. Duration of treatment is also controversial. Some physicians would treat patients for 4 weeks, some would continue a maintenance dose for 2 or 3 months, and others would substitute a corticosteroid for ACTH and continue treatment for up to 12 months. However, I standardly give 30 to 40 units of ACTH for a period of 1 month. If this treatment is ineffective, it is discontinued. If effective, treatment is continued for a further month and then ACTH is withdrawn gradually. Relapses are relatively few among the cryptogenic group; treatment failures and relapses have occurred principally among the symptomatic patients.

A further variable determining response is the treatment lag. Most authors agree that the longer the elapsed time between the onset of seizures and the institution of therapy, the less favorable the outcome.

There continues to be a significant disparity between the outcome in terms of cessation of sizures (which can be achieved quite regularly) and ultimate intelligence. The intellectual outcome is considerably less certain than seizure outcome, even in those whose seizures cease rapidly after institution of ACTH treatment and whose electroencephalogram returns to normal and remains normal. Here again it has been claimed that a more favorable intellectual outcome is obtained when therapy is instituted early. The most striking correlation, however, appears to be with premorbid neurologic development. Those children with normal development and a cryptogenic seizure pattern do considerably better (25% to 30% with satisfactory school attainment) than those whose seizures are symptomatic (10% or less doing reasonably well in school). Children who relapse usually do not respond well to subsequent courses of treatment, and the EEG likewise does not achieve even transient recovery.

Side effects of steroid therapy are quite significant. A large proportion of patients develop Cushing's syndrome; hypertension is a frequent development and mandates termination of therapy in a significant portion of cases. In this context, a blood pressure of 140/90 represents significant hypertension in this age group. Apart from further attention and electrolyte disturbances, susceptibility to infection is raised; septicemia occasionally occurs and may lead to death. Hypokalemia has been reported as a troublesome side effect.

The present status of therapy then is that children who have infantile spasms caused by severe structural neurologic disease tend to respond poorly to medication and those who do respond tend to relapse; in any event, the prognosis for intellectual development is grim indeed. On the other hand, children whose infantile spasms occur on the background of a premorbidly normal neurologic development are classified as idiopathic or cryptogenic and show a rapid early cessation of seizures with treatment, have a considerably more favorable long-term outlook, particularly if treated early. The side effects of steroidal therapy are sufficiently severe and frequent to make research for alternative therapy ethically valid.

Adrenocorticotropic hormone therapy has been shown to cause changes in the CT scan (Willig et al 1980). These changes consist of reversible brain changes, including enlargement of the ventricular system, the sulci, and the basal cisterns, accompanied by decrease of brain substance; this appearance resolves to a normal appearance after discontinuation of therapy. This suggests transient changes in fluid content, but the relationship of these two clinical changes is quite uncertain at this time.

Alternative treatment modes include the administration of drugs of the benzodiazepine group and valproic acid. The benzodiazepine drugs that have been used include clonazepam and nitrazepam (Dummermuth and Kovacs 1973, Markham 1964, Volzke and Doose 1967). Clonazepam has been used in doses of 0.1 to 0.3 mg/kg/day. A good response has been obtained in approximately 20% of the patients (Vassella et al 1973). Unfortunately a tolerance develops to this drug, and side effects, including somnolence and increased salivation, have been frequent. Nitrazepam in a dose of 0.5 to 1.0 mg/kg/day has resulted in a 50% satisfactory response rate (Hrachovy et al 1980b). Again, a tolerance frequently develops after approximately 2 months of therapy. The side effects of nitrazepam have been similar but rather less pronounced than with clonazepam. At the present time, no definite comparisons exist between the benzodiazepines and the steroids.

Recent reports indicate that valproic acid may prove beneficial in the therapy of infantile spasms (Bachman 1982).

Ultimately the resolution of this devastating problem will have to wait for further elucidation of the underlying mechanism, which is presumbly a disturbance of the central neural transmitter regulation.

BIBLIOGRAPHY

Aicardi J, Chevrie JJ, Rousselie F: Le syndrome spasms en flexion, agénésie calleuse, anomalies choriorétiniennes. *Arch Fr Pediatr* 1969;26:1103–1120.

Bachman DS: Use of valproic acid in the treatment of infantile spasms. *Arch Neurol* 1982; 39:49–52.

Charlton MH, Mellinger JF: Infantile spasms and hypsarrhythmia. *Electroencephalogr Clin Neurophysiol* 1970;29:413.

Chevrie JJ, Aicardi J: Convulsive disorders in the first year of life: Neurological and mental outcome and mortality. *Epilepsia* 1978;19:67–74.

Coleman M: Infantile spasms associated with 5-OH tryptophane administration in patients with Down's syndrome. *Neurology* 1971;21:911–919.

Crichton J: Infantile spasms in children of low birth weight. *Dev Med Child Neurol* 1969;10: 36–41.

Dennis J, Bower BD: The Aicardi syndrome. *Dev Med Child Neurol* 1972;14:382–390.

Druckman R, Chao D: Massive spasms in infancy and childhood. *Epilepsia* 1964;4:61–72.

Dummermuth G, Kovacs E: The effect of clonazepam (RO5-4083) in the syndrome of infantile spasms and hypsarrhythmia and in petit mal variant or the Lennox syndrome. *Acta Neurol Scand* [suppl 53]1973;49:26–28.

Feldman RA, Schwartz JF: Possible association between cytomegalovirus infection and infantile spasms. *Lancet* 1968;1:180–181.

Freidman IE, Pampiglione G: Prognostic implications of electroencephalographic findings of hypsarrhythmia in the first year of life. *Br Med J* 1971;4:323–325.

Frost JD Jr, Hrachovy RA, Kellaway P, et al: Quantitative analysis and characterization of infantile spasms. *Epilepsia* 1978;19:273–282.

Gamstorp I: *Pediatric Neurology*. New York, Meredith, 1970, pp 75–78.

Gastaut H, Roger J, Soulayrol R, et al: L'Encephalopathie myoclonique infantile avec hypsarrythmie (syndrome de West). Paris, Masson and Cie, 1964.

Gibbs FA, Gibbs EL: *Atlas of Electroencephalography*. Cambridge, MA, Addison-Wesley Publishing Co, 1952.

Gibbs EL, Fleming MM, Gibbs FA: Diagnosis and prognosis of hypsarrhythmia and infantile spasms. *Pediatrics* 1954;33:66–72.

Hanson RA, Menkes JH: A new anticonvulsant in the management of minor motor seizures. *Dev Med Child Neurol* 1972;14:3–14.

Hrachovy RA, Frost JD Jr, Kellaway P, et al: A controlled study of ACTH therapy in infantile spasms. *Epilepsia* 1980a;21:631–636.

Hrachovy RA, Frost JD Jr, Kellaway P, et al: A controlled study of prednisone therapy in infantile spasms, in Wada JA, Penry JK (eds): *Advances in Epileptology*. New York, Raven Press, 1980b.

Janz D: *Die Epilepsien*. Stuttgart, Georg Thieme Verlag, 1969.

Jeavons PM, Harper JR, Bower BD: Long-term prognosis of infantile spasms: A follow-up on 112 cases. *Dev Med Child Neurol* 1970;12:413–421.

Jeavons PM, Bower BD: Infantile spasms, a review of the literature and a study of 112 cases, in *Clinics in Developmental Medicine*, no 15. London, William Heinemann Medical Books, 1964.

Jeavons PM, Bower BD, Dimittrakoudi M: Long-term prognosis of 150 cases of West syndrome. *Epilepsia* 1973;14:153–164.

Jeavons PM, Bower BD: Infantile spasms, in Vinken PJ and Bruyn GW (eds): *Handbook of Clinical Neurology*, vol 15. Amsterdam, North Holland Publishing, 1974, pp 219–234.

Lennox WG, Davis JP: Clinical correlates of the fast and slow spike-wave electroencephalogram. *Pediatrics* 1950;5:626–644.

Levin NC, Pearce WG: Diagnostic and genetic aspects of infantile spasms. *J Med Genet* 1968; 5:273–279.

Livingstone S, Eisner V, Pauli L: Minor motor epilepsy: Diagnosis, treatment and prognosis. *Pediatrics* 1958;21:916–928.

Low NL: Electroencephalographic studies following pertussis immunizations. *J Pediatr* 1955; 47:35–39.

Markham CH: The treatment of myoclonic seizures of infancy and childhood with LA-1. *Pediatrics* 1964;34:511–518.

Pampiglione G: West's syndrome (infantile spasms)—A polymyographic study. *Arch Dis Child* 1964;39:2078.

Pollack MA, Zion T, Kellaway P: Long-term prognosis of patients with infantile spasms following ACTH therapy. *Epilepsia* 1979;20:255–260.

Rizzuto N, Ferrari G: Familial infantile myoclonic epilepsy in a family suffering from tuberous sclerosis. *Epilepsia* 1968;9:117–125.

Roth JC, Epstein CJ: Infantile spasms and hypopigmented macules: Early manifestations of tuberous sclerosis. *Arch Neurol* 1971;25:547–551.

Singer WD, Rabe EF, Haller JS: The effect of ACTH treatment upon infantile spasms. *J Pediatr* 1980;96:485–489.

Sorel L, Dusaucy-Bauloye A: A propos de 21 cas d'hypsarrhythmie de Gibbs: Son traitement spectaculare par l'ACTH. *Acta Neurol Psychiatr Belg* 1958;58:130–141.

Trojaborg W, Plum P: Treatment of "hypsarrhythmia" with ACTH. *Acta Paediatr Scand* 1960;49:572–582.

Vassella F, Pavlincova E, Schneider HJ, et al: Treatment of infantile spasms and Lennox-Gastaut syndrome with clonazepam (Rivotril). *Epilepsia* 1973;14:165–175.

Volske E, Doose H, Stephan E: The treatment of infantile spasms with Mogadon. *Epilepsia* 1967;8:64–70.

West WJ: On a peculiar form of infantile convulsions. *Lancet* 1841;1:724–725.

Willig RP, Langenstein I, Kuhne D: Hints on direct action of ACTH on cerebral function and morphology during treatment of infantile seizures. *Epilepsia* 1980;21:201.

Zellweger H: Blitz-Nick und Salaam Krämpfe. In Krämpfe im Kindesalter. *Helv Paediatr Acta* 1948 [suppl 5].

CHAPTER 7

Myoclonic Seizures

Fritz E. Dreifuss

Myoclonic jerks (single or multiple) are sudden, brief, shock-like contractions that may be generalized or confined to the face and tongue, or to one or more extremities, or even to individual muscles or groups of muscles. Myoclonic jerks may be rapidly repetitive or relatively isolated. They may occur predominantly around the hours of going to sleep or of awakening from sleep. They may be exacerbated by volitional movement and are then known as action myoclonus. At times they may be regularly repetitive.

Many instances of myoclonic jerks and action myoclonus are not classified as epileptic seizures. The myoclonic jerks of myoclonus due to spinal cord disease, dyssynergia cerebellaris myoclonica, subcortical segmental myoclonus, paramyoclonus multiplex, and opsoclonus-myoclonus syndrome must be distinguished from epileptic seizures (Commission on Classification and Terminology 1981).

Myoclonus is frequently associated with a giant evoked potential in response to a somatosensory stimulus. In association with a cortical giant evoked potential, there is frequently enhancement of the response at the thalamic level (Dawson 1946, 1947, Halliday 1972). Many types of myoclonus may be produced at the spinal level (Luttrell et al 1959, Swanson et al 1962). However, in the majority of experimental situations, impulses responsible for myoclonus travel to the cerebral hemispheres (Ingvar and Hunter 1955) and then caudally to the spinal level, producing the appropriate latencies in the record (Halliday 1972, Harriman and Millar 1955). The latency is usually characteristic of the modality involved, be this photic, auditory, or somatosensory. At times, stimulus-sensitive myoclonus may be asymmetrical (Dawson 1947). In some cases of hemiplegia, a reflex myoclonic jerk in response to tapping the affected limb may be unilateral and associated with a large cortical potential in the opposite hemisphere. Halliday (1972) describes "pyramidal" myoclonic discharges that follow with a fixed characteristic latency cortical spike discharge involving the contralateral motor area. In addition to pyramidal myoclonic discharges, he describes so-called "extrapyramidal" myoclonus in which there is no concomitant surface EEG but that may occur following an arousal stimulus. Some myoclonus may occur locally at the spinal cord or brain stem level (Luttrell et al 1959). Here myoclonic jerking develops in muscles innervated by a locally affected segment of spinal cord. Luttrell describes this phenomenon as a response to spinal cord infection, but it has also been seen clinically in patients with local spinal cord deformities such as tumors.

Myoclonic seizures with associated EEG spikes are seen in cases with progressive myoclonic epilepsy with (Diebold et al 1967, Janeway 1967, Van Heycopten Ham

1963) and without Lafora bodies (Horenko and Toivakka 1961), cerebral lipidoses, infantile hemiplegia, viral encephalitis, and hypoxic encephalopathy (Lance and Adams 1963), as well as in cases of massive myoclonic jerking seen in patients with epilepsy. Although most myoclonic jerks in these conditions are associated with cortical spike discharges, the association does not necessarily imply that the cortex is the pacemaker for the myoclonus, which may occur at subcortical levels including brain stem structures and in which the impulses travel rostrally and caudally simultaneously. Some patients in fact may have increased excitability at the spinal level, and most patients with myoclonic seizures have pathological changes in the region of the dentate nucleus, red nucleus, or inferior olive (Greenfield 1954).

Some patients with progressive myoclonic epilepsy appear to have the "extrapyramidal" type of myoclonus without spike discharges in the EEG.

Some myoclonic jerking is seen in association with 3-Hz spike-and-wave discharges that appear as a manifestation of absence seizures. This condition is termed absence with mild clonic components (Gibbs and Gibbs 1952). It is usually associated with clouding of consciousness, and the rhythmic myoclonic jerking occurs in concert with the spike-wave discharge seen in the EEG. Atonic drop attacks may be associated with brief myoclonic jerks prior to loss of muscle tone because a polyspike-slow wave complex frequently accompanies such an attack. Similar findings have been described by Lance and Adams (1963) in anoxic myoclonus, in which a jerk followed by muscle hypotonia was associated with a spike followed by a slow wave. However, it seems clear that motor inhibitory or atonic seizures do occur independently of myoclonus.

DISORDERS ASSOCIATED WITH MYOCLONUS

Myoclonic jerks are associated with several pathological conditions (Table 7-1).

Table 7-1
Disorders Associated with Myoclonus

A. As part of other forms of corticoreticular epilepsy
   1. Absence with clonic components
   2. Adolescent myoclonus
   3. As a component of generalized tonic-clonic seizures

B. As part of progressive neurologic disease, not primarily epileptic
   1. Progressive myoclonic epilepsy
      a. with Lafora bodies
      b. without Lafora bodies
   2. Dyssynergia cerebellaris myoclonica (Ramsay Hunt)

C. As part of generalized diseases of the cerebral gray matter
   1. Lipid storage diseases
   2. Infections such as SSPE Creutzfeldt-Jakob disease
   3. Progressive poliodystrophy (Alpers disease)

D. As part of systemic disease
   1. Metabolic encephalopathies, eg, uremia, hyperosmolar states
   2. Paraneoplastic syndromes such as infantile polymyoclonia and opsoclonus
   3. Postanoxic

E. As part of the infantile spasm syndrome

Association with Other Forms of Corticoreticular Epilepsy

Myoclonic jerks may occur in association with generalized or corticoreticular epilepsies.

ABSENCE WITH CLONIC COMPONENTS (Gibbs and Gibbs 1952, Penry et al 1975). One of the subgroups of the absence seizure syndrome is characterized by clonic components that are usually mild but that occasionally form a major manifestation of the seizure. In its mildest form, the seizure consists of eyelid blinking; in other cases there may be mild rhythmic jerking of the shoulders more or less synchronously with the rhythmicity of the spike-wave discharge. In more severe cases the trunk may be flexed, the arms raised, and the myoclonic excursions pronounced. Myoclonus is a prominent feature in the atypical absence seizures associated with the Lennox-Gastaut syndrome (see Chapter 8).

ADOLESCENT MYOCLONUS. Myoclonus is the most prominent feature in the condition of bilateral massive myoclonus described as impulsions, secousses, commotions epileptiques (Herpin 1867), or impulsiv petit mal (Janz 1969). Characteristically, this condition occurs during adolescence in patients who frequently have generalized tonic-clonic seizures. Classically, the attacks occur predominantly at first waking in the morning. They consist of a sudden shocklike contraction, mainly of the shoulder girdles and upper extremities, frequently in the presence of totally preserved consciousness. Because of the time of occurrence, they may catch the victim holding a coffee cup or other breakfast utensil, which gets unceremoniously flung across the room during such an attack. If an attack occurs while the patient is taking a shower, the patient may be flung to the ground and may be injured on projecting edges, such as the soap dish. A jerk may be single or multiple. The EEG during such an attack is characterized by sudden, bilateral, synchronous, multiple, spike-and-wave complexes (usually more marked anteriorly). The attack is from a fraction of a second to 3 seconds in duration. The rapidly repetitive polyspike component is characteristic. Sometimes the jerks may be provoked by photic stimulation. At times a repetitive series of jerks may lead into a generalized tonic-clonic convulsive seizure, at which time consciousness is lost. Some patients can predict the imminent occurrence of a generalized tonic-clonic seizure by noting an increase in the number of massive myoclonic jerks over a period of several days, after which the massive myoclonic jerks culminate in a convulsive seizure. The convulsive seizure having occurred, the myoclonic jerking may then be in abeyance for a matter of days or weeks. Recurrence of the myoclonic jerking is assumed to herald further convulsive episodes.

There is frequently a family history of this kind of attack; the prognosis is frequently for a favorable outcome with increasing age.

Therapy for this type of seizure is complicated by the fact that the adolescent age group in which these seizures frequently occur is predisposed to poor compliance and sleep deprivation, which tends to be a precipitating factor in this type of seizure. Valproic acid is frequently effective in controlling massive myoclonic seizures as well as the generalized tonic-clonic seizures to which these patients are heir. Phenytoin is frequently effective in controlling the generalized tonic-clonic seizures but appears to be less effective in the prevention of the myoclonus, as are carbamazepine and phenobarbital. Primidone is frequently effective but is likely to be associated with undesirable personality changes, an effect that limits its usefulness in the treatment of persons in this age group. Ethosuximide is rather less effective than valproic acid in the massive myoclonic seizures.

112

COMPONENT OF GENERALIZED TONIC-CLONIC SEIZURES. Myoclonus may be part of the syndrome of generalized tonic-clonic seizures. Individual tonic-clonic seizures may be ushered in by a short series of massive myoclonic jerks, which then take the characteristic of "clonic-tonic-clonic" seizures. Again, the electroencephalographic characteristic is that of multiple polyspikes or polyspike-and-wave discharges.

Association with Progressive Neurologic Diseases

Myoclonus may be seen as part of progressive neurologic diseases that may or may not be characterized by primary epileptic symptomatology.

PROGRESSIVE MYOCLONIC EPILEPSY. Those neurologic diseases with predominantly epileptic symptomatology include the progressive myoclonic epilepsies. These syndromes comprise two principal subdivisions: syndromes with Lafora bodies and syndromes without Lafora bodies.

Lafora body encephalitis is a condition thought to be controlled by an autosomal recessive gene. The patients usually begin their clinical course during the second or third decade of life. The first symptom may be a generalized tonic-clonic convulsion or myoclonic jerks, at first capriciously irregular and ultimately more and more frequent. The myoclonic jerks are often action-induced and may occur during physical exertion. Later they become more and more frequent and interfere with most motor activities. The prominence of generalized tonic-clonic seizures varies from person to person. The disease is slowly progressive, and during its course intellectual deterioration frequently occurs. Sometimes deterioration in school performance is the very first symptom to bring the patient to the attention of the physician. Coordination becomes impaired, and cerebellar symptomatology is a frequent accompaniment to the deteriorating clinical condition. Generalized tonic-clonic seizures vary in frequency and may punctuate the downhill course with increasing frequency. The patient ultimately becomes quite incapable of self-care; after a period of decreasing mobility, the patient is limited to a wheelchair and ultimately becomes bedridden. The myoclonic jerks become more and more obtrusive, both in the form of large-amplitude contractions and in the form of smaller and almost continuous activity involving the facial musculature.

Concentric amyloid bodies are found in the cytoplasm of cells throughout the nervous system, particularly in the dentate nucleus, the red nucleus, and the substantia nigra and hippocampus. They have the staining characteristics of a mucopolysaccharide–protein complex. These PAS-positive deposits are found in skeletal muscle, in the liver, sweat glands and, on occasion, in the renal tubules.

The electroencephalogram associated with Lafora body encephalitis is characterized by generalized slowing with superimposed bilateral synchronous spikes, which are sometimes associated with irregular spike-wave complexes. There is frequently evidence of exacerbation by photic stimuli.

No medication satisfactorily inhibits the progression of the disease. However, valproic acid is effective in ameliorating the seizures, and some patients who were bedridden become mobile and are able to care for themselves after treatment with valproic acid. Benzodiazepines, including diazepam and clonazepam, have been useful adjuncts in the management of the myoclonic jerks.

Progressive myoclonic epilepsy without Lafora bodies also seems to be controlled by an autosomal recesive gene (Horenko and Toivakka 1961). The clinical course of this condition is similar to that of Lafora body encephalitis. However, the progression is less dramatic, the condition is considerably more benign, and survival is more prolonged. Apart from these quantitative differences, the symptomatology is qualitatively identical with that of Lafora body encephalitis. Biopsies of the muscle, liver, and brain fail to disclose Lafora bodies, however. It is thought that dementia and significant cerebellar dysfunction are considerably less prominent in progressive myoclonic epilepsy of the non-Lafora type.

DYSSYNERGIA CEREBELLARIS MYOCLONICA. This condition was first described by Ramsey Hunt in 1921 and is characterized by progressive cerebellar ataxia and a progressive myoclonus. It has also been referred to as dentatorubral atrophy. The onset of this disease is later than that of the progressive myoclonic epilepsies. The condition is considerably more benign, and it is not usually classified under the epilepsies because, apart from myoclonic jerks, there is very little evidence of cortical epileptic involvement either clinically or electroencephalographically. Convulsive seizures do not as a rule punctuate the clinical course, which is a slowly progressive ataxia punctuated by myoclonus—frequently action-induced.

The initial symptoms are frequently "flinching," ie, when the patient is suddenly confronted by a change in direction or by an unexpected event, a jerk takes place, which initially may be quite mild and which ultimately becomes sufficiently severe to cause a lightning-like movement. As the condition progresses, the induction of movement in itself will be sufficient to cause "flinching." On examination, it is frequently difficult to distinguish a cerebellar ataxia from an ataxia induced by the frequent interruption of a smooth movement by repetitive myoclonic jerks.

Intellectual functions remain preserved, in contrast to the condition seen in the progressive myoclonic epilepsies, particularly those associated with Lafora bodies. There is degeneration of the dentate nucleus, the red nucleus, the dentatorubral fibers, and the spinocerebellar tracts as well as the superior cerebellar peduncle.

A further nonepileptic myoclonic disturbance is paramyoclonus multiplex, or essential myoclonus (Korten et al 1974). This condition is controlled by an autosomal dominant gene and is characterized by myoclonic jerking that is usually precipitated by sensory stimuli.

Association with Generalized Disease of the Cerebral Gray Matter

Myoclonus may occur as part of generalized disease of the cerebral gray matter. These conditions include 1) lipid storage disease, 2) infections such as subacute sclerosing panencephalitis (SSPE) and Creutzfeldt-Jakob disease, and 3) progressive polio dystrophy (Alpers disease).

LIPID STORAGE DISEASES (Menkes et al 1971, O'Brien 1969, Okada and O'Brien 1968, 1969, Pilz et al 1966, Suzuki and Suzuki 1970). This group of diseases includes some recessively inherited disorders in which excessive ganglioside deposition occurs as a result of enzyme defects that inhibit ganglioside metabolism. The conditions are subdivided according to the nature of the deposited material. GM_2 gangliosidosis or Tay-Sachs disease is the best known of the lipidoses. Neurons are distended with GM_2 ganglioside. The condition appears during the first year of life. In the involved neurons the deposited substance appears to be "membranous cytoplasmic inclusion bodies" consisting of ganglioside, cholesterol, and some protein. In the majority of patients, hemoxaminidase A is absent or grossly defective. In a variant (Sandhoff's disease), both hexosaminidase A and B are grossly reduced, and viscera other than the nervous system may be involved.

The disease usually begins within the first decade of life with listlessness, irritability, and an undue sensitivity to noise that leads to a myoclonic-type startle response. Thereafter a regression in previously attained developmental milestones occurs and is associated with evidence of diminution of vision. Physical examination reveals hypotonia and a typical cherry-red macular spot. As the disease progresses, frequent myoclonic jerks occur independently of noise or startle, first as low-amplitude repetitive jerks and later as much more prominent jerking movements. Generalized tonic-clonic convulsive seizures are frequently supervened and may become a prominent part of the illness. Generalized gangliosidosis with GM_1 ganglioside is similar to the preceding disease. However, it has a later onset. Children with this generalized gangliosidosis have an appearance similar to that of children with Hurler's disease and with an enzyme defect in β-galactosidase. Visceral involvement here is prominent; the liver and the spleen are enlarged. Again myoclonic jerks are quite prominent, as are generalized convulsive seizures.

Cerebromacular degenerative diseases with onset occurring between the ages of 2 and 4 years are again characterized by progressive deterioration of previously attained developmental milestones. Inclusions vary between so-called curvilinear bodies and lipofuschin-like material. Patients with these diseases have largely unknown enzymatic defects (Zeman et al 1970). All are characterized by macular changes of the retinal pigments and prominent myoclonic seizures that become ever more prominent and that are interspersed with generalized tonic-clonic attacks. The late-infantile and juvenile lipidoses run a considerably slower course than the GM_2 and GM_1 gangliosidoses. The victims may survive for many years. In Niemann-Pick disease (Crocker and Farber 1958), the stored lipid is sphingomyelin, and a cherry-red macular spot is frequently observed. Sphingomyelin is deposited in the bone marrow and in the viscera as well as in the brain. The onset is some time in the first decade of life, and the progress of the disease, while inexorable, may be quite slow. Again, myoclonic jerks are exceedingly prominent throughout the course of this condition until the final stages.

INFECTIONS OF THE NERVOUS SYSTEM WITH MYOCLONUS AS A PROMINENT FEATURE. Subacute sclerosing panencephalitis (SSPE) (Brain et al 1948, Cobb 1966, Dawson 1933, Freeman 1969, Horta-Barbosa et al 1969) is a condition characterized by a demyelinating leukoencephalopathy in association with a polio dystrophy characterized by type A intranuclear inclusions with virus particles suggestive of measles virus. The condition is thought to be a slow virus infection with a curious host–virus immune relationship. Measles antibody titers are elevated in the serum and in the cerebrospinal fluid, and the nervous system contains large quantities of IgG. There is usually a history of measles infection earlier in life. The affected child, usually between the ages of 4 and 15 years, begins to show deterioration of previously acquired intellectual attainments and may show personality changes with behavior problems that frequently are noticed first by a teacher. Over the course of subsequent weeks or months, convulsive seizures may develop, the child may become clumsy and have a tendency to stumble or fall and to drop things from the hand. The patient is then noticed to be suffering from myoclonic jerks, which may begin insidiously and occasionally unilaterally. Sometimes a hemiparetic appearance may give the impression of focal neurologic involvement. In the early stages, the electroencephalogram may not be considered to be abnormal or may just show some generalized slowing. As the disease progresses, typical, periodic, high-voltage, slow-wave bursts occur at regular intervals throughout the tracing (approximately every 2 to 6 seconds), may be associated with myoclonic jerks when these assume prominence in the clinical picture. The disease may plateau for long periods of time or may be inexorably progressive. The myoclonic jerks become less prominent as the child becomes more severely rigid and decerebrate. Macular degenerative changes indicating viral infection in the ganglion cells may be noted during the course of the illness (Figure 7-1).

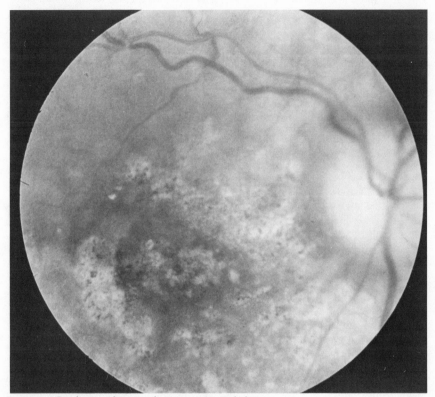

Figure 7-1 Fundus in subacute sclerosing panencephalitis.

Creutzfeldt-Jakob disease is the result of a slow virus infection and is mentioned here for the sake of completeness. It is a condition similar to SSPE in its propensity for producing myoclonus as a very prominent part of its clinical course, but it is not seen in childhood (Burger et al 1972, Creutzfeldt 1920, Gonatas et al 1965).

PROGRESSIVE POLIO DYSTROPHY (ALPERS DISEASE) (Alpers 1931, Christensen and Krabbe 1949, Dreifuss and Netsky 1964). This condition is characterized by progressive deterioration of the cerebral gray matter. It probably does not represent a single entity but may consist of a condition controlled by an autosomal recessive gene on the one hand and of a sporadic inflammatory condition on the other. Alpers disease usually has an onset between 3 and 6 years of age. The child deteriorates from previously attained levels intellectually and in motor performance skills. The downhill course may be quite rapid. It may be punctuated by convulsive seizures and especially by prominent myoclonus, which is the major neurologic diagnostic feature pointing to deterioration of the cerebral gray matter.

Pharmacologic therapy of myoclonic seizures depends on the cause of the disorder. When myoclonus is associated with absence seizures, treatment of the latter with ethosuximide or valproate is usually successful in abolishing all the manifestations of the seizures. In light-sensitive absence with myoclonus, valproic acid is also the drug of choice. This is administered in a dose of 15 mg/kg, which is then gradually increased until a therapeutic blood level of 50–100 μg/mL is obtained. The maximum dose is 60 mg/kg. Occasionally, clonazepam is used and is quite successful in abolishing the myoclonus. However, the side effects of this drug, including behavioral change and a tendency for development of tolerance, render this a less desirable agent than valproic acid.

In cases of myoclonus due to massive myoclonic seizures of adolescence (impulsiv petit mal), valproic acid is again the drug of choice. In the case of the progressive myoclonic epilepsies, therapy is difficult. Valproic acid is the drug of choice in retarding the disability imparted to this progressive condition by the severe frequent myoclonic jerks, which are the most devastating feature of this disorder. Benzodiazepines, such as diazepam and clonazepam in quite large doses, should ameliorate the myoclonus.

Valproic acid is administered in the usual dose. Diazepam is given in as big a dose as 60 or 80 mg a day, and clonazepam doses may reach 10–20 mg a day. If generalized tonic-clonic seizures continue, carbamazepine or phenytoin may be helpful, though phenytoin may actually exacerbate the tendency to myoclonus, possibly by its effect on the cerebellum. Cerebellar ataxia is, of course, a significant feature of this group of diseases.

In postanoxic myoclonus, 5-hydroxytryptophan has been found to be a useful agent in the amelioration of the myoclonus. Here, too, valproate may be beneficial.

Primidone may play a useful role in some instances of epilepsy associated with myoclonus. Janz (1969) found this drug to be effective in massive adolescent myoclonic jerks. I have found it to be beneficial in progressive myoclonic epilepsy.

The Syndrome of Polymyoclonia with Opsoclonus

In 1962, Kinsbourne reported an unusual infantile myoclonic encephalopathy with truncal and extremity ataxia and with an abnormal chaotic ocular motility disturbance described as opsoclonus (Cogan 1969). This condition usually comes on gradually. The abnormal movements become more pronounced when the child is upset. At that time a rapid tremulous myoclonus-like extremity movement is seen. There is an associated jerky movement of the eyes that interrupts smooth eye movements in both the horizontal and vertical plane and that becomes particularly pronounced when the eyes cross the midline, which they do in a series of jerks. The condition has also been referred to as "dancing eyes, dancing feet" (Dyken and Kolar 1968). Several authors have noted that the condition may be ameliorated by the administration of ACTH.

The syndrome is related to the presence of neural crest tumors, particularly neuroblastomas (Brissaud and Beaubias 1969, Martin and Griffith 1971). These are most frequently located in the thorax in these children, but it should be stressed that the tumors may be difficult to locate and may come to light a considerable time after the appearance of the polymyoclonia. Skeletal x-rays, computerized tomography, and urine VMA or HVA determinations have been useful in the diagnosis of neural crest tumors when these have been present. There have been reports of improvement after removal of the tumors. On the other hand, polymyoclonia may respond favorably to ACTH when a neuroblastoma is present. The cerebrospinal fluid frequently shows a pleocytosis. Tumors are frequently associated with a similar syndrome in adults. However, in adults, carcinoma of lung, breast, or ovary are encountered rather than neural crest neoplasms.

The dosage of ACTH employed is 40 units daily for 6 to 8 weeks; withdrawal is gradual. The polymyoclonias not associated with tumors usually remit spontaneously with age, but children with this condition frequently demonstrate some delay in reaching developmental milestones.

Because of the relationship of polymyoclonia to neoplasms, this condition is classed as a paraneoplastic syndrome. It is most likely a disorder of the immune system induced by the tumor, although it could be a toxicity phenomenon.

BIBLIOGRAPHY

Alpers B: Diffuse progressive degenerations of the gray matter of the cerebrum. *Arch Neurol Psychiatr* 1931;25:469–505.

Brain WR, Greenfield JG, Russell DS: Subacute inclusion encephalitis (Dawson type). *Brain* 1948;71:365–385.

Brissaud HE, Beaubias P: Opsoclonus and neuroblastoma. *N Engl J Med* 1969;280:1242.

Burger LJ, Rowan AJ, Goldensohn ES: Creutzfeldt-Jakob disease, an electroencephalographic study. *Arch Neurol* 1972;26:428–433.

Christensen E, Krabbe KH: Poliodystrophia cerebri, progressive infantilis. *Arch Neurol Psychiatr* 1949;61:28–43.

Cobb W: The periodic events of subacute sclerosing leucoencephalitis. *Electroencephalogr Clin Neurophysiol* 1966;21:278–294.

Cogan DG: Opsoclonus, body tremulousness and benign encephalitis. *Arch Ophthalmol* 1969;79:545–551.

Commission on Classification and Terminology, International League against Epilepsy: Proposed revisions of clinical and electroencephalographic classification of epileptic seizures. *Epilepsia* 1981;22:489–501.

Creutzfeldt HG: Uber eine eigenartige herdformige Erkrankung des Zentralnervensystems. *Z Gesamte Neurol Psychiatr* 1920;57:1–18.

Crocker AC, Farber S: Niemann-Pick disease: A review of 18 cases. *Medicine (Baltimore)* 1958;37:1–95.

Dawson GD: The relation between the electroencephalogram and muscle action potentials in certain convulsive states. *J Neurol Neurosurg Psychiatry* 1946;9:5–22.

Dawson GD: Investigations on a patient subject to myoclonic seizures after sensory stimulation. *J Neurol Neurosurg Psychiatry* 1947;10:141–162.

Dawson JR: Cellular inclusions in cerebral lesions of lethargic encephalitis. *Am J Pathol* 1933;9:7–16.

Diebold K, Hafner H, Vogel F: Zur Klinik der progressiven Myoklonusepilepsien. *Dtsch Z Nervenheilk* 1967;190:199–240.

Dreifuss FE, Netsky MG: Progressive poliodystrophy: Degenerations of the cerebral gray matter. *Am J Dis Child* 1964;107:649–656.

Dyken P, Kolar O: Dancing eyes, dancing feet: Infantile polimyoclonia. *Brain* 1968;91:305–310.

Freeman JM: The clinical spectrum and early diagnosis of Dawson's encephalitis. *J Pediatr* 1969;75:590–603.

Gibbs FA, Gibbs EL: *Atlas of Electroencephalography.* Cambridge, MA, Addison-Wesley Publishing Co, 1952, vol 2.

Gonatas NK, Tery RD, Weiss M: Electromicroscopic study in two cases of Jakob-Creutzfeldt disease. *J Neuropathol Exp Neurol* 1965;24:575–598.

Greenfield JG: *The Spinocerebellar Degenerations.* Oxford, Blackwell, 1954.

Halliday AM: The electrophysiological study of myoclonus in man. *Brain* 1972;90:241–284.

Harriman DGF, Millar JHD: Progressive familial myoclonus epilepsy in 3 families: Its clinical features and pathological basis. *Brain* 1955;78:325–348.

Herpin T: Des acces incomplets d'epilepsie. Paris, Balliere, 1867.

Horenko A, Toivakka E: Myoclonic epilepsy in Finland. *Acta Neurol Scand* 1961;37:282–296.

Horta-Barbosa L, Fuceillo D, Sever JL, et al: Subacute sclerosing panencephalitis: Isolation of measles virus from brain biopsy. *Nature* 1969;221:974.

Hunt JR: Dyssynergia cerebellaris myoclonica—Primary atrophy of the dentate system. *Brain* 1921;44:490–538.

Ingvar DG, Hunter J: Influence of visual cortex on light impulses in the brainstem. *Acta Physiol Scand* 1955;33:194–218.

Janeway R, Ravens JR, Pearce LA: Progressive myoclonic epilepsy with Lafora bodies: Clinical, genetic, histopathological and biochemical study. *Arch Neurol* 1967;16:565–582.

Janz D: Die Epilepsien: Spezielle Pathologie und Therapie. Stuttgart, Georg Thieme Verlag, 1969.

Kinsbourne M: Myoclonic encephalopathy of infants. *J Neurol Neurosurg Psychiatry* 1962;25:271–276.

Korten JJ, Nortemans SLH, Frenoken GWGM, et al: Familial essential myoclonus. *Brain* 1974;97:131–138.

Lance JA, Adams RD: The syndrome of intention or action myoclonus as a sequel to hypoxic encephalopathy. *Brain* 1963;86:111–136.

Luttrell CN, Bang FB, Luxenberg K: Newcastle disease encephalomyelitis in cats. II. Physiological studies on rhythmic myoclonus. *Arch Neurol Psychiatr* 1959;81:285–291.

Martin ES, Griffith JF: Myoclonic encephalopathy and neuroblastoma. *Am J Dist Child* 1971;122:257–258.

Menkes J, O'Brien JAS, Okada S, et al: Juvenile GM_2 gangliosidosis: Biochemical and ultrastructural studies on a new variety of tsd. *Arch Neurol* 1971;25:14.

Moe PG, Nellhaus G: Infantile polymyoclonia: Opsoclonus syndrome and neural crest tumors. *Neurology* 1970;20:756–764.

Mountcastle VB, Powell TPS: Central nervous mechanisms subserving position sense and kinesthesis. *Bull Johns Hopkins Hosp* 1959;105:173–200, 201–232.

O'Brien JS: Five gangliosidoses. *Lancet* 1969;2:805.

Okada S, O'Brien JS: Generalized gangliosidosis β-galactosidase deficiency. *Science* 1968;160:1002.

Okada S, O'Brien JS: Tay-Sachs disease: Generalized absence of a β-D-n-acetylhexosaminidase component. *Science* 1969;165:686.

Penry JK, Porter RJ, Dreifuss FE: Simultaneous recording of absence seizures with video tape and electroencephalography. *Brain* 1975;98:427–440.

Pilz H, Sandhoff K, Jatzkewitz G: A disorder of ganglioside metabolism with storage of ceramide lactoside, monosialoceramide lactoside and tsd ganglioside in brain. *J Neurochem* 1966;13:1273–1282.

Suzuki Y, Suzuki K: Partial deficiency of hexosaminidase A in juvenile GM_2 gangliosidosis. *Neurology* 1970;20:848–851.

Swanson PD, Luttrell CN, Magladery JW: Myoclonus—A report of 67 cases and review of the literature. *Medicine (Baltimore)* 1962;41:339–356.

Van Heycopten Ham MW, De Jager H: Progressive myoclonic epilepsy with Lafora bodies: Clinical and pathological features. *Epilepsia* 1963;4:95–119.

Zeman W, Donahue S, Dyken P, et al: The neuronal ceroid lipofuscinosis (Batten-Vogt syndrome), in Vinken PJ, Bruyn GW (eds): *Handbook of Clinical Neurology*. Amsterdam, North-Holland Publishing Co, 1970, vol 10, pp 588–679.

CHAPTER 8

Lennox-Gastaut Syndrome

Fritz E. Dreifuss

CHILDHOOD EPILEPTIC ENCEPHALOPATHY
WITH DIFFUSE SLOW SPIKE-WAVE DISCHARGES

In the international classification of epileptic seizures, atypical absence seizures are defined as those seizures in which are seen changes in tone that are more pronounced than in classic absence seizures; whose onset and/or cessation is not as abrupt as those of classic absence seizures; and whose EEG findings are more heterogeneous and include irregular spike-and-slow-wave complexes, or fast activity, or other paroxysmal activity including slow spike-wave discharges that are bilateral but often irregular and asymmetrical. In the *Dictionary of Epilepsy* (Gastaut 1973), atonic epileptic seizures are described

> . . . in which the decrease of abolition of postural tone is of very brief duration (generally a fraction of a second). Depending on whether the loss of tone involves all the postural muscles or only those of the head and neck, the subject either slumps to the ground or his head suddenly falls onto his chest (epilepsia nutans). He gets up again immediately after the fall, which may be violent enough to cause injury, particularly when his head strikes an object in its path. Such epileptic drop attacks coincide with the slow waves of polyspike-wave complexes on the EEG and are very typical in young people, in whom they may occur in association, and sometimes in combination, with epileptic myoclonus (in which case they are called myoclonic-atonic epileptic seizures). Epileptic drop attacks are sometimes described as akinetic petit mal because they are accompanied by a polyspike-wave discharge. . . . They are only observed, alone or in association with either myoclonus or tonic seizures in children with chronic encephalopathy and some degree of mental retardation, especially the Lennox-Gastaut syndrome.

The existence of a severe childhood epileptic encephalopathy that is characterized clinically by a variety of intractable seizure forms in which varieties of absence and drop attacks are common and that frequently is associated with mental retardation has been well recognized and described (Aicardi and Chevrie 1971, Chevrie and Aicardi 1972, Doose 1964ab, Gastaut et al 1966, Kruse 1968, Lennox and Davis 1950, Sorel 1964). The existence of an irregular, slow spike-wave EEG pattern, described variously as the diffuse, slow, spike-wave activity or "petit mal variant," has been recognized almost as long as has the 3-Hz spike-and-wave pattern of absence seizures. The association of the clinical pattern with a specific EEG pattern has led to the recognition that a single syndrome has been variously described as petit mal variant epilepsy, astatic seizures, epileptic encephalopathy with diffuse spike-wave discharges, myoclonic-astatic petit mal, the minor-motor seizure syndrome, the Lennox syndrome, and the Lennox-Gastaut syndrome. There is, in most series, a male preponderance, which varies from 1.5 to 1 (Chevrie and Aicardi 1972) to 3.3 to 1 (Kruse 1968). In my experience, the preponderance is approximately 3 to 1. Within the syndrome there are probably several statistical populations. This may account for the variation in age of onset—between 4 months and 11 years.

CLINICAL MANIFESTATIONS

The clinical manifestations vary tremendously. In children who have onset before the age of 2 years, seizures comprise frequent head drops, eye blinking, and, occasionally, laughing and flushing. When onset occurs after 2 years, frequent eye blinking, head nodding, and drop attacks are more commonly seen. The frequency of attacks gradually increases. Classic absence seizures do not usually begin before the age of 4 years, and absence seizures prior to this age frequently herald the more severe epileptic encephalopathy under discussion.

The drop attacks may be of several varieties. Head drops (epilepsia nutans) are a mild form of seizure. Further loss of muscle tone may cause the patients to buckle and, as it were, collapse into themselves. Almost as soon as this has occurred, patients regain their senses and pick themselves up. On other occasions patients may fall like a tree and may be injured severely by hitting projecting surfaces or the ground, with subsequent damage to the head, face, and teeth (Figure 8-1). Such falls occasionally lead to broken bones, usually in an upper extremity. Consciousness is usually disturbed during a fall; however, the fall may be so rapid as to deprive the observer of the opportunity to observe loss of consciousness. Occasionally tone is lost in the midst of a series of persistent absence seizures, with upward rotation of the eyes, blinking, and mild clonic components; in this case there is very evident disturbance of the conscious state.

At times there is a very obvious myoclonic jerk associated with the beginning of the fall; this form of attack is called *astatic-myoclonic attack*. The myoclonic jerk is particularly noticeable when the patient is sitting; the attack is characterized by head drop and very frequently by extension of the arms and shoulders. Here again the attack may be heralded by the eye blinking reminiscent of absence. Prolonged absence seizures with mild clonic components may be the most characteristic part of the syndrome; we have seen children who have been in absence status for years at a time. The child can be momentarily aroused to smile, to follow commands, and to attend to feeding and occasionally to toilet needs; but the child spends most of its waking hours in a state of petit mal obnubilation, unable to perform complex sequential tasks to a successful conclusion. Prolonged, confused behavior, apparently senseless laughter or crying, and apparent lack of a sense of self-preservation are frequent concomitants of this condition.

Genralized tonic-clonic seizures, tonic seizures, or clonic seizures occur in over 60% of patients with Lennox-Gastaut syndrome. Generalized tonic-clonic seizures are frequently nocturnal, occurring particularly around the time of going to sleep or awakening. They tend to occur in clusters and for a time may be seen almost every night.

In some of the older patients, the syndrome begins with a generalized tonic-clonic seizure or a series of seizures. The history may be one of slow development and sometimes includes "staring spells" or eye blinking episodes earlier in life. In the late-

123

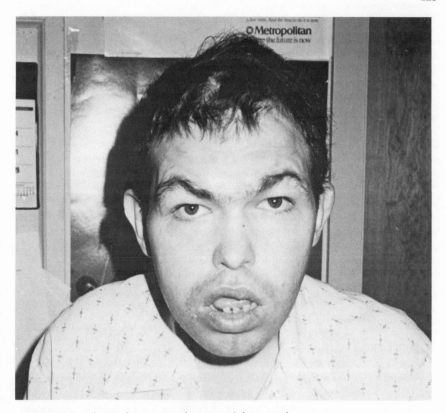

Figure 8-1 Facial scars from repeated trauma of drop attacks.

onset seizures, severe drop attacks are seen more frequently.

In all the patients there is frequently a periodicity in the seizure frequency, with episodes of prolonged repetitive seizures interspersed with periods of relative freedom from attacks. Such a periodicity makes evaluation of anticonvulsant drug therapy rather difficult and frequently results in a sense of achievement that is rudely shattered by the occurrence of the next episode of seizures.

ANTECEDENT HISTORY

Lennox and Davis (1950) found a family history of epilepsy in approximately one-quarter of their cases. However, it is much lower in most series [2.5% in the series of Chevrie and Aicardi (1972)]. Kruse (1968) obtained a family history of epilepsy in 16%.

A patient may have a past history of infantile spasms. The occurrence of Lennox-Gastaut syndrome is one of the consequences of infantile spasms, both the idiopathic and the symptomatic varieties. It is therefore not surprising that tuberous sclerosis is occasionally seen in patients with Lennox-Gastaut syndrome.

PRIMARY AND SECONDARY VARIETIES

Lennox-Gastaut patients can be divided into primary, or idiopathic, and secondary, or symptomatic, groups. In the secondary group, antenatal causative factors, such as cerebral malformations, phacomatosis, congenital infections such as toxoplasmosis, and other fetal abnormalities may be identified. A history of difficult delivery, with a low Apgar score at birth, is present in approximately 10% of the secondary group, and postnatal factors including neonatal hypoglycemia, meningitis, and hemiconvulsive hemiplegic syndrome (including those secondary to exanthematous diseases) may play a role in approximately 20%. So-called primary cases make up between 30% and 70% of different reported series (Gastaut et al 1966, Doose 1964ab). With the development of more sophisticated diagnostic techniques, the distinction between so-called primary and so-called secondary seizures becomes less clear, as in both groups there is a high frequency of abnormality on the CT scan—mainly cerebral atrophy, which in the case of the Lennox-Gastaut syndrome is predominantly subcortical (Gastaut et al 1980). Other diagnostic studies, including biochemical evaluation of cultured fibroblasts and brain biopsy evaluation, have yielded instances of metabolic lesions such as lipidosis or subacute encephalopathies (including Lafora encephalitis). Two of my patients with otherwise typical Lennox-Gastaut syndrome were found to have nonketotic hyperglycinemia.

If one is going to use the distinction between the primary and the secondary syndrome for purposes of prognostication, every attempt has to be made to exclude causative factors having an influence on such prognosis; I suspect that the primary group ultimately will turn out to be quite small.

NEUROLOGIC FINDINGS

Neurologic examination of children with Lennox-Gastaut syndrome reveals abnormalities in approximately one-half the cases. A small head circumference (not amounting to microcephaly), esotropias and exotropias, symmetrical or asymmetrical increase in deep tendon reflexes, and ankle clonus and extensor plantar responses are seen in approximately 30% to 50% of patients with Lennox-Gastaut syndrome. Many of the children have not developed a definite hand preference at the time they are seen, and clumsiness, delay in speech acquisition and communication skills, and coordination defects are frequent.

Encephalographic features were first described by Gibbs and co-workers (1939) as "petit mal variant" characterized by slow spike-wave formations with a duration of $\frac{1}{15}$ second or longer. The spike may be negative or triphasic. The spike-wave discharge may vary among different head regions. It may be only a spike in one lead and only a wave in another, with constancy or shifting hemisphere emphasis. The background is characteristically slow and relatively unresponsive to eye opening; the spike-wave discharges may be superimposed as solitary complexes or discontinuous chains. During sleep, 10-Hz discharges occurring in runs may be seen. In less than one-quarter of the cases, the EEG background is normal. Not all drop attacks are accompanied by spike-wave discharges. In some of them, the record may flatten into low-voltage fast activity. The majority of attacks, however, are characterized by recurrence of regular or irregular high-voltage, sharp, slow-wave complexes with a frequency of 2 to 2.5 per second. In those children where spike-wave stupor persists for prolonged periods of time, the record is virtually continuously abnormal, with irregular polyspike-and-wave discharges or spike-and-wave discharges interspersed with 1- to 2-Hz high-voltage slow waves throughout the recording. Frequently the discharges are asymmetrical, and they may be synchronous or asynchronous between the two hemispheres. Hyperventilation does not change the EEG pattern of patients with Lennox-Gastaut syndrome with nearly the regularity with which activation can be produced during absence seizures. Only relatively infrequently can photic stimulation induce spike-wave discharges.

PROGNOSIS

The prognosis for Lennox-Gastaut syndrome is variable and to some extent has to be linked with the underlying cause. Thus, a patient whose intellectual development was lagging at the time of the first seizure has a poor outlook with respect to ultimate intellectual development. Prognosis is also unfavorable for those patients whose seizures are caused by significant structural neurologic abnormalities such as prenatal, perinatal, or postnatal insults, massive infantile spasms, or metabolic disease. The seizures themselves may persist as episodes of absence interspersed with atonic or myoclonic attacks. On the other hand, generalized tonic-clonic seizures (particularly of the nocturnal variety) and the emergence of partial seizures (particularly complex-partial seizures) is quite frequent with increasing age, with subsequent amelioration of the atonic and myoclonic events.

Patients in whom no underlying cause is apparent tend to achieve greater intellectual development. According to Chevrie and Aicardi (1972), those patients whose Lennox-Gastaut syndrome follows infantile spasms have the highest incidence of severe retardation and patients with so-called secondary seizures have the second highest incidence of severe retardation. Those with predominantly myoclonic seizures of late onset fare much better; of course, their conditions may represent a different genre of syndrome altogether, as there is certainly an overlap here between these and the massive myoclonus syndrome of adolescence, which is a significantly more benign condition. Ohtahara et al (1977) discerned the poor intellectual prognosis (84.5%) and poor prognosis for cessation of seizures. Although, in general, the earlier the onset the worse the prognosis, there were a number of patients with Lennox-Gastaut syndrome in whom onset occurred in the second half of the first decade and who appeared to be suffering from a progressive and deteriorating condition that then reached a plateau without further deterioration of intellectual function; however, the patient was still severely mentally impaired. The influence of anticonvulsant medication should be considered in those patients in whom progressive intellectual impairment occurs during the course of the illness, particularly in those patients to whom the sedative drugs such as barbiturates and benzodiazepines are administered. When phenytoin is administered, a progressive encephalopathy may occur. A further complicating factor is the social isolation in which patients with this condition find themselves. This isolation occurs because of the danger inherent in sudden unheralded falls. Frequently the parents are overprotective and exclude the child from normal childhood activities, including normal educational opportunities.

TREATMENT

The intractability of the seizures associated with the Lennox-Gastaut syndrome is attested to by the number of anticonvulsant drugs that have been used in the management of the syndrome. Through the Comprehensive Epilepsy Program, I have seen patients who have been subjected to as many as six, simultaneously administered, antiepileptic drugs.

Therapy with as few simultaneously administered drugs as possible should be the aim of pharmacotherapy.

When the child has head nodding, eye blinking, laughing, or flushing episodes in infancy, the drug most often used is phenobarbital, which is not usually successful in changing the frequency or character of these episodes. Sodium valproate is becoming the most frequently prescribed drug and may lead to considerable amelioration of the seizures (Jeavons et al 1977). Occasionally dramatic improvement results, even in children whose seizures have proved intractable for a number of years. In my experience, sodium valproate is the drug of choice and is more likely to be successful than any other available agent. Whether improvement is attributable to administration of valproate or to discontinuation of a previously administered medication (usually in doses and combinations sufficient to produce toxicity) is not clear at this time. The reduction of ineffective medication, particularly of the sedatives, has in and of itself frequently benefited previously incapacitated children (Sutula 1981). Other drugs useful in the treatment of absence seiures associated with spike-wave EEG patterns are not usually successful in controlling the seizures of Lennox-Gastaut syndrome, even when combined with valproate, if valproate by itself is ineffective. Such drugs include ethosuximide, methosuximide, and trimethadione, though we have had two patients in whom the Lennox-Gastaut was characterized predominantly by absence-like episodes and for whom trimethadione was effective; reduction of the dose of trimethadione led to a recurrence of clinical attacks. Acetazolamide alone or in combination with valproate has occasionally been of benefit. Where generalized tonic-clonic or partial seizures are a prominent feature of the attacks, carbamazepine and phenytoin have been effective in controlling these components, though they have not been of major benefit in controlling the atonic or myoclonic components of the syndrome. Use of the ketogenic diet has a long tradition in the therapy of seizures associated with Lennox-Gastaut syndrome. Ketosis is achieved by the administration of a diet consisting predominantly of fat (fat constitutes about three-fourths of the administered calories). The beneficial component of the diet (either ketone bodies or free fatty acids) is undetermined. It is conceivable that a certain amount of valproic acid is administered in this manner. The diet is difficult to achieve. The compliance level is quite low, and in many cases the diet is not economically feasible. Since the introduction of valproate, the administration of the ketogenic diet has become less popular. It is still occasionally helpful and, when successful, should be administered for as long as a year. Prolonged administration is not generally recommended because of growth and wound-healing problems associated with this nutritional travesty.

Benzodiazepine drugs, particularly clonazepam, have proved beneficial in controlling drop attacks, myoclonic seizures, and absence seizures associated with the Lennox-Gastaut syndrome (Browne and Penry 1973). Unfortunately most benzodiazepine drugs elicit the development of tolerance during their administration. With increasing doses, side effects are frequent, and a subsequent reduction of dose frequently leads to the emergence of generalized tonic-clonic seizures that may be quite intractable. Moreover, in some patients with Lennox-Gastaut syndrome, tonic seizures have been precipitated by the administration of benzodiazepines (Tassinari 1972). The introduction of benzodiazepines was greeted with enthusiasm. However, as for most drugs, this enthusiasm rapidly subsided because favorable results could not be sustained in this syndrome (Dreifuss and Sato 1982).

Here as much as in any other type of epilepsy, attention to the needs of the child as a whole is of paramount importance. Because of the dramatic nature of the seizures, the frequent injuries, the resulting deformities, and the limitations induced by such attacks, the child is limited to a small number of activities, with a consequent loss of the normal childhood opportunities to explore and to learn by expanding his or her horizons. Protective head gear, removal of sharp corners from furniture, and other protective measures help to some extent to give the child more freedom. Improvement in anticonvulsant regimen and a sympathetic multidisciplinary approach to management will help to lessen the disadvantages of this syndrome. The child should, insofar as possible, be allowed to function in a peer environment, including attending school at a level and with an educational plan appropriate to the child's abilities and individual needs. These children enjoy sporting and supervised summer camp activities and experience personality growth in such settings, responding to the dignity of risk.

BIBLIOGRAPHY

Aicardi J, Chevrie JJ: Myoclonic epilepsy of childhood. *Neuropaediatrie* 1971;3:177-190.

Browne TR, Penry JK: Benzodiazepines in the treatment of epilepsy: A review. *Epilepsia* 1973; 14:277-310.

Chevrie JJ, Aicardi J: Childhood epileptic encephalopathy with slow spike-wave. *Epilepsia* 1972;13:259-271.

Doose H: Das akinetische Petit Mal. I. Das klinische und elektroenzephalographische Bild der akinetischen Anfälle. *Arch Psychiatr Nervenkr* 1964a;205:625-636.

Doose H: Das akinetische Petit Mal. II. Verlaufsformen und Beziehungen zu den Blitz-Nick-Salaamkrampfen und den Absencen. *Arch Psychiatr Nervenkr* 1964b;205:637-654.

Dreifuss FE, Sato S: Clonazepam, in Woodbury D, Penry JK, Pippenger C (eds): *Antiepileptic Drugs.* New York, Raven Press, 1982.

Gastaut H: *Dictionary of Epilepsy. Part 1: Definitions.* Geneva, World Health Organization, 1973.

Gastaut H, Pinsard N, Genton P: Electrical correlations of CT scans in secondary generalized epilepsies, in Canger R, Angeleri F, Penry JK (eds): *Advances in Epileptology.* New York, Raven Press, 1980, pp 45-52.

Gastaut H, Roger J, Soulayrol R, et al: Childhood epileptic encephalopathy with diffuse slow spike-wave (otherwise known as "petit mal variant" or Lennox syndrome). *Epilepsia* 1966;7:139-179.

Gibbs FA, Gibbs EL, Lennox WG: The influence of the blood sugar level on the wave and spike formation in petit mal epilepsy. *Arch Neurol Psychiatr* 1939;41:1111-1116.

Jeavons PM, Clark JE, Meshwari WC: Treatment of generalized epilepsy of childhood and adolescence with sodium valproate. *Dev Med Child Neurol* 1977;19:9-25.

Kruse R: *Das Myoklonisch-Astatische Petit Mal.* Berlin, Springer Verlag, 1968, p 131.

Lennox WG, Davis JP: Clinical correlates of the fast and slow spike-wave electroencephalogram. *Pediatrics* 1950;5:626.

O'Donohoe NV: *Epilepsies of Childhood.* London, Butterworths, 1979.

Ohtahara S, Yamatogi Y, Ohtsuka Y: Prognosis of the Lennox syndrome. A clinical and electroencephalographic study. *Epilepsia* 1977;18:130-131.

Sorel R: L'épilepsie myokinetique grave de la première enfance avec pointe-onde lente (petit mal variant) et son traitement. *Rev Neurol (Paris)* 1964;110:215-223.

Sutula TP, Sackellares JC, Miller JQ, et al: Efficacy of prolonged hospitalization and intensive monitoring in refractory epilepsy. *Neurology* 1981;31:243-247.

Tassinari CA, Dravet C, Roger J, et al: Tonic status epilepticus precipitated by intravenous benzodiazepine in five patients with Lennox-Gastaut syndrome. *Epilepsia* 1972;13: 421-435.

CHAPTER 9

Partial Seizures: Simple Partial Seizures

Fritz E. Dreifuss

Hughlings Jackson (1931) recognized two classes of seizures that were generalized from the beginning. One class he called "epilepsy proper," and he included vertigo, petit mal, and grand mal in this group. The second class of seizures began focally; these he called "epileptiform or epileptoid." In this second group he included convulsions beginning unilaterally, unilateral dysesthesia, and epileptiform amaurosis. He recognized that convulsions began from excessive discharges of nerve cells and that these were concerned "with excessive (primary) discharges as constituting discharging lesions," and sometimes of them as making up a 'physiological fulminate,' or occasionally, using Horseley's term, of their being together an 'epileptogenous focus.'

Jackson distinguished between 1) seizures that begin in the "highest centers" and result in loss of consciousness and 2) seizures that begin at a lower level, frequently involve face, hand, or foot, either remain localized or spread, and are frequently followed by postictal paralysis.

Fritsch and Hitzig (1870) and, shortly thereafter, Ferrier (1873) showed experimentally that electrical stimulation of areas of the motor cortex led to focal convulsive seizures in the contralateral limbs and that these sometimes progressed to generalized convulsions. Thus, 100 years ago, the functional organization of the brain was reasonably delineated and causative lesions were related to specific seizure types. Electroencephalography and further stimulation studies tended to confirm a fundamental distinction between "focal" and "generalized" seizures and the concept then arose that the former were due to a focus of origin in the cerebral cortex and the latter was related to a deep-seated "centrencephalic" or diffuse disorder (Penfield and Jasper 1954). Further studies have shown that a large number of so-called generalized seizures and even seizures with a so-called generalized electroencephalographic pattern may be due to secondary bilateral synchronous discharge resulting from a primary focal and localized hemispheric origin. Moreover, in focal cortical seizures, there may be widespread participation of central structures; in so-called generalized seizures, participation by subcortical or centrencephalic structures may be missing.

Secondary, bilateral synchrony may be seen in experimental epilepsy caused by focal cortical influences such as alumina-creme, cobalt, freezing, penicillin, or electrical stimulation. Moreover, such stimuli may lead to the development of a contralateral "mirror focus." This mirror focus may develop its own independent epileptogenicity, which may remain even after the primary focus is removed. Though in the mirror focus an apparently unscathed portion of the brain appears to become epileptic, histological and biochemical analyses reveal that changes do occur and that these changes are associated with changes in dendritic spine formation and with biochemical alterations. Two principal theories have been formulated to explain the epileptogenic instability of aggregates of neurons. One is an extension of Cannon's theory of denervation hypersensitivity to neurotransmitters such as acetylcholine (Cannon 1929). The other suggests disinhibition rather than deafferentation as a mechanism leading to system instability; disinhibition is an inherent property of the neuronal network. Some of the cortical projections may play a role in epileptic hyperexcitability, and the generation of epileptic activity may be related to antidromic discharge. Epileptic firing is also a property of in vitro cortical slices, which are becoming an important investigative model (Schwartzkroin and Prince 1976, 1977).

The finding of increased extracellular concentrations of potassium during interictal and ictal activity has led to the theory that glia may play a major role in focal epileptogenesis (Dichter et al 1972, Fisher et al 1976, Pollen and Trachtenberg 1970). Both cyclic AMP and cyclic GMP may exert nervous system effects during seizures. The level of cyclic AMP is elevated during increased neuronal activity. Cyclic GMP is thought to accumulate because of influx of calcium ions during seizures. The relationship of calcium to the epileptic process appears to be a complex one in that the calcium ion may be the main initiator of dendritic action potentials in the tissue culture model (Ferrendelli et al 1979, Greengard 1968).

The development of a focus of epileptic activity leads to the theoretical possibility of kindling. Kindling occurs in an experimental situation where the application of a subepileptic stimulus to appropriate brain sites, such as the amygdaloid nucleus or the hippocampus, will ultimately result in the development of afterdischarge and later of seizures. Finally the seizures occur without the intermediation of an electrical stimulus (Goddard et al 1969, Morrel 1979, Wada et al 1975, McNamara et al 1980). Once kindling has developed, it remains for a prolonged period of time. Although there is no evidence that a similar mechanism operates in the human epileptic cortex, such a phenomenon would explain why epileptic seizures constitute a risk factor for further seizures or epilepsy. Such a mechanism might also explain the development of the mirror focus (Morrell 1959, 1979). Moreover, the development of late posttraumatic epilepsy following early posttraumatic epilepsy might be the result of altered brain function as the result of early seizures.

The occurrence of an epileptic discharge appears to evoke an inhibitory response. Following a burst of spikes, a hyperpolarization occurs at the site and may be, in part, the result of inhibitory interneurons fired by the axonal spike discharge (Prince 1978). Most partial seizures remain localized, possibly because of the hyperpolarization and possibly because of excitation of an inhibitory surround in the vicinity of the focus, which limits the spread of activity into adjacent brain areas. It is interesting to note that kindling of seizures might result in an increased number of benzodiazepine receptors (Valdes et al 1982) in certain areas of the brain and that these might then potentiate γ-aminobutyrate-mediated interneuron input of an inhibitory nature.

Focal postictal, or Todd's paralysis might be the result of enhanced focal inhibitory activity (Efron 1961) rather than the result of neuronal exhaustion, such as had been initially postulated by Todd and by Jackson (1931). This suggestion is to some extent supported by the finding that some of the most severe Todd's paralyses occur in patients who have only sensory seizures.

GENETICS OF SIMPLE PARTIAL SEIZURES

Although inheritance plays a significant role in generalized seizure disorders, it does not appear to play a major part in partial seizures, particularly of the simple partial variety (Andermann 1972, Eisner et al 1959) except in those patients with rolandic epilepsy (Blom et al 1972, Nayrae and Beaussart 1958), where inheritance was found to be approximately 25%.

CLINICAL TYPES OF SIMPLE PARTIAL SEIZURES

WITH MOTOR SIGNS. Seizures may remain relatively restricted to part of the body, such as the face, the hand, or the foot, or they may spread to other areas of the same side. The patient remains fully conscious. Subsequently, the seizure may involve the whole of one side of the body. If a simple partial seizure begins to involve those structures on whose integrity the state of consciousness depends, consciousness will be impaired and the seizure will become a complex partial seizure. At any time, a simple partial seizure may become a generalized tonic-clonic seizure or may arrive at this state via sufficient limbic participation to clearly define a complex partial seizure. A simple partial seizure with a march is known as a Jacksonian seizure. The majority of patients suffering from Jacksonian seizures have purely motor symptomatology, but others may have sensory or psychic symptoms.

WITH SENSORY SYMPTOMS. Sensory symptoms accompanying simple partial seizures are usually paresthesiae and, on occasion, shock-like sensations and numbness (Mangniere and Courjon 1978). Rarely, pain may be experienced, but this is an exceptional epileptic symptom. Some patients with sensory symptoms experience an impression of distortion of parts of the body such as a feeling of change in size or occasionally a feeling of missing a part of the body. The latter feeling is particularly likely to occur when the right hemisphere is the source of seizure discharge. Because of the nature of cortical representation, the majority of the cortical surface is occupied by cortex representing the thumb, forefinger, and face. For this reason, partial seizures affect these areas predominantly. In seizures commencing in the parasagittal region the proximal limb may be first involved. As a rule, each patient has a particular repertoire of symptoms that is reproduced in each attack.

Occasionally, atonicity rather than motor activity may occur in a portion of a limb. The seizure is then characterized by an inhibitory phenomenon or a sudden loss of function rather than a positive motor or sensory symptom. When the lower extremity is affected in this way, the child may suddenly fall; the use of the limb is gradually regained over the next several minutes. If the seizure discharge originates in the supplementary motor area, there is frequently a movement of the contralateral upper extremity with abduction of the shoulder and flexion at the elbow. These movements are accompanied by rotation of the head toward the affected limb, actions that give the impression that the patient is looking at the flexed arm. Occasionally, such a movement is seen ipsilateral to the focus. In supplementary motor seizures, the movement is predominantly tonic rather than clonic jerking.

As a rule, focal cortical seizures are quite short, lasting for seconds to a few minutes. However, they may become generalized tonic-clonic seizures of longer duration, and on occasion they may persist as epilepsia partialis continua for hours or days.

Apart from seizures that may lead to loss of motor function, simple partial seizures may be followed by Todd's paralysis, as previously mentioned. The paralysis may in part be the result of neuronal exhaustion but may be predominantly caused by excessive inhibition.

Very localized seizures may present with masticatory movements, which are occasionally associated with unintelligible vocalization or arrest of speech when the person is speaking at the time of the seizure. Vocalization and occasionally repetitive utterances are more likely to occur when the focus is in the nondominant hemisphere. Speech arrest is more likely to occur when the focus is in the dominant hemisphere. However, foci in either hemisphere may be associated with unintelligible dysarthric utterance resulting from uncontrolled movements of the muscles subserving speech, including muscles of the tongue, the pharynx, the lips, and the jaws. Occasionally uncontrolled coughing may be an epileptic phenomenon; this has been referred to as "Charcot's laryngeal epilepsy" (Charcot 1876, Janz 1969). Laryngeal epilepsy is sometimes confused with loss of consciousness induced by vigorous coughing, which causes impairment of venous return as a result of prolonged increased intrathoracic pressure. This condition occurs in patients with obstructive pulmonary disease.

WITH SPECIAL SENSORY PHENOMENA. Special sensory phenomena associated with a simple partial seizure may include distortions in the sense of smell. Olfactory sensations associated with a seizure are usually unpleasant, difficult to categorize, thoroughly disagreeable odors. Onion or garlic is a common designation for a pungent sensation. Although this olfactory sensation may be the only seizure manifestation, it is followed commonly by focal motor activity and occasionally by a dreamy state (an alteration of consciousness). The attack then becomes a complex partial seizure. Olfactory hallucinations frequently are a warning of a neoplastic cause of the seizure. Gustatory hallucinations are also quite frequent, and again the taste is difficult to describe and usually is designated as "metallic." The localizational significance is similar to that of the olfactory hallucination and both may be subserved under the rubric of "uncinate fits" (Jackson 1931).

Auditory seizures vary from rushing, hissing, or crescendo noises to quite elaborate auditory hallucinatory phenomena such as hearing music, either a familiar or a long-forgotten tune or snatches of a melody. One of my patients experienced the recurrent auditory sensation of a race course crowd shouting the name of a horse. This was frequently followed by spread of the seizure into a generalized tonic-clonic convulsion.

Vertiginous seizures are rare and are usually characterized by a sensation of vague dizziness rather than true vertigo (Kogeorgos and Scott 1981). However, a severe paroxysmal vertigo may occur, and it has been described as "tornado epilepsy."

Visual phenomena vary in their degree of elaboration, depending on the site of origin of the seizure. In occipital seizures, there is usually a rather unstructured, scintillating, bright or colored, spectral sensation in the half field opposite the focus. Occasionally a negative phenomenon, such as a sensation of darkness, rather than a positive phenomenon (namely, flashing lights) may occur. This type of sensation is quite frequently encountered in children with infantile hemiparesis who have a porencephaly in the distribution of the posterior cerebral artery. In seizures originating in the visual association areas, rather more elaborate hallucinatory phenomena occur, including visions with distinct shapes, objects, people, animals, or parts of people or animals. In its most elaborate form, panoramic hallucinations may be seen. At any time during the evolution of the seizure, a complex partial seizure may occur with diminution of consciousness. Or the seizures may become a generalized tonic-clonic seizure, either directly or via the intermediation of a complex partial seizure.

Adversive seizures are defined as seizures in which the head and eyes turn. Usually, these movements are part of a complex partial seizure, and the patient is unaware of the occurrence. Occasionally, however, consciousness is preserved, and the patient is aware of a jerking movement of the head and eyes to the side. One of my patients was awakened from sleep with a sensation as if someone had grabbed his head and was pulling it to the side. This was a recurrent dream and on awakening he would find himself in an adversive epileptic seizure that frequently involved the upper extremity and that on occasion resulted in a generalized tonic-clonic attack. Head and eye deviation do not constitute a valuable localizing sign, for although the movement is generally contraversive, it may on occasion be an ipsilateral phenomenon or true adversion. Some persons experience a sensation as if someone were behind them and just off to one side, and they would then turn in that direction as a portion of an adversive seizure. In some children, this is the beginning of a rotatory seizure in which the child then continues to turn in a twirling manner.

WITH AUTONOMIC PHENOMENA. Autonomic phenomena may be seen in partial seizures (Gastaut et al 1959, 1960, Solomon 1977). Pupil dilatation is probably most common. Pupil dilatation accompanies many seizure types and has on occasion been the only outward manifestation of recurrent epileptic activity; this conclusion is based on intensive monitoring with prolonged EEG recording. On rare occasions, a transient Horner's syndrome may be seen on the side opposite a discharging parietal lobe focus.

Recurrent abdominal discomfort and vomiting may occur as a seizure manifestation in children. Here it has to be distinguished from other "recurrent" syndromes such as migraine, cyclical vomiting, or recurrent acidosis. If a focal paroxysmal EEG discharge can be identified during an attack, it is convincing evidence of the epileptic nature of the disturbance. Focal, unilateral, piloerection (or goose flesh) may occur. In children it is not unusual to see pallor, flushing, or even unilateral color change as part of a partial seizure (a harlequin phenomenon). Such seizures are sometimes associated with incongruous laughter as a gelastic seizure (Daly and Mulder 1971, Gastaut and Broughton 1972, Loiseau et al 1971). Increased salivation may be an autonomic phenomenon. Patients with partial seizures occasionally have an uncontrollable gush of saliva, which may prove extremely discomfiting to the patient who cannot wipe it up quickly enough to prevent the formation of a puddle.

WITH PSYCHIC SYMPTOMS (DISTURBANCE OF HIGHER CEREBRAL FUNCTION). Psychic symptoms usually occur with impairment of consciousness (ie, complex partial seizures).

DYSMNESIC SYMPTOMS. A distorted memory experience may occur. These experiences include a distortion of the time sense, a dreamy state, a flashback, or a sensation as if a new experience had been experienced before (known as déjà vu), or as if a previously experienced sensation had not been experienced (known as jamais vu). Similar auditory experiences are known as déjà entendu or jamais entendu, respectively. Occasionally, as a form of forced thinking, the patient may experience a rapid recollection of episodes from his past life; this is known as panoramic vision.

COGNITIVE DISTURBANCES. Cognitive disturbances include dreamy states; distortions of the time sense; and sensations of unreality, detachment, or depersonalization.

AFFECTIVE SYMPTOMATOLOGY. Sensation of extreme pleasure or displeasure, as well as fear and intense depression with feelings of unworthiness and rejection may be experienced during seizures. Unlike the feelings of psychiatrically induced depression, these symptoms tend to come in attacks lasting for a few minutes. Anger or rage is occasionally experienced; but unlike temper tantrums, epileptic anger is apparently unprovoked, and it abates rapidly. Fear or terror is the most frequent symptom; it is sudden in onset, usually unprovoked, and may lead to running away. Associated with the terror are frequently objective signs of autonomic activity, including pupil dilatation, pallor, flushing, piloerection, palpitation, and hypertension.

Epileptic or gelastic seizure laughter should not, strictly speaking, be classed as an affective symptom because the laughter is usually without affect and hollow. Like other forms of pathological laughter, it is often unassociated with true mirth.

ILLUSIONS. These take the form of distorted perceptions in which objects may appear deformed. Polyoptic illusions such as monocular diplopia and distortions of size (macropsia or micropsia) and of distance may occur. Distortions of sound, including microacusia and macroacusia, also may be experienced. Depersonalization, as if the person were outside his body, may occur. Altered perception of size or weight of a limb may be noted.

STRUCTURED HALLUCINATIONS. Hallucinations may occur as manifestations or perceptions without a corresponding external stimulus and may affect the somatosensory, visual, auditory, olfactory, and gustatory senses. If the seizure arises from the primary receptive area, the hallucination tends to be rather primitive. Flashing lights may be seen or rushing noises may be heard. In more elaborate seizures involving visual or auditory association areas with participation of mobilized memory traces, formed hallucinations occur. These hallucinations may include scenery, persons, spoken sentences, or music. The character of these perceptions may be normal or distorted.

SPECIFIC SYNDROMES IN THE PARTIAL SEIZURE CATEGORY

BENIGN FOCAL EPILEPSY (ROLANDIC SEIZURES, SYLVIAN SEIZURES, OR BENIGN MID-TEMPORAL SPIKE EPILEPSY OF CHILDHOOD). Since the first description of this type of seizure in 1958 (Nayrac and Beaussart 1958) clinicians have recognized its frequent occurrence in children, beginning during the second half of the first decade of life and usually ending spontaneously in the early teens. Seizures may occur in either sex, but males are affected more frequently than females. The attacks are usually quite stereotyped. Characteristically, seizures occur during the night when the child awakes with twitching of one side of the face and possibly of the arm. When the child starts to speak, he or she makes unintelligible gurgling noises. The child may feel as if the tongue is too large for the mouth and he or she seemingly becomes quite distressed. When the attack is over, the child goes back to sleep and may have no memory of the seizure upon awakening the next morning. When the attacks occur during the daytime, they are recollected much better. In some children, the attacks occur only during sleep and in others they may occur either during sleep or in the waking state. The duration of attacks is usually less than 2 minutes. The electroencephalographic features consist of midtemporal or centrotemporal spiking, which is usually unilateral and which is sometimes seen only during sleep (Beaussart 1972, Beaussart and Faou 1978, Blom et al 1972, Lombroso 1967).

The importance of recognition of this type of seizure is that it is self-limited with a benign outcome. It is rare that seizures persist beyond puberty or that they are the harbinger of a more severe seizure disorder. The attacks respond quite well to medication as a rule, and the drug of choice is carbamazepine, though other anticonvulsants such as valproic acid or phenytoin are also effective.

There is a significant genetic incidence in this seizure disorder.

EPILEPTIC APHASIA. Aphasia may occur under several conditions in association with partial seizures. As an ictal phenomenon, the speech disturbance will depend on the region of the brain involved in the epileptic discharge. When seizures arise from the dominant hemisphere, speech arrest is common; this is similar to what is observed with stimulation of the frontal and temporal regions of the brain at craniotomy. When seizures arise from the nondominant hemisphere, speech arrest may also occur, but there may be speech perseveration or the iteration of repetitive utterances. For example, a patient may cry out, "Here it comes, here it comes, here it comes." One of my patients would regularly start to count as soon as he entered an attack and would then repeat a short series of numbers with great rapidity. In some cases, humming and mumbling takes the place of speech, and on occasion a distinct receptive or expressive aphasia occurs.

In addition to transient ictal aphasias, speech disturbance may take the form of a prolonged acquired aphasia occurring during the course of a seizure disorder. In these cases, hearing deficit is common; aphasia develops in relation to an epileptic disturbance, but the aphasia may precede or follow the seizures; and aphasia persists for prolonged periods of time and may even be permanent, with a fairly rapid progression followed by a plateau or very gradual improvement over the course of months or years (Goldstein et al 1960, Ingrams 1959, Victor et al 1972). Focal electroencephalographic disturbances, and on occasion generalized electroencephalographic disturbances, are frequently seen, and seizures may be a prominent part of the illness or may occur just from time to time, though seizures usually are seen at the onset of the disturbance. The nature of this is not clear, though it is suspected that a form of encephalitis is the precipitating factor.

Finally, a seizure disorder may be associated with a developmental expressive aphasia in which a seizure disorder is the only finding and mental deficiency, pseudobulbar palsy, auditory imperceptions or autism are not complicating features. Occasionally, treatment of the electroencephalographic disturbance results in amelioration of the aphasia, but as a rule there is no improvement after the administration of anticonvulsant drugs. In these cases, the electroencephalographic disturbance is usually predominantly unilateral but secondary bilateral spread frequently occurs (Sato and Dreifuss 1973).

The relationship between speech disturbances and epilepsy is thus a rather complex one without a definite cause and effect relationship.

UNILATERAL SEIZURES. The rubric of unilateral seizures includes a variety of childhood epileptic syndromes with different causes. Some infants and young children have seizures characterized by their unilaterality, their clonic nature, and occasionally a variation from side to side in different attacks of the convulsion, producing what Gastaut et al (1974) have referred to as "see-saw seizures." They regarded this type of seizure as a variant of generalized seizures; however, with less impairment of consciousness and with the epileptic discharge confined at any one time to a single hemisphere. In one variety—the unilateral tonic-clonic seizures— the diminution of consciousness and the tonic seizure giving way to clonic jerking near the end of the seizure is suggestive of what is seen in generalized tonic-clonic seizures. According to Gastaut et al (1974) the interictal EEG is characterized by bilaterally synchronous and symmetrical or sometimes asymmetrical spike-and-wave or polyspike-and-wave activity. On the other hand, unilateral clonic seizures do not generally impair consciousness, and the attacks last longer. They may be followed by a postictal hemiparesis, and the EEG is quite variable as this type of seizure has several outcomes including a protracted hemiparesis. On occasion this type of seizure is indistinguishable from epilepsia partialis continua.

Another variety of unilateral epileptic seizures is that associated with infantile hemiplegia (Aicardi et al 1969, Freud 1897, Gastaut et al 1959, 1960, Gold and Carter 1976). Hemiplegia of early onset is a condition characterized by the development of a hemiplegia in a previously well child and is probably due to a number of causes; thus, it represents a clinical syndrome. The onset may be with a convulsive seizure followed by a flaccid hemiplegia. At other times, the hemiplegia follows a vague period of malaise with or without convulsions. Convulsions, when they do occur, may be unilateral or generalized. According to Solomon et al (1970), the majority of children with this syndrome are less than 2 years of age. Known causes include sudden vascular occlusions, either spontaneous or traumatic. Thus, a middle cerebral artery thrombosis may occur or the carotid artery may be involved. In one of my patients, a popsicle stick injury in the pharynx resulted in traumatic carotid artery occlusion with the infantile hemiplegia syndrome. The condition may complicate encephalitis, collagen vascular disease, sickle cell anemia, retropharyngeal abscess, moya-moya disease (Susuki and Takatu 1969), or congenital heart disease.

The initial seizure or series of seizures usually subsides rapidly, but seizures frequently recur within the first year in approximately 50% of the cases and later in the other 50%; in fact, they may not occur until adolescence (Solomon 1977). They are then typically hemicorporeal or they may remain focal to the upper or lower extremity. The sequence of hemiplegia with seizure followed by a seizure-free interval and the recurrence of seizures at a later time have been designated by Gastaut et al (1959, 1960) as the hemiconvulsion, hemiplegia, and epilepsy syndrome (HHE). As in most cases of hemisphere destruction of early onset, porencephaly is common, as is unilateral ventricular dilatation and displacement toward the atrophic side. Compensatory skull thickening occurs on the affected side and the development of the limbs on the hemiparetic side is frequently hypoplastic (Dyke et al 1933, Dreifuss 1956).

A special variety of the syndrome is the condition associated with cutaneous angiomatosis in the form of the Sturge-Weber syndrome (Alexander 1972). The cutaneous angioma is part of a congenital ectodermal disorder. It occurs in the distribution of one or more of the divisions of the fifth cranial nerve; the cerebral hemisphere is characteristically shrunken, with intracranial calcification in the cortex and telangiectasia of the meninges.

ETIOLOGY OF SIMPLE PARTIAL SEIZURES

Despite the fact that simple partial seizures are the paradigm of the symptomatic epilepsies, a focal structural cause is rarely identified. In adults, where causative factors such as brain tumors and cerebrovascular disease loom large, an identifiable cause is rather more common than among children. Different series estimate that the cause will be unknown in approximately 30–50% of cases, and that in others the putative cause cannot be substantiated, particularly in those pediatric patients with vague histories of "difficult birth" and various degrees of head trauma.

Prenatal and perinatal causes constitute the majority of causative factors for seizures in the first few years of life. However, during the second decade, cerebral trauma becomes considerably more prominent, and after puberty brain tumors begin to appear to a larger degree in the differential diagnosis.

Inborn errors of metabolism may present with focal seizure disturbances early or they may be delayed. Thus, maple syrup urine disease, phenylketonuria, galactosemia, and hyperglycinemia may present with seizures very early in life, whereas the neuronal storage disease, which also may be associated with partial seizure disturbances, may occur later in infancy or early childhood. These conditions are characterized by the early onset of seizures that are very prominent, particularly in the diseases of the cerebral gray matter. In the leukodystrophies, seizures are somewhat less prominent and spasticity of muscles with progressive paresis may be relatively more obtrusive. In the neonatal period, abnormalities in the blood levels of electrolytes, calcium, and glucose are frequent causes of partial seizures, which are often multifocal. Why a generalized metabolic disorder, such as hypoglycemia, manifests itself multifocally rather than in a generalized manner is not clear. Hypocalcemia may be seen in infants who are premature, small for age, or born of diabetic mothers or mothers suffering from toxemia. Galactosemia, maple syrup urine disease, and glycogen storage diseases may also present as hypoglycemia. Hyponatremia may result from excessive water intake or from inappropriate secretion of antidiuretic hormone secondary to intracranial infection or bleeding, or it may complicate the adrenogenital syndrome. Hypernatremia is seen in hypertonic dehydration, in diabetes insipidus, or in injudicious administration of salt solution. Both these conditions may result in multifocal cortical seizures. Hypocalcemia is common in the newborn period as a condition secondary to severe cerebral compromise, or after the third day of life, as primary neonatal tetany. Again, multifocal cortical seizures frequently occur on the background of a jittery child with increased extensor tonus.

Congenital, natal, and perinatal factors include brain malformations and antenatal infections that affect brain development, including toxoplasmosis, cytomegalic inclusion disease, rubella, and syphilis. These children frequently show stigmata of intracranial infection in utero, including chorioretinitis, microcephaly, and intracranial calcifications.

Vascular causes for partial seizures include vascular malformation, the previously mentioned encephalofacial angiomatosis (Sturge-Weber disease; Figure 9-1), diseases involving the intracranial vessels, such as fibromuscular hyperplasia, moya-moya disease, and cerebral embolization from congenital heart disease.

Postnatal infections such as meningitis, particularly in infants, may be heralded, accompanied, or followed by seizures. Convulsions in meningitis may be due to the direct irritating effect of the inflammation or may occur as a result of focal cortical venous occlusions or even abscess formation. Occasionally, seizures may occur after meningitis as a complication of postmeningitis hydrocephalus. Viral encephalitides may present with simple partial seizures, as may the postinfectious encephalomyolitides. Parasitic infections, including cysticercosis and enchinococcosis, deserve diagnostic consideration in parts of the world where these are endemic.

Toxic causes for partial seizures include conditions such as lead encephalopathy,

138

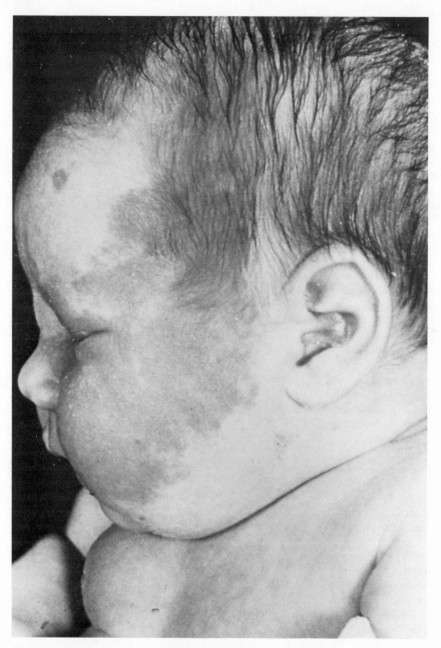

Figure 9-1 Encephalofacial angiomatosis (Sturge-Weber syndrome).

(which is the most common manifestation of lead poisoning in small children), withdrawal from sedative medications (which may be seen in newborn infants or later in life when children are withdrawn rapidly from drugs such as barbiturates), and burn encephalopathy.

Brain tumors in small children are usually represented by subtentorial lesions, but occasionally supratentorial tumors occur during the first decade of life. However, brain tumors become relatively more frequent as a cause of simple partial seizures with increasing age. Such tumors are gliomas, A-V malformations, and metastatic tumors. In small children, neuroblastomas, rhabdomyosarcomas, and complication of proliferative diseases such as leukemia may present in this manner.

HEAD TRAUMA AND PARTIAL SEIZURES

One of the important consequences of head injury is the development of convulsive seizures. The incidence of epilepsy after head injury depends on many factors. One of these factors is the severity of the injury as defined by the degree of penetration of the brain as well as by the duration of unconsciousness or amnesia following the injury. Epilepsy occurs much more frequently when there is penetration of the brain; under this condition it may occur in as many as 40% of the cases (Caveness et al 1962, Jennett 1975). An open head wound is defined as one in which the intracranial contents are exposed to the exterior environment. These wounds can be brought about either by a penetrating injury or by a fracture through one of the air sinuses or mastoid cells. The distinction between open and closed head injuries is significant, because the latter, through exposure of the intracranial contents to the outside, leads to a high incidence of infection, with devastating results. In the case of a penetrating or missile injury, the penetrating object is forced into the cranial cavity at the point of entry, together with bone fragments, and hair. If the dura is torn, the fragments are forced into the nervous system itself, causing laceration and brain damage. Interestingly, in many of these cases, consciousness may not be lost, and the patient may walk away from the scene of the accident with brain matter issuing from the wound. Most civilian head injuries result from trauma without penetration and are caused by external blows to the cranium which may or may not be sufficient to fracture the skull. The effect of closed head injuries depends on the mechanical factors involved. For example, the patient's head may be crushed and the skull fractured like an egg shell; yet the patient may remain conscious. On the other hand, if the head is in motion and strikes a stationary object or if a fast-moving object strikes a stationary head, sudden acceleration or deceleration of the nervous system within the skull occurs and causes contusion of the brain at the point of impact between brain and skull and an acute kinking at the site where the brain is relatively tightly anchored to the skull, such as in the region of the brain stem, where the latter is invested by the membranous tentorium of the cerebellum and the bony foramen magnum. Compression occurring here leads to immediate loss of consciousness, which is referred to as concussion. If the patient does not regain consciousness or if he suffers from permanent brain damage, then something more than concussion has occurred. This further injury is usually a contusion of the brain or a laceration with hemorrhage into the brain or hemorrhage that causes compression of the brain. The patient who is rendered unconscious by a head injury usually suffers from a period of amnesia that extends beyond the period during which he appears to be unconscious. Thus, the patient may apparently regain consciousness, take food, perform purposeful acts, and yet after finally regaining his faculties, have no memory for the period during which he has performed these acts. This is known as the period of posttraumatic amnesia.

In children, the most frequent causes of epilepsy after nonpenetrating head wounds are associated with linear or depressed skull fractures. On the other hand, children frequently have early traumatic epilepsy after relatively trivial head injuries not associated with fractures. However, apart from these, the incidence of epilepsy is more or less proportional to the length of the posttraumatic amnesia.

Early epilepsy is usually in the nature of simple partial seizures with motor phenomena, and in more than half the cases, it arises within 24 hours of injury (Jennett 1975). In children under the age of 5, status epilepticus is common after severe head injuries. By and large, the prognosis of patients suffering with immediate or early posttraumatic epilepsy is favorable, though 25% will develop later seizures. Later posttraumatic epilepsy represents the majority of posttraumatic seizures. Although in children the onset may be delayed for many years (Courjon 1970), the majority of posttraumatic epilepsy occurs within 3 years of the injury, and the seizures are either of the generalized tonic-clonic or of the simple or complex partial variety, with the overwhelming majority of patients suffering from generalized tonic-clonic seizures. This is somewhat surprising in view of the high incidence of focal brain damage in these patients. The development of late epilepsy is of sinister significance because there is a high percentage of persistence of occasional seizures in this instance. The pathogenesis of posttraumatic epilepsy is still largely unknown. Foerster and Penfield (1930) and Penfield and Jasper (1954) emphasized the role of the meningocerebral circatrix and of focal ischemic factors. Involvement of neurons in the region of the epileptic focus is shown by a characteristic focal EEG disturbance, with focal spiking and potential shifts. The persistence and recurrence of slow wave foci in the EEG are found to be associated with the risk of traumatic epilepsy (Creutzfeldt 1969, Scherzer and Wessely 1978). Experimental models of epilepsy, such as the penicillin focus or the alumina-creme focus, may be used as a study of the epileptogenic effects of focal cerebral lesions. These experiments have shown that neurons in the affected region are not only electrically, but also structurally, abnormal with changes in the dendritic spine density (Ward 1969). The hyperexcitability of these cells has been documented (Echlin 1959). As mentioned previously, changes in glial cells may result in changes in potassium ion concentration, with epileptogenic consequences.

Abnormal neurotransmitter concentrations, such as acetylcholine and GABA are observed in epileptogenic areas (Tower 1969), and these may be associated with changes in neuronal excitability.

Willmore et al (1978) have suggested that head injury with contusion or cortical laceration causes extravasation of blood and deposition of hemoglobin within the neuropil; and the development of posttraumatic epilepsy may be related to red blood cell and hemoglobin breakdown with hemosiderin deposition. They suggest that the ions stimulate peroxidation of lipids of microsomes and mitochondria and that peroxidative injury may be critical in the development of seizure discharge (Rubin and Willmore 1980).

The significance of genetic predisposition in the development of traumatic epilepsy is not at all clear, but it is felt by some (Caveness et al 1979, Anderman 1972) that an individual's seizure susceptibility may be an interacting factor with multiple environmental factors in the development of seizures in any one individual.

A specific form of traumatic epilepsy in children relates to seizures in response to the placement of ventricular shunts. Seizures resulting after the placement of ventricular shunts for the patient's hydrocephalia are nearly always simple partial seizures (Ines and Markand 1977). These seizures have to be differentiated from intermittent obstruction attacks due to shunt malfunction. They occur usually several months to years after the introduction of the shunt, and frequent shunt revisions increase the tendency to such seizures.

BIBLIOGRAPHY

Aicardi J, Amsili J, Chevrie JJ: Acute hemiplegia of infancy and childhood. *Dev Med Child Neurol* 1969;11:162–173.

Alexander GL: Sturge-Weber syndrome, in Vinken PJ, Bruyn GW (eds): *Handbook of Clinical Neurology.* Amsterdam, North-Holland Publishing Co, 1972, vol 14.

Andermann ED: Focal epilepsy and related disorders: Genetic, metabolic and prognostic studies, thesis. McGill University, Montreal, 1972.

Beaussart M: Benign epilepsy of children with rolandic (centro-temporal) paroxysmal foci: A clinical entity. Study of 221 cases. *Epilepsia* 1972;13:793–796.

Beaussart M, Faou R: Evolution of epilepsy with rolandic paroxysmal foci: A study of 324 cases. *Epilepsia* 1978;19:337–342.

Blom S, Heijbel J, Bergfass IG: Benign epilepsy of children with centrotemporal electrographic foci. *Epilepsia* 1972;13:609–619.

Cannon WB: A law of denervation. *Am J Med Sci* 1929;198:737–750.

Caveness WF: Epilepsy: A product of trauma in our time. *Epilepsia* 1976;17:207–215.

Caveness WF, Meirowsky AM, Rish BL, et al: The nature of post-traumatic epilepsy. *J Neurosurg* 1979;50:545–553.

Caveness WF, Walker AR, Ascroft PB: Incidence of post-traumatic epilepsy in Korean War veterans as compared with those from World War I and World War II. *J Neurosurg* 1962;19:122–129.

Charcot JM: Discussion. *Gaz Méd Paris* 1876;5:588.

Courjon JA: A longitudinal electro-clinical study of 89 cases of post-traumatic epilepsy observed from the time of the original trauma. *Epilepsia* 1970;2:29–36.

Creutzfeldt OD: Neuronal mechanisms underlying the EEG, in Jasper HH, Ward AA, Pope A (eds): *Basic Mechanisms of the Epilepsies.* Boston, Little Brown & Co, 1969, pp 397–410.

Daly DD, Mulder DW: Gelastic epilepsy. *Neurology* 1971;7:189–192.

Dichter MA, Herman CJ, Selzer M: Silent cells during interictal discharges and seizures in hippocampus penicillin foci. *Brain Res* 1972;48:173–183.

Driefuss FE: Proposal for a revised classification of epileptic seizures. *Epilepsia* 1981;22: 489–501.

Dreifuss FE: Bone changes in hemiplegia of early onset. *Br J Radiol* 1956;29:601–604.

Dyke CG, Davidoff LM, Mason CB: Cerebral hemiatrophy with homolateral hypertrophy of skull and sinuses. *Surg Gynecol Obstet* 1933;58:588.

Echlin FA: The supersensitivity of chronically isolated cerebral cortex as a mechanism of focal epilepsy. *Electroencephalogr Clin Neurophysiol* 1959;11:697–772.

Efron R: Post-epileptic paralysis: Theoretical critique and report of a case. *Brain* 1961;84: 381–394.

Eisner V, Pauli LL, Livingstone S: Hereditary aspects of epilepsy. *Bull Johns Hopkins Hosp* 1959;105:245–271.

Ferrendelli JA, Gross RA, Kinscherf DA, et al: Effects of seizures and anticonvulsant drugs on cyclic nucleotide regulation in the central nervous system, in Palmer GC (ed): *Neuropharmacology of Cyclic Nucleotides.* Baltimore, Urban and Schwarzenberg, 1979, pp 211–227.

Ferrier D: Experimental researches in cerebral physiology and pathology. *West Riding Lunatic Asylum Medical Reports* 1873;3:30–96.

Fisher RS, Pedley TA, Moody WJ Jr, et al: The role of extracellular potassium in hippocampal epilepsy. *Arch Espurol* 1976;33:76–83.

Foerster O, Penfield W: The structural basis of traumatic epilepsy and results of radical operation. *Brain* 1930;53:99.

Freud S: *Die infantile Cerebrallahmungen.* Vienna, Holder, 1897.

Fritsch G, Hitzig EL: Uber elektrische Erregbarkeit des Grosshirns. *Arch Anat Physiol* 1870; 37:310–320.

Gastaut H, Broughton R: *Epileptic seizures: Clinical and Electrographic Features, Diagnosis and Treatment.* Springfield, IL, Charles C Thomas Publisher, 1972, pp 123–124.

Gastaut H, Broughton R, Tassinari CA, et al: Unilateral epileptic seizures, in Vinken PJ, Bruyn GW (eds): *Handbook of Clinical Neurology.* Amsterdam, North-Holland Publishing Co, 1974, pp 235–245.

Gastaut H, Poirier F, Salamon G, et al: H.H.E. syndrome. *Epilepsia* 1959/60;1:418–447.

Goddard GV, McIntyre DC, Leech CK: A permanent change in brain function resulting from daily electrical stimulation. *Exp Neurol* 1969;25:295–330.

Gold AP, Carter S: Acute hemiplegia of infancy and childhood. *Pediatr Clin North Am* 1976; 23:413–433.

Goldstein R, Landau WM, Kleffner FR: Neurological observations in a population of deaf and aphasic children. *Ann Otol Rhinol Laryngol* 1960;69:756–764.

Greengard P: Cyclic Nucleotides, Phosphorylated Proteins and Neuronal Function. New York, Raven Press, 1968.

Hosking GP: Fits in hydrocephalic children. *Arch Dis Child* 1974;49:633–635.

Ines DF, Markand OM: Epileptic seizures and abnormal electroencephalographic findings in hydrocephalus and their relation to shunting procedures. *Electroencephalogr Clin Neurophysiol* 1977;42:761–768.

Ingrams TSS: Specific developmental disorders of speech in childhood. *Brain* 1959;82: 450–467.

Jackson JH: On convulsive seizures, in Taylor J (ed): *Selected Writings of John Hughlings Jackson.* London, Holder & Staughton, 1931, vol 1, pp 412–457.

Janz D: *Die Epilepsien.* Stuttgart, W. Thieme, Georg Thieme Verlag, 1969.

Jennett B: *Epilepsy after Non-Missile Head Injuries,* ed 2. London, William Heinemann Medical Books, 1975.

Kogeorgos J, Scott DF, Swash M: Epileptic dizziness. *Br Med J* 1981;1:687–689.

Llinas R, Hess R: Tetrodotoxin resistant dendritic spikes in avian Purkinje cells. *Proc Natl Acad Sci USA* 1976;73:2520–2523.

Loiseau P, Cohadon F, Cohadon S: Gelastic epilepsy: A review and report of 5 cases. *Epilepsia* 1971;12:313–323.

Lombroso CT: Sylvian seizures and midtemporal spike foci in children. *Arch Neurol* 1967; 17:52–59.

Mangniere F, Courjon J: Somatosensory epilepsy: A review of 127 cases. *Brain* 1978;101: 307–332.

McNamara JO, Byrne MC, Dasheiff RM, et al: The kindling model of epilepsy: A review. *Prog Neurobiol* 1980;15:139–159.

Morrell F: Secondary epileptogenic lesions. *Epilepsia* 1959/60;1:538.

Morrell F: Human secondary epileptogenic lesions. *Neurology* 1979;29:558.

Nayrac P, Beaussart M: Les pointes-ondes prerolandiques: Expression EEG tres particuliere. Etude electroclinique de 21 cas. *Rev Neurol (Paris)* 1958;99:201–206.

Penfield W, Jasper H: *Epilepsy and the Functional Anatomy of the Human Brain.* Boston, Little Brown & Co, 1954.

Pollen DA, Trachtenberg MJ: Neuroglia: Gliosis and focal epilepsy. *Science* 1970;167:1252.

Prince DA: Neurophysiology of epilepsy. *Annu Rev Neurosci* 1978;1:392–416.

Rubin JJ, Willmore LJ: Prevention of iron-induced epileptiform discharges in rates by treatment with antiperoxidants. *Exp Neurol* 1980;67:472–480.

Sato S, Dreifuss FE: Electroencephalographic findings in a patient with developmental expressive aphasia. *Neurology* 1973;23:181–185.

Scherzer E, Wessely P: EEG in post-traumatic epilepsy. *Eur Neurol* 1978;17:38–42.

Schwartzkroin PA, Prince DA: Microphysiology of human cerebral cortex studied in vitro. *Brain Res* 1976;155:497–200.

Schwartzkroin PA, Prince DA: Penicillin-induced epileptiform activity in the hippocampal in vitro preparation. *Ann Neurol* 1977;1:463–469.

Shu S: Polyphasic spike or spike and wave complex occurring in the rolandic region in children. *J Nagoya Med Assoc* 1975;97:141–146.

Solomon GE, Hilal SK, Gold AP: Natural history of acute hemiplegia of childhood. *Brain* 1970;92:102–120.

Solomon G: Diencephalic autonomic epilepsy caused by a neoplasm. *J Pediatr* 1977;83: 277–280.

Susuki J, Takatu A: Cerebrovascular moya-moya disease: A disease showing abnormal net-like vessels in base of brain. *Arch Neurol* 1979;20:288–289.

Sypert GW, Ward AA Jr: Unidentified neuroglia potentials during propagated seizures in endocortex. *Exp Neurol* 1971;33:239–255.

Tower D: Neurochemical mechanisms, in Jasper HH, Ward AA, Pope A (eds): *Basic Mechanisms of the Epilepsies.* Boston, Little Brown & Co, 1969.

Valdes F, Dashieff RM, Birmingham F, et al: Benzodiazepine receptor increase following repeated seizures. *Proc Natl Acad Sci USA* 1982;79:193–197.

Victor D, Gascon G, Goodglass H: The syndrome of acquired aphasia, EEG abnormality without convulsive seizures in children. *Arch Neurol* 1972; :   – .

Wada JA, Osawa T, Mizoguchi T: Recurrent, spontaneous seizure state induced by prefrontal kindling in Senegalese baboons, Papio papio. *Can J Neurol Sci* 1975;21:477–492.

Ward AA Jr: The epileptic neurone: Chronic foci in animals and man, in Jasper HH, Ward AA, Pope A (eds): *Basic Mechanisms of the Epilepsies.* Boston, Little Brown & Co, 1969, pp 263–288.

Willmore LJ, Sypert GW, Munson JB: Recurrent seizures induced by cortical iron injection: A model of post-traumatic epilepsy. *Ann Neurol* 1978;4:329–336.

CHAPTER **10**

Partial Seizures: Complex Partial Seizures

Fritz E. Dreifuss

This type of seizure has been known as petit mal intellectuel (Falret 1860, 1861), automatismes ambulatoires (Charcot 1877-1889), dreamy state (Jackson 1931), psychomotorische Äquivalente, or psychomotor epilepsy (Gibbs et al 1937). Jackson introduced the concept of the "dreamy state"—a condition in which consciousness was altered and in which there was frequently a type of "mental diplopia" with a curious feeling of unreality on the one hand and a heightened awareness of an illusory or hallucinatory experience on the other. The elaborate hallucinations of complex partial seizures are frequently associated with crude experiences such as smell or taste disturbances, unlike any previously experienced.

The cardinal point that separates complex partial seizures from simple partial seizures is the impairment, distortion, or loss of the conscious state. The presence of so-called psychical phenomena is not sufficient to impart to the seizure the concept of complexity but represents the result of the epileptic discharge in a region where a discharge evokes an elaborate sensory aura in the same manner as a similar discharge in a parietal lobe would excite sensory hallucination, in the occipital lobe a visual hallucination, and in the frontal lobe an abnormal movement. When the limbic structures subserving memory, consciousness, emotion, and visceral symptomatology are affected, a different order of sensation is experienced. A dreamy state supervenes and may be associated with a visceral sensation, autonomic manifestations, affective disturbance, and, frequently, automatic behavior.

Illusory seizures may cause visual, auditory, labyrinthine, or mnestic illusions that are misinterpretations of real experiences, unlike the experiences without a stimulus associated with hallucinations. Thus, there may be disturbances in distance and size, in loudness of noise, in spatial position, in the time sense as in déjà vu phenomenon; and there may be illusions of unreality as if the person were outside of himself regarding himself at a distance, as if he were in an audience looking at himself on a stage. Similar phenomena were described under the heading of simple partial seizures; however, in the case of complex partial seizures, an alteration of the conscious state occurs either near the onset or somewhere during the course of the seizure. At any time, consciousness may be completely lost and the seizure may spread to involve motor function and may even become secondarily generalized.

As in the case of simple partial seizures, hallucinatory phenomena may occur. These may be visual, auditory, vertiginous, olfactory, gustatory, and somatosensory, or they may affect several systems. The elaborateness of hallucinations will depend on the association areas involved, as was described for simple partial seizures. Visual hallucinations frequently include animals or parts of animals, occa-

146

sionally people, sometimes "little people." One of my patients saw little people coming in through the ward window. Some of them climbed over her bed and ended up in the middle of the ward lighting a fire. This child had a right temporal lobe vascular malformation with a small subarachnoid hemorrhage. In more elaborate hallucinations, such as panoramic scenes, the content may to some extent be predicated on a person's previous experiences and cultural milieu, which no doubt accounts for many of the religious visions that have been described. Similarly, auditory hallucinations involving music nearly always involve previously experienced music and not new tunes. It is as if the bureau drawer of memories had been spilled and some of these had landed face up. In the attacks described by Jackson as "uncinate fits" (for which he implies the involvement of a specific anatomical locus because he found lesions there), the experiences of smell and taste are frequently unfamiliar though they are described in familiar terms such as "peaches," "lemons," "resin," and (frequently) cooking odors, particularly garlic. Some people experience what Daly (1975) described as multimodal hallucinations. I have treated a child who suffered from postencephalitic complex partial seizures. During these seizures she always saw herself in a semidarkened room, which would then be pervaded by sickly sweet smell, which in turn heralded the arrival of a lady dressed in red. The lady was an extremely frightening apparition whose face the child was never able to discern and who never spoke. A pervading sense of dread was associated with a slowing of the passage of time, and observers described staring, pupil dilatation, flushing, sweating, and unresponsiveness lasting for approximately 2 minutes.

The affective symptoms are frequently fear, extreme loneliness (Penfield and Jasper 1954), and occasionally depression or sadness, anger, joy, and even sexual excitement. Ecstasy was reported by Dostoievsky (Gastaut 1978). The most frequently experienced symptom is fear. Unlike the child with the "lady in red" hallucination, the fear is often not in relation to anything specific but is an all-pervading sensation of dread. Some children will run during such a seizure and may end up a long way from where they started without knowing how they got there, completely spent. Such a phenomenon is then regarded as a "cursive seizure." Sometimes the sensation of fear is afterward forgotten and only the running element of the fit remains for the telling.

Anger is a rare epileptic symptom in a child and is more commonly experienced as a postictal symptom when someone tries to restrain the patient during the postictal confused state. On the other hand, some patients do experience the phenotypic changes of anger, including piloerection, pallor, or flushing; they will frequently knock objects to the floor, though the facial expression is frequently one of fear. Many instances of reported anger may be the result of a reaction to a sensation of fear, though this can only be surmised in the majority of patients, as they are unable to verbalize this.

Visceral sensations, including epigastric discomfort, borborygmi, tachycardia, pupil dilatation, and skin color changes are quite commonly observed in children.

PSYCHOMOTOR AUTOMATISMS

Automatisms in the course of seizures have been described for over three centuries (Temkin 1971). Jackson introduced the term to describe mental disorders after paroxysms, although he did not exclude the possibility of automatisms occurring during seizures. Thus, he allowed that "it sometimes replaces a fit" and stated "I think it probable that there is a transitory epileptic paroxysm in every case of mental automatism occurring in epileptics before their mental automatism sets in." He felt that these resulted from overaction of lower nervous centers because the highest or controlling centers "have been thus put out of use." This was in keeping with his hypothesis of dissolution of the nervous system from the most voluntary to the most automatic levels of functioning; he postulated that the "epileptic discharge removes control by temporarily paralyzing the highest centers." He recognized that "if a slight fit occurs while the patient is already employed in something which is largely automatic as, for example, playing a well-practiced tune, he may well go on doing that automatic thing, may continue playing correctly while unconscious."

Automatisms have been described (Gastaut 1973) as

> more or less coordinated and adapted involuntary motor activity occurring during a state of clouding of the consciousness, either in the course of, or after, an epileptic seizure, and usually followed by amnesia for the event. The automatism may be simply a continuation of an activity going on when the seizure occurred or, conversely, a new activity that developed in association with the ictal impairment of consciousness. Usually, the activity is common-place in nature, often provoked by the subject's environment or by his sensations during the seizure.

A distinction has been made between "forced automatisms" (such as mastication or swallowing, which are thought to be due to the epileptic discharge itself) and "reactive motor activities" (which are thought to be the result of unrecalled psycho-sensory manifestations) (Ajmone Marsan and Ralston 1957, Paillas 1958). The following types of automatisms have been distinguished:

1. *Oroalimentary automatisms.* Includes chewing, lip and tongue smacking, and swallowing.
2. *Automatisms of mimicry.* Includes fear, anxiety, anger, joy. As previously mentioned, expression of anxiety or fear are particularly common. Such expression is sometimes accompanied by cursive behavior and occasionally by a fearful utterance.
3. *Gestural automatisms.* Includes clapping, scratching, and stereotyped hand movements or more elaborate quasi-purposeful activities including cleaning, polishing, or playing music.
4. *Ambulatory automatisms.* Includes walking, driving, or riding a bicycle (and apparently the ability to avoid obstacles). This behavior may seem to be goal-directed or may be completely disorganized. The patient may find himself far from the intended goal of the itinerary.
5. *Verbal automatisms.* These may be in response to sensations experienced during the height of the seizure and at other times are stereotyped repetitive utterances. Speech automatisms may be the result of discharges in the nondominant temporal lobe (Serafetinides and Falconer 1969).

Penry and Dreifuss (1969) have studied the nature of automatisms that occur in association with absence seizures. They recognized two principal types:

1. *Perseverative automatisms,* which are a continuation of activity engaged in prior to the onset of the seizure following transient interruption.

2. *An automatism that began de novo during the course of the seizure* and that could be regarded as "reactive" to external or internal environmental stimuli and as "released," ie, actions are carried out that would be normally eschewed, eg, scratching, undressing, and indecorous exhibition. In psychomotor automatisms, postictal disorientation is a prominent feature of the attack.

Automatisms have some localizational significance. Penfield (1954) produced automatisms by stimulation of the gray matter of the medial temporal lobe adjacent to the insula, but Penfield and Jasper (1954) early pointed out that automatic behavior and amnesia could be produced from the frontal lobe and that automatisms could occur during discharges involving the centrencephalic system. Fornix stimulation, stimulation of the circuminsular temporal cortex, the amygdaloid nucleus, the hippocampal gyrus, and the periamygdaloid region and temporal insular cortex deep in the anterior part of the Sylvian fissure have all resulted in automatisms.

Postictal amnesia usually follows automatisms. Sometimes automatisms are not recognized as such; the amnesia is then the cardinal sign of the seizure. Thus, one of my patients was sent for popcorn and a soda during the intermission in a movie. He took the money, bought the refreshments, threw them untouched into the trash can, and returned to the movie, completely unaware of the fact that he had left it.

There is great variation in the natural history of complex partial seizures. In the case of static lesions, the symptomatology remains fairly stereotyped; however, the seizures frequency may vary, and in the course of time may gradually increase. Clustering of seizures is frequent; clusters may be related to hormonal changes, to emotional, precipitating factors, sometimes to the exertion of playground activities, and occasionally to the stress of examinmations, family disputes, and grief.

Occasionally, complex partial seizures may occur in status epilepticus form. This may occur as a "continuous aura" (Scott and Masland 1953) or an episodic dreamy state (Dreyer 1965). This is one of the causes of a prolonged confusional state, which may have manifestations rather similar to those of absence status and which may last for minutes, hours, or even days. During psychomotor status, the patient appears as if in a daze, is slow to register and to respond, is frequently unable to communicate with speech, and may appear restless and disoriented. Occasionally, psychomotor status is discontinuous, with short periods of relatively good orientation. Thus, complex partial seizure or psychomotor status enters into the differential diagnosis of so-called epileptic fugue states and resembles the so-called spike-wave stupor. Diagnosis has to be made electroencephalographically during an attack. In patients with complex partial seizures, acute confusional or psychotic states are more frequently related to conditions other than status epilepticus.

Another condition that is a relatively rare manifestation of complex partial seizures is a seizure with impairment of consciousness only, which may be difficult to distinguish except electroencephalographically from an absence seizure. Approximately 4% of complex partial seizures are of this type (Caffi 1973). The distinction is critical for the institution of appropriate pharmacologic management. On clinical grounds, the most important distinguishing feature from absence is the frequent presence of postictal confusion following the complex partial seizure.

ELECTROENCEPHALOGRAPHIC MANIFESTATIONS
OF COMPLEX PARTIAL SEIZURES

The EEG findings in complex partial seizures were first described by Gibbs and co-workers (1937) and were subsequently elaborated by others. Electroencephalographic descriptions have paralleled the classification changes of the seizures, which have been variously described as psychomotor, temporal lobe, or limbic.

In the interictal period, an anterior temporal lobe spike discharge is the most frequently encountered EEG abnormality, though in a certain portion of patients similar abnormalities arise from outside the temporal lobe (Gastaut 1953, Penfield and Jasper 1954). The EEG changes may occur at a distance and of course frequently arise from areas of brain peripheral to the actual lesion. Interictal discharges are frequently bilateral, and such bilaterality may be temporally independent or relatively synchronous. Klass (1975) noted that bilateral independent temporal spikes render a brain tumor diagnosis unlikely. Occasionally, a temporal lobe EEG discharge may trigger secondary bilateral synchrony. In this case, the focal EEG discharge may precede the bilateral synchronous activity. These patients frequently also have generalized seizures (Gabor and Ajmone Marsan 1969).

Apart from the spike discharge, slow-wave foci may be recorded from a temporal lobe in the interictal period. This is frequently the consequence of lesions in the posterior temporal region and may represent a deeply situated lesion or may represent a destructive or progressive lesion.

The interictal EEG is frequently normal at any one time. If activating techniques such as sleep deprivation and nasopharyngeal or sphenoidal electrodes are used in addition, a much smaller portion of patients with complex partial seizures will have normal interictal recordings.

Ictal activity may take the form of an increase in the number of spikes or of low-voltage fact activity (Jasper 1951). A third method of representation is that of sinusoidal rhythms (Klass et al 1973). Most complex partial seizures are followed by postictal changes of focal or generalized, 2- to 3-Hz slow-wave activity. Of course, if a complex partial seizure becomes secondarily generalized, both ictal and postictal EEG abnormalities will be those of generalized seizures, although the slow-wave activity may predominate on the side of the origin of the seizure. This observation may be helpful in localization. Postictal activity may be absent (Ajmone Marsan and Ralston 1957, Klass et al 1973).

Ictal recordings are extremely important for accurate localization of the seizure focus. The interictal and the ictal EEG foci may not coincide and may even occur on different sides. Ictal recordings, furthermore, help to distinguish between complex partial seizures and phenotypically similar pseudoseizures.

Activation techniques include hyperventilation, which may be successful in evoking a complex partial seizure. However, the success rate of this technique is not nearly as high as it is for absence seizures. Sleep is a potent activator of epileptiform discharge in the interictal period in patients with complex partial seizures. This is true of spontaneous sleep and of sleep induced by prolonged sleep deprivation. Sleep deprivation is a particularly potent activator of seizure discharge in this epileptic syndrome (Pratt et al 1968). Pentylenetetrazol or barbiturates such as methohexital administered intravenously may be used as pharmacologic activating agents but are not used frequently now.

ETIOLOGY OF COMPLEX PARTIAL SEIZURES

Complex partial seizures are not seen as heritable syndromes as frequently as are age-related attacks such as absence seizures. However, they are apparently more frequently familial than are simple partial seizures, perhaps because etiologically they may be consequentially related to a familial seizure form such as febrile convulsions. Complex partial seizures are caused by the same factors that cause other partial seizures, eg, prenatal, natal, and postnatal causes, trauma, tumors, and inflammatory diseases. Complex partial seizures, however, are frequently preceded by febrile seizures (Falconer et al 1964) although complex partial seizures are not a common consequence of febrile seizures (Nelson and Ellenberg 1981). The early onset of the causative factors is attested to by the frequent radiological finding of hemispheric asymmetries, with focal atrophy and ventricular dilatation. Early childhood status epilepticus may feature in the history.

The temporal lobes are quite susceptible to anatomical damage in closed head injuries of the acceleration or deceleration type, and head trauma is an antecedent to many complex partial seizures. Any event that rapidly raises intracranial pressure and causes compromise in the distribution of the posterior cerebral artery circulation may also be followed by the development of complex partial seizures as a result of compromise of the integrity of the posterior portion of the temporal lobes unilaterally or bilaterally. When tumors are responsible for complex partial seizures in children, radiological appearances of the skull include thinning and bulging on the side of the tumor, findings that indicate its long-standing presence. The presence of olfctory or gustatory hallucinations suggests the presence of a tumor, whereas dreamy states are relatively less common in this context. Encephalitis is etiologically important (Ounsted et al 1966, Matthes 1961) and some encephalopathies, such as those caused by herpes simplex, have a predilection for a temporal lobe localization. Thrombophlebitis associated with or following mastoiditis frequently has a temporal lobe localization.

The age of onset of complex partial seizures in children is sometimes related to the cause, occurring earlier in those children whose epilepsy follows febrile seizures or status epilepticus (Ounsted et al 1966).

INTERICTAL MANIFESTATIONS OF COMPLEX PARTIAL SEIZURES

The theme of interictal disturbances in complex partial seizures pervades much of the complex partial seizure literature written in the past 50 years. Most of the attention has been focused on behavior changes in persons with complex partial seizures and on the prevalence of psychosis, which occurs more commonly in persons with complex partial seizures (some authors have postulated a cause and effect relationship between the two). These topics represent major sources of controversy in the literature on complex partial seizures and present outstanding challenges for objective prospective research endeavors.

Personality development and coping style are predicated on various factors including age of onset of epilepsy, side and site of the causative lesion, inherent personality characteristics, presence or absence of other seizure types, presence or absence of other signs of major neurologic dysfunction, and effects produced by medication and by the psychosocial consequences to which the person with epilepsy is subjected.

A major problem with previous studies is the lack of a clear distinction between associations and consequences and an invocation of cause and effect relationships. Complex partial seizures have come in for particular scrutiny in this regard as they are the final common path for other forms of epilepsy. Gibbs and co-workers (1938) recognized various neurotic and psychotic symptoms associated with complex partial seizures, but even in 1938 they recognized that the nature of these disturbances varied as to whether the person was suffering from only one type of seizure or from several seizure types.

Relationship to Intelligence

It would appear that there is no direct relationship between seizure type or seizure frequency and intelligence. Thus, a child with numerous absence seizures is frequently of normal or superior intelligence; yet persons with rare seizures may be severely intellectually handicapped. Epileptics as a group tend to have somewhat lower mean IQ scores than control subjects (Collins and Lennox 1946, Dikmen and Matthews 1977, Klove and Matthews 1966). Factors that appear to relate to this include age of onset (Dikmen et al 1977) and frequency of major seizures, particularly the presence of generalized seizures in addition to partial seizures (Dikmen et al 1977, Wilkurs and Dodrill 1976, Matthews and Klove 1967). Milner (1975) suggested that disparity in subtest scores between verbal and visiospatial function was related to the site of the seizure focus, ie, in the left or the right hemisphere; this has been amply substantiated.

Memory Function

The limbic system and the temporal lobe cortex are important mediators of memory, including recording and retrieval functions. Persons with complex partial seizures frequently complain of difficulty with memory. Milner (1975) recognizes a difference between loss of verbal and loss of nonverbal memory function, a difference depending on whether the focus is in the left or right temporal lobe. This is a rather complex subject because of the potential effects of medication and the relationship of memory to other modalities. Memory recording might be interfered with by distractability and short attention span, which are common manifestations of children with cerebral hemispheric disorders. Or memory dysfunction may be more highly correlated with structural neurologic dysfunction than with the location of the seizure focus. Thus, Rutter and co-workers (1970) found that such characteristics were particularly frequent in children with supratentorial cerebral lesions. Specific difficulties with memory are not nearly as frequently encountered in children with complex partial seizures as in adults (Matthes 1961).

Changes in Mood and Affect

Episodic disturbances in mood may last for hours or days. These disturbances usually consist of depression; more rarely, excitation. Rage attacks have been reported (Ounsted 1969), and suicide is considerably more frequent in the epileptic population than in the general population. MacIntyre and co-workers (1976) found that patients with left hemisphere discharges were considerably more reflective or ruminative, whereas those whose discharges were lateralized to the right side were given to impulsivity. Ounsted found that children who had a tendency to rage had seizures of early onset and an associated hyperkinetic syndrome, again evidence for structural neurologic dysfunction.

Personality Changes

Whether or not a distinctive personality characterizes persons with complex partial seizures is one of the most controversial topics in epileptology (Stevens 1975). Gastaut described irritability, aggressiveness, and relative lack of inhibition in the behavior of persons with complex partial seizures. Glaser (1964) described delusional behavior with paranoid and depressive reactions and excessive religiosity. Falconer (1973) added aggression as a component of the personality of persons with complex partial seizures. Bear (1977) and Fedio (Bear and Fedio 1977) described specific aspects of behavior, including irritability, hostility, loss of libido, self-recrimination, hypermoralism, circumstantiality, and a certain viscosity, hypergraphia, and religiosity. Control studies are lacking, and each one of these factors may occur in patients with chronic diseases other than epilepsy. In the series of Dewhurst and Beard (1970), religious conversions were seen in patients who had generalized seizures more often than in those who had only complex partial seizures. Bear and Fedio (1977) suggested that in terms of behavioral profiles, those with right temporal lobe disturbances were seen as more externally emotive, whereas persons with left temporal foci developed an internal, ideational pattern of behavior, such as religiosity, philosophical interest, and hypergraphia. Tizard (1962) suggested that the sociopsychological background of a patient was more impressive in the cause of the psychopathology than the site of the lesion. It is likely that an evaluation of persons from a general outpatient clinic would yield somewhat different results than the evaluation of persons seen in psychiatric hospitals and psychiatric clinics. The bulk of the reported series, including that of Ounsted et al (1966), are based on evaluation of persons in psychiatric hospitals and clinics, who are mainly children.

Considerable work remains to be done in this area. There has been too little research on personality development prior to the onset of seizures and on the reaction of the child to its own seizures. There has been little study of those patients who do not exhibit changes in their personality despite seizures that are identical with those in persons who do exhibit such alleged changes. Persons with cerebral lesions without seizures may, on the other hand, have characteristics similar to those described in patients with complex partial seizures. The most absurd extrapolation occurs when a diagnosis of complex partial seizures is affixed to a person who had the alleged personality characteristics and who has never experienced a seizure. This has major medical–legal implications (Delgado-Escueta et al 1981, Pincus 1980).

Psychotic Manifestations in Complex Partial Seizures

The occurrence of schizophreniform psychoses in complex partial seizures is well recognized (Bruens 1974, Flor-Henry 1969, Scott 1978, Slater et al 1963, Taylor 1977, Blumer 1975). This association occurs more frequently in adults than in children. It is rarely associated with epilepsy caused by mesial temporal sclerosis and is more frequently seen in temporal lobe lesions caused by "alien tissue." Schizophreniform psychoses may begin assiduously with apathy, depersonalization, and lassitude with illusions and auditory hallucinations in patients with long-standing seizures. Landolt (1958) described "alternative psychoses with forced normalization" in which there appears to be an inverse relationship between complex partial seizures and psychotic manifestations, ie, when the former are controlled, the latter become more prominent. Paranoid symptoms with ideas of reference as well as auditory hallucinations and depersonalization experiences are manifestations of the psychotic disorder. Flor-Henry (1969) suggested that schizophreniform psychoses were more common in patients with left temporal lobe abnormalities and that depressive symptoms were more common in patients with right temporal lobe abnormalities. The majority of psychotic patients have the onset of their disease around the time of puberty; there is a preponderance of females over male. The schizophrenia is relatively benign, with preservation of affect, and the patient may retain some insight.

Although it is sometimes recommended that anticonvulsant medication be reduced to allow seizures to occur (these seizures in turn can be pharmacologically ameliorated) in order to prevent a chronic psychotic condition from setting in, modern recommendations are to treat the psychosis and the epilepsy separately, each on its own merit.

The relationship between seizures and psychiatric disorders is a complex one. Stevens (1975) suggests that "epileptic seizures themselves are not often the cause of the interictal disorders when these are present but that the psychological disturbance relates to interactions between environmental causes and the neurological disorder underlying the epilepsy." One of the more important environmental factors may be the limbic neurochemical environment upon which the epilepsy–psychosis association is predicated.

PHARMACOLOGIC MANAGEMENT OF PARTIAL SEIZURES

Carbamazepine

The drugs of choice in the treatment of partial seizures include carbamazepine, phenytoin, phenobarbital, and primidone. Until recently, carbamazepine was used predominantly as adjunctive therapy, but it is evident that this drug is effective as monotherapy in most forms of partial seizures, particularly those of the complex partial variety. A blood level of 6–12 μg/mL is generally regarded as the therapeutic range. Institution of treatment with carbamazepine should be gradual, starting with 100 mg twice a day and gradually building up to a dose of 20–25 mg/kg or until the therapeutic blood level is reached. Carbamazepine half-life is approximately 14 hours. In some individuals, blood levels vary greatly throughout the day unless the drug is given in at least two divided doses. The maximum tolerated blood level is usually lower when it is given together with other anticonvulsants because of drug interactions. Carbamazepine induces its own metabolic enzymes, and the dose may have to be increased when the patient has not taken this drug for a period of time. Toxic side effects include nausea, loss of appetite, gastrointestinal complaints, drowsiness, disturbance of vision, ataxia, and impaired psychomotor function. These effects are usually dose-related and often occur during initiation of therapy. They can frequently be largely obviated by the gradual increase in dose. Allergic reactions are not common; they include skin eruptions and acute eosinophilic myocarditis. Reactions that may be either allergic or dose-related include bone marrow depression, manifested as leukopenia or aplastic anemia. Hepatotoxicity has been reported, as has the development of inappropriate levels of antidiuretic hormone, with water retention. The latter complication may be successfully treated with phenytoin.

Serious side effects are relatively infrequent with carbamazepine. In relation to central nervous system toxicity, such as impairment of cognitive function, carbamazepine is a very benign drug compared with phenytoin and phenobarbital.

Primidone

Primidone is a useful drug in the treatment of most seizure types other than absence. It has a reputation for being particularly useful in complex partial seizures, though it is doubtful whether it has any particular specificity. It is structurally and functionally similar to phenobarbital and is to a large extent metabolized to phenobarbital, though primidone itself has antiepileptic properties. The desired blood level is 5–10 $\mu g/mL$, which may be attained by the administration of approximately 20 mg/kg/day in divided doses. The half-life of primidone is quite short, and multiple daily doses are therefore recommended. After chronic use, peak blood concentrations after a single oral dose occur sometime after 3 hours. The side effects include ataxia, vertigo, nausea, and vomiting. These side effects may be to some extent dose-related and can be avoided to a large degree by starting the drug in low doses and then increasing the dosage.

Primidone is associated with a high instance of behavioral disorders in children. Unlike phenobarbital, these are not the common variety of hyperactivity but are frequently manifested as rather severe and intransigent behavioral disturbances.

Phenytoin

Phenytoin has for 40 years been the first-line drug in the treatment of most types of seizures. Phenytoin is quite slowly absorbed, and several days may be required to attain therapeutic plasma levels, which range from 10 to 20 $\mu g/mL$. The recommended dose in children is 5–8 mg/kg/day. In children the half-life is 20–24 hours; in most instances, phenytoin may be administered in a single daily dose. One advantage of phenytoin is that it can be given intravenously and may therefore be the drug of choice following the treatment of status epilepticus. Because the drug is quite well tolerated, treatments often commence with a loading dose of 15 mg/kg, followed by the usual daily maintenance dose.

Toxicity from the drug includes acute overdose effect of ataxia, nausea, vomiting, and vertigo. Increased seizure frequency has been reported as a result of phenytoin toxicity, and cerebellar symptoms may persist for some time after the dose has been reduced. On long-term administration, cosmetic side effects (including hirsutism, gum overgrowth, thickening and coarsening of facial features) may prove extremely burdensome. Other long-term side effects include some affliction of nearly every organ system, including folic acid metabolism, vitamin D metabolism, adrenal metabolism, interference with the immune system, progressive encephalopathy, peripheral neuropathy, as well as teratogenic effects.

Phenobarbital

Phenobarbital continues to be a useful and relatively safe drug in the treatment of partial and generalized tonic-clonic seizures, though the effects on childhood behavior and potential learning problems make it a less desirable drug than primidone or phenytoin for first-line use in partial seizures.

The usual dose is 5-7 mg/kg, with an expected blood level of 15-30 μg/mL.

Valproate and Clorazepate

Valproate has been recommended in the treatment of complex partial seizures and has been said to reduce attacks by as much as 60% (compared with placebo) in various studies. Clorazepate (Tranxene) is a useful adjunct in the treatment of complex partial seizures in a dose of 3.75-7.5 mg two or three times a day. It is usually employed as an adjunctive agent; in my experience, a combination of carbamazepine and clorazepate is quite effective in most patients with partial seizures, particularly those with complex partial seizures.

BIBLIOGRAPHY

Ajmone Marsan C, Ralston BL: *The Epileptic Seizure.* Springfield, IL, Charles C Thomas Publisher, 1957.

Bear DM: The significance of behavioral change in temporal lobe epilepsy, in Blumer D, Levin K (eds): *The Psychiatric Complications of the Epilepsies: Current Research and Treatment.* Belmont, MA, McLean Hospital Journal, June, 1977, pp 9-21.

Bear DM, Fedio P: Quantitative analysis of interictal behavior in temporal lobe epilepsy. *Arch Neurol* 1977;34:454-467.

Blumer D: Temporal lobe epilepsy and its psychiatric significance, in Benson DF, Blume D (eds): *Psychiatric Aspects of Neurological Disease.* New York, Grune & Stratton Inc, 1975.

Bruens JH: Psychosis in epilepsy, in Vinken PJ, Bruyn GW (eds): *Handbook of Clinical Neurology.* Amsterdam, North-Holland Publishing Co, 1974, pp 593-610.

Caffi J: Zur Frage klinischer Anfallsformen bei psychomotorischer Epilepsie. *Schweiz Med Wochenschr* 1973;103:469-475.

Charcot JM: *Lectures on Diseases of the Nervous System,* Sigerson G. (trans). London, New Sydenham Society, 1877-1889.

Collins AL, Lennox WG: The intelligence of 390 private epileptic patients. *Res Publ Assoc Res Nerv Ment Dis* 1946;26:586-603.

Daly DD: Ictal clinical manifestations, in Penry JK, Daly DD (eds): *Advances in Neurology.* New York, Raven Press, 1975, vol 2, pp 57-83.

Delgado-Escueta AV, Mattson RH, King L, et al: The nature of aggression during epileptic seizure. *N Engl J Med* 1981;12:711-716.

Dewhurst K, Beard AW: Sudden religious conversions in temporal lobe epilepsy. *Br J Psychiatry* 1970;117:497-507.

Dikmen S, Matthews CG: The effects of major motor seizure frequency upon cognitive-intellectual functions in adults. *Epilepsia* 1977;18:21-29.

Dikmen S, Matthews CG, Harley JP: Effect of early versus late onset of major epilepsy on cognitive-intellectual performance: Further considerations. *Epilepsia* 1977;18:31-36.

Dreyer R: Zur Frage des Status epilepticus mit psychomotorischen Anfallen. Ein Bertrag zum temporalen Status epilepticus und zu atypischen Dammerzustanden und Verstimmungen. *Nervenarzt* 1965;36:221,1.

Falconer MA: Reversibility by temporal lobe resection of the behavioural abnormalities of temporal lobe epilepsy. *N Engl J Med* 1973;289:451-455.

Falconer MA, Serafetinides MA, Corsellis JAN: Etiology and athogenesis of temporal lobe epilepsy. *Arch Neurol* 1964;10:233-248.

Falret J: De l'etat mental des epileptiques. *Arch Gen Med* 1860, 1861;16:669-679, 17:461-491, 18:423-443.

Flor-Henry P: Psychosis and temporal lobe epilepsy. *Epilepsia* 1969;10:363-395.

Gabor AJ, Ajmone Marsan C: Coexistence of focal and bilateral diffuse paroxysmal discharges in epileptics: Clinical-electrographic study. *Epilepsia* 1969;10:453–472.

Gastaut H: *Dictionary of Epilepsy: Part 1: Definitions.* Geneva, World Health Organization, 1973.

Gastaut H: So-called "psychomotor" and "temporal lobe" epilepsy—A critical study. *Epilepsia* 1953;2:59–76.

Gastaut H: Fyodor Dostoievsky's involuntary contribution to the symptomatology and prognosis of epilepsy. *Epilepsia* 1978;19:186–201.

Gibbs FA, Gibbs EL, Lennox WG: Epilepsy. A paroxysmal cerebral dysrhythmia. *Brain* 1937; 60:377–388.

Gibbs FA, Gibbs EL, Lennox WG: The likeness of the cortical dysrhythmias of schizophrenia and psychomotor epilepsy. *Am J Psychiatry* 1938;95:255–269.

Glaser GH: The problem of psychosis in psychomotor epileptics. *Epilepsia* 1964;5:271–278.

Jackson JH: On epilepsy and epileptiform convulsions, in Taylor J (ed): *Selected Writings of J Hughlings Jackson.* London, Hodder & Stoughton, 1931, vol 1.

Jasper H, Pertuisset B, Flanigin H: EEG and cortical electrograms in patients with temporal lobe seizures. *Arch Neurol Psychiatr* 1951;65:272–290.

Klass DW, Espinosa RE, Fischer-Williams M: Analysis of concurrent electroencephalographic and clinical events occurring sequentially during partial seizures. *Electroencephalogr Clin Neurophysiol* 1973;34:728.

Klass DW: Electroencephalographic manifestations of complex partial seizures, in Penry JK, Daly DD (eds): *Advances in Neurology.* New York, Raven Press, 1975, vol 2, pp 113–140.

Klove H, Matthews CG: Psychometric and adaptive abilities in epilepsy with differential etiology. *Epilepsia* 1966;7:330–338.

Landolt H: Serial electroencephalographic investigations during psychotic episodes in epileptic patients during schizophrenic attacks. *Folia Psychiatr Neurol Neurochir Neerlandica* 1958;suppl 4:91–133.

Matthes A: Die psychomotorische Epilepsie im Kindesalter. *Z Nervenheilk* 1961;84:472.

Matthews CG, Klove H: Differential psychological performances in major motor, psychomotor and mixed seizure classifications of known and unknown etiology. *Epilepsia* 1967; 8:117–128.

McIntyre M, Pritchard PB III, Lombroso CT: Left and right temporal lobe epileptics: A controlled investigation of some psychological differences. *Epilepsia* 1976;17:377–386.

Milner B: Psychological aspects of focal epilepsy and its neurosurgical management, in Purpura DP, Penry JK (eds): *Advances in Neurology.* New York, Raven Press, 1975, vol 8, pp 299–321.

Nelson JKB, Ellenberg JH: *Febrile Seizures.* New York, Raven Press, 1981.

Ounsted C: Aggression and epilepsy: Rage in children with temporal lobe epilepsy. *J Psychosom Res* 1969;13:237–242.

Ounsted C, Lindsay J, Norman R: *Biological Factors in Temporal Lobe Epilepsy; the Spastics Society.* London, William Heinemann Medical Books, 1966.

Paillas JE: Aspects cliniques de l'épilepsie temporale: Constatations faites sur une série de 50 malades opérés, in Baldwin M, Bailey P (eds): *Temporal Lobe Epilepsy.* Springfield, IL, Charles C Thomas Publishing, 1958, pp 411–439.

Penfield W, Jasper H: *Epilepsy and the Functional Anatomy of the Human Brain.* Boston, Little Brown & Co, 1954.

Penry JK, Dreifuss FE: Automatisms associated with the absence of petit mal epilepsy. *Arch Neurol* 1969;21:142.

Pincus JH: Can violence be a manifestation of epilepsy? *Neurology* 1980;30:304–307.

Pratt KL, Mattson RH, Weikers NJ, et al: EEG activation of epileptics following sleep deprivation: A prospective study of 114 cases. *Electroencephalogr Clin Neurophysiol* 1968;24: 11–15.

Rutter M, Graham P, Yule W: A neuropsychiatric study in childhood. *Clinics in Developmental Medicine.* London, William Heinemann Medical Books, 1970.

Scott DF: Psychiatric aspects of epilepsy. *Br J Psychiatry* 1978;132:417–430.

Scott JG, Masland RL: Occurrence of continuous symptoms in epilepsy patients. *Neurology* 1953;3:297–301.

Serafetinides EA, Falconer MA: Speech disturbances in temporal lobe seizures: A study in 100 epileptic patients submitted to anterior temporal lobectomy. *Brain* 1969;86:333.

Slater E, Beard AW, Githero E: The schizophrenia-like psychosis of epilepsy. *Br J Psychiatry* 1963;109:95–150.

Stevens JR: Interictal clinical manifestations of complex partial seizures, in Penry JK, Daley DD (eds): *Advances in Neurology.* New York, Raven Press, 1975, vol 11, pp 85–112.

Taylor D: Epileptic experience, schizophrenia and the temporal lobe, in *Psychiatric Complications in the Epilepsies.* Belmont, MA, McLean Hospital Journal, June, 1977, pp 22–39.

Temkin O: *The Falling Sickness. A History of Epilepsy from the Greeks to the Beginnings of Modern Neurology,* ed 2. Baltimore, Johns Hopkins Press, 1971.

Tizard B: The personality of epileptics: A discussion of the evidence. *Psychol Bull* 1962;559: 196–210.

Wilkurs RJ, Dodrill CB: Neuropsychological correlates of the electroencephalogram in epileptics. *Epilepsia* 1976;17:89–100.

11

Neonatal Seizures

John M. Freeman

Asphyxia neonatorum . . . is very apt to be accompanied with, and to be succeeded by, convulsions at variable periods after birth. It will be borne in mind that convulsions at birth, or subsequently to it, are but a symptom of lesion of a nervous center (Little 1862).

[I am able] to look back upon a considerable number of children who had been born semi-asphyxiated, in consequences of difficulty involving resort to the forceps or turning, many of these children were healthy, and did not appear to bear any trace of the difficulties that attended their birth. . . . [I have] observed that occasionally children born with difficulty were liable to convulsions for a short time, but if they survived, they commonly did well (Barnes 1862).

Neonatal seizures are a major prognostic indicator of children who will later have both severe mental retardation and cerebral palsy (Nelson and Broman 1977). Although chronic hypoxia-asphyxia is more common in children who later have severe mental retardation and cerebral palsy, most children who have prolonged and severe asphyxia, as indicated by 10- and 15-minute Apgar scores of 3 or less, do well. However, the combination of very low 10- and 15-minute Apgar scores *and* neonatal seizures carries a poor prognosis (Nelson and Ellenberg 1981). Although most children with neonatal seizures do well, the Apgar score, the need for resuscitation after 5 minutes of age, and the duration of seizures are the early predictors of later cerebral palsy and mental retardation (Holden et al 1981, Mellits et al 1981).

The preceding studies look at outcomes of children with neonatal seizures from different points of view. However, they all suggest that neonatal seizures are a better indicator of more severe or more prolonged asphyxia than is the Apgar score and that prolonged seizures or seizures repeated on a number of days may be further evidence of the degree of cerebral damage caused by the asphyxia-ischemia. Thus, "convulsions at birth are but a symptom of lesion of a nervous center" (Little 1862), and "children born with difficulties are liable to convulsions . . . but if they survive, they commonly do well" (Barnes 1862).

Although it has been customary to discuss neonatal seizures as if they were a single entity or a series of entities, it is apparent that there are two distinct epochs within the neonatal period and, therefore, two classes of neonatal seizures: seizures that occur during the first 3 days of life and that are primarily secondary to hypoxia-ischemia, and seizures that occur after the third day and that have other etiologies and a different prognosis (Mellits et al 1981, Brown et al 1972).

INCIDENCE AND RECOGNITION

The incidence of seizures in the newborn period ranges from 0.2–1.4%. A large prospective study found that 0.5% of neonates had recognizable seizures (Mellits et al 1981).

However, the true incidence is unknown. Some studies have included stimulus-provoked seizures (Keen 1969), which we would class as "jitteriness." Most subtle seizures, which are characterized by minor eye movements, alterations of respiration, or facial grimacing, are probably missed.

Seizures in the newborn rarely take the form of generalized tonic-clonic activity but are more commonly in the form of multifocal jerks, opisthotonic posturing, intermittent apneic episodes, and focal tonic or clonic activity. On most occasions these activities are accompanied by nystagmus, by tonic deviation of the eyes, by sucking motions of the lips, or by eyelid blinking or fluttering.

Any type of bizzare or unusual transient event may be a seizure. If these events are stereotyped, if they recur periodically, or if there are combinations of unusual events, seizures should be suspected. Unlike the older child or adult, classification of seizures seems to be of little prognostic importance. With the exception of tonic seizures of the small infant, there seems to be no relationship between cause or outcome and seizure type (Mellits et al 1981). Tonic stiffening is statistically related both to later cerebral palsy and to mental retardation. However, this posturing may not be a true seizure, but rather may represent the opisthotonus associated with an intraventricular hemorrhage (Mellits et al 1981).

Seizures may be differentiated from jitteriness, which is characterized by large-amplitude, high-frequency, rhythmic movements that may be decreased or abolished by flexion of the limb. Jitteriness may also be provoked by stimuli. Seizures, on the other hand, are unprovoked, nonrhythmic, low-frequency activity and have a fast and a slow component. This differentiation is seen in Table 11-1.

ETIOLOGY

The multiple causes of seizures in the newborn are shown in Table 11-2. Although there is obvious overlap, the causative factors change with time.

Days 0-4

Seizures during the first 3 days of life are almost always due to hypoxia, ischemia, or intracranial bleeding. Hypocalcemia, hypoglycemia, and hypomagnesemia are often emphasized as treatable causes of seizures, but during the first 3 days of life they are usually secondary to perinatal stress and distress. These metabolic problems will be discussed separately; however, their contribution, if any, to an ensuing cerebral deficit is unclear. Asphyxia and ischemia produce an ongoing process, and that process may be the most important determinant of outcome.

Hypoxic-ischemic encephalopathy has two major mechanisms. Asphyxia causes more than 90% of the encephalopathy (Volpe 1977). This asphyxia is primarily due to a disturbance of gas exchange across the placenta and may be exacerbated by respiratory failure at the time of birth. Postnatal respiratory insufficiency and severe right-to-left cardiac shunts are postnatal events that cause less than 10% of the seizures. Ischemia is secondary to intrauterine asphyxia with cardiac insufficiency both in utero and at the time of birth. Postnatal events such as severe congenital

Table 11-1
Comparison of Jitteriness and Seizures

Characteristic	Jitteriness	Seizures
Movement	High frequency Large amplitude Equal rate	Low frequency Amplitude variable Fast and slow component
Stimulus sensitive	Yes	No
Response to flexion of extremity	Abolished	No effect

heart disease, recurrent apneic spells, or cardiovascular collapse secondary to sepsis are uncommon causes of ischemia.

The animal model of hypoxia-ischemia developed by Myers (1977) and Brann (1980) suggests that chronic tissue hypoxia leads to local cerebral edema. This edema further compromises local circulation, causing further ischemia, further edema, and further compromise of circulation. Thus, this is an ongoing process over hours or the first several days of life.

The Apgar score is an indicator of the degree of hypoxia in the brain and the body. However, the fact that most babies with a low Apgar score do well, even when that low Apgar score (3 or less) persists for 10 or 15 minutes, suggests that the score does not indicate the presence of permanent damage. Perhaps the Apgar score is an indication of short and recent asphyxia. However, when the low Apgar score is followed by seizures, the prognosis for mental and motor impairment is far worse (Nelson and Ellenberg 1981). Therefore, the seizures may be an indicator of a more severe or a more prolonged degree of intrauterine hypoxia-ischemia, with a higher likelihood of permanent damage. Because seizures that are prolonged (more than 30 minutes) or that are recurrent during the neonatal period are more likely to be accompanied by death or by severe neurologic damage, they probably represent even more severe or prolonged anoxia or ischemia (Holden et al 1981, Mellits et al 1981). There is some question (Gilles 1977) whether the cerebral swelling seen in Meyer's animal model and in the asphyxiated newborn represents edema with increased water content in the brain or whether it represents swelling due to necrosis of cells. This argument is as yet unsettled. Nevertheless, seizures in the child with a low Apgar are the best early indicator of a potential for later damage.

Hypoglycemia during the first 4 days of life is most commonly found in children who have had a traumatic birth or who are stressed by hypoxic-ischemic injury (Hopkins 1972). Although the role of the hypoglycemia in the genesis of seizures in these infants is undetermined, there is growing evidence that hypoglycemia may add additional insult to that already present and that maintenance of a normal, or perhaps even above-normal blood sugar concentration could, at least theoretically, be beneficial. Hypocalcemia, with or without hypomagnesemia, in the first few days of life is also a reflection of a distressed baby (Hopkins 1972). Although treatment of hypocalcemia is advised, there is little evidence that treatment alters the child's prognosis. However, it is possible that actively firing cells further compromise neuronal

Table 11-2
Major Causes of Neonatal Seizures

Category	Day 0–4	Day 5–14	Day 14–28
Anoxia	Fetal perintal primary secondary to trauma		
Developmental anomalies		Incontinentia pigmenti	Cerebral dysgenesis
Infection		Encephalitis Coxsackie B Cytomegalic-inclusion disease Herpes simples Toxoplasmosis Meningitis ± sepsis Sepsis ± meningitis, bacterial	
Metabolic amino acidurias		Arginosuccinic aciduria Hyperammonemia I and II Hyperglycinemia Isovaleric acidemia Methylmalonic acidemia Propionic acidemia Maple syrup urine disease	Phenylketonuria
Bilirubin		Kernicterus	
Drug withdrawal		Alcohol Barbiturates (addiction or anticonvulsants) Heroin Methadone	
Hypocalcemia	Hypomagnesemia Intracranial trauma Maternal hyperpara- thyroidism	High phosphate (cow's milk) load Neonatal hypopara- thyroidism	
Hypoglycemia	Diabetic mother Intracranial bleeding Low birth weight Meningitis	Fructosemia Galactosemia Glycogen storage disease Idiopathic Islet cell tumor Leucine sensitivity	
Hypomagnesemia	With hypocalcemia Without hypocalcemia		
Hyponatremia or hypernatremia		Inappropriate anti- diuretic hormone	

Table 11-2 *(Continued)*

Category	Day 0–4	Day 5–14	Day 14–28
		Inappropriate fluid therapy	
		Salt substituted for sugar	
Pyridoxine	Deficiency		Deficiency
	Dependency		
Trauma, birth	Periventricular bleeding secondary to anoxia		Subdural hematoma
	Subarachnoid bleeding		
	Subdural bleeding		
	Thrombosis		

function by increasing the metabolic requirements of damaged cells at the same time that homeostasis is impaired by the effects of edema and impaired circulation.

The hypoglycemic infant of a diabetic mother clearly warrants therapy, and early therapy is correlated with outcome (Senior 1973, Milner 1972).

Days 4–14

During the last part of the first week of life and during the second week, the primary cause of seizures is infection. Metabolic abnormalities, hypoglycemia, hypocalcemia, and hypomagnesemia may occur independently of perinatal stress. Other metabolic abnormalities such as amino acidurias, abnormalities of glucose metabolism, and genetic problems are more common. Specific diagnosis and appropriate therapy may abolish the seizures. Evaluation and management of the problems listed in Table 11-2 are to be found in standard texts.

Days 14–28

Seizures beginning in the last 2 weeks of the neonatal period have diverse causes. They are far less common than seizures with earlier onset. Infection, cerebral dysgenesis, subdural hemotomas, trauma, and metabolic factors may each play a role and require evaluation.

ARE SEIZURES IN THE NEWBORN HARMFUL?

Seizures at any age are aesthetically unpleasant and indicate that the brain is malfunctioning. Prolonged generalized seizures in newborn rats (equivalent to 6-month-old to 1-year-old humans) and in older animals increase cellular metabolism and result in a fall in the level of high energy phosphate (ATP) and an increase in the level of cellular lactate (Plum et al 1974). Prolonged seizures may cause local or generalized cerebral edema. After repeated seizures in the newborn experimental animal, there is a fall in the level of brain glucose and a reduction in the levels of brain DNA, RNA, protein, and cholesterol (Wasterlain and Plum 1973). There may be a reduction in cell number but not in cell size. These alterations may or may not be reversible. Whether any of these findings have relevance to the human newborn is debatable. In most human infants, seizures are secondary to anoxia and asphyxia. Therefore, the effects of the seizures per se cannot be isolated from the effects of the primary insults. Because most neonatal seizures are brief or subtle and do not cause hypoxia, the pathological correlation with findings in more mature experimental animals who have experienced prolonged tonic-clonic seizures is uncertain.

Treatment should be given for prolonged generalized seizures, and perhaps for constant multifocal seizures and seizures associated with apnea. However, there is no evidence that less severe seizures *cause* damage. Evaluation of the seizing child should proceed rapidly to uncover the cause of the seizures and, where possible, to enable specific therapy. This approach is far more important than the administration of anticonvulsant medication.

EVALUATION OF THE NEONATE WITH SEIZURES

The initial evaluation of an infant with neonatal seizures is usually performed in a stereotyped fashion and is done hand-in-hand with empirical therapy. A history and physical examination should have been done prior to the onset of seizures.

History

Important points to be stressed in the history are

1. *The 5-minute Apgar score.* An Apgar score of less than 6 indicates asphyxia; a score below 3 indicates severe asphyxia. Asphyxia, particularly in premature infants, is often accompanied by germinal matrix hemorrhage, which may rupture into the ventricle and cause intraventricular hemorrhage (Brann and Dykes 1977, Volpe 1976).
2. *The delivery.* Precipitous delivery, prolonged labor, and abnormal presentations are often associated with asphyxia, low Apgar scores, and seizures beginning in the first 3 days. Full-term infants with seizures starting on the second or third day and with a history of a traumatic birth may have a subdural hematoma or subarachnoid hemorrhage (Hopkins 1972). Prolonged rupture of membranes suggests a risk of later sepsis.
3. *Family history.* A history of a previous child with neonatal seizures or of a child who died in the neonatal period without obvious cause should alert the clinician to possible metabolic abnormalities such as pyridoxine dependency, amino acidopathies, or parathyroid disease in the mother.
4. *Drugs.* Withdrawal from narcotic-analgesics is likely to produce an infant who is jittery and irritable for the first 3–4 days, but this withdrawal only occasionally causes seizures (Zelson et al 1971, Herzlinger et al 1977). The occurrence of seizures on the second and third days of life should raise the suspicion of maternal addiction to a short-acting barbiturate such as secobarbital.

Physical Examination

The physical examination contributes relatively little to the process of determining the cause of neonatal seizures. Intraventricular hemorrhage may be suspected in an infant who suddenly lapses into coma and progresses to hypoventilation and respiratory arrest with generalized tonic seizures, "decerebrate" posturing, pupils fixed to light, and eyes fixed to all vestibular stimulation, and, finally to a flaccid quadriparesis. The course of this deterioration may be minutes to hours. A bulging fontanelle and a falling hematocrit accompany the deterioration. A slower, stuttering course over hours or days may also occur (Volpe 1977). However, there are no findings in the examination that reliably predict either the presence or the severity of the hemorrhage (Lazzara et al 1978).

Physical stigma such as wide-set eyes or other craniofacial abnormalities may suggest developmental abnormalities of the cortex. A large liver and a large spleen and petechiae may be early signs of congenital infections. Vesicular lesions on the skin may be early evidence of incontinentia pigmenti, herpes simplex, or other viral diseases.

From the history and physical examination, an educated guess as to the cause of the seizures can frequently be made. Despite that educated guess, laboratory evaluation and therapeutic intervention should proceed.

Laboratory and Therapeutic Evaluation

A lumbar puncture and blood chemistries should be carried out in every child with neonatal seizures, regardless of the age of onset.

1. *Lumbar puncture* is performed to rule out meningitis and to evaluate intracranial bleeding. A sample of spinal fluid should be centrifuged, if bloody, and compared with water to evaluate xanthochromia. Xanthochromia results from breakdown of hemoglobin and thus is proportional to the serum bilirubin and the CSF protein. With a bilirubin level of less than 0.01/mg/dL xanthochromia is detectable at a protein level of 100 mg/dL. When there has been bleeding into the subarachnoid space, with breakdown of hemoglobin, xanthochromia increases disproportionately to the CSF protein level.

   Evaluation of the red cell count in the first and third tubes of CSF collected may also help in evaluating a traumatic tap.

2. *Blood* should be drawn for the determination of serum levels of glucose and electrolytes prior to the lumbar puncture. An estimate of the blood glucose should be made immediately by Dextrostix, and the remaining blood should be sent to the laboratory for the determination of serum levels of glucose, electrolytes, calcium, phosphorus, magnesium, and urea nitrogen.

THERAPY

Hypoglycemia

A blood glucose concentration less than 20 mg/dL in the premature infant or of less than 30 mg/dL in the full-term infant is defined as hypoglycemia. Despite the lack of evidence that blood glucose levels in this range are necessarily harmful (Pildes et al 1974, Oh and Vohr 1980) and because of some evidence that a normal blood glucose level, or even hyperglycemia (Wasterlain and Duffy 1975), may be beneficial, glucose should be administered to the infant with seizures in sufficient amounts to maintain the blood glucose level in the normal range. Approximately 0.5 to 1 g/kg of glucose (25% solution) should be given as an immediate intravenous dose and administration should be maintained at a rate of 0.5 g/kg/hour. Further evaluation and therapy should await the results of the lumbar puncture and the blood chemistries previously obtained (Dodson 1977).

Hypocalcemia and Hypomagnesemia

Hypocalcemia, defined as a serum calcium concentration below 7 mg/dL, is more common in low-birth-weight infants and is often associated with perinatal trauma (Hopkins 1972). It is rarely the sole cause of seizures during the first few days of life (Volpe 1977). Late onset hypocalcemia, occurring at the end of the first week and during the second week, is often related to the ingestion of a high phosphate load such as is found in cow's milk. The effects, if any, of hypocalcemia and the seizures caused by hypocalcemia on later brain function are unknown. When an infant has hypocalcemia in the absence of other prenatal or perinatal problems, the mother's serum calcium and serum phosphorus concentrations should be evaluated as a means of identifying parathyroid adenoma.

A 5% solution of calcium gluconate given intravenously is used for treatment of hypocalcemia; 4 mL/kg (200 mg/kg) should be given slowly, and the cardiac rate carefully monitored. Because calcium is a cerebral depressant, cessation of seizures does not prove that the seizures were caused by hypocalcemia.

Hypomagnesemia

A serum magnesium level of less than 1 mg/dL is usually associated with hypocalcemia and its causes (Volpe 1977). Persistent hypocalcemia despite the administration of calcium suggests hypomagnesemia; administration of magnesium may reverse the hypocalcemia. Magnesium (0.2–0.3 mL/kg) may be given intramuscularly as a 50% magnesium sulfate solution. Excess magnesium may result in neuromuscular blockade and transient weakness with hypotonia and respiratory depression.

Pyridoxine Dependency

Pyridoxine dependency is a rare cause of seizures, which may even begin in utero (Swaiman and Millstein 1970). These seizures are persistent and, if recognized late, may cause mental retardation or death. Early recognition and therapy enables these children to be normal. Because there is no specific diagnostic test for pyridoxine dependency, a child with persistent seizures should be given 50 mg of pyridoxine intravenously. If seizures cease within minutes, dependency should be suspected. If seizures recur, pyridoxine should be readministered during a simultaneous EEG. Prompt normalization of the EEG and cessation of seizures confirms the diagnosis. The dependent child should be maintained on 10 mg of pyridoxine orally, indefinitely.

Other Metabolic Abnormalities

Amino acidurias may occasionally be the cause of seizures in the newborn. Screening tests with ferric chloride or nitroprusside should be confirmed with chromatography. Ketonuria in the perinatal period suggests hyperglycinemia, methylmalonic aciduria, glycogen storage disease, or maple syrup urine disease.

Reducing substance in the urine by Benedict's reagent in the absence of a positive test by the glucose oxidase method suggests glactosemia. Early attention to these metabolic abnormalities may mean the difference between a normal and a damaged child (Nyhan 1977).

Meningitis and Sepsis

Meningitis or sepsis should be suspected in any infant with seizures, particularly the infant whose seizures begin after 4 days of age or where there has been rupture of the membranes for an extended interval. Signs of infections in the newborn may be subtle; and although seizures occur in one-third to one-half of patients with neonatal meningitis, they are not commonly the initial symptom of this disease. However, to rule out sepsis or meningitis (as well as to evaluate subarachnoid hemorrhage), a child with neonatal seizures should have a lumbar puncture, with complete examination of the cerebral spinal fluid. Pleocytosis may follow a subarachnoid hemorrhage, but cerebral spinal fluid glucose concentration usually remains normal. Although gram-negative organisms are common causes of neonatal meningitis, other infectious agents such as gram-positive bacteria (particularly *Streptococcus*), cytomegalic inclusion disease, toxoplasmosis, and herpesvirus should be considered. The evaluation and therapy for these infections may be found in standard text books.

THE ELECTROENCEPHALOGRAM

For patients in whom seizures are merely suspected, an electroencephalogram with simultaneous clinical observation of the paroxysmal phenomena by trained nursery personnel are helpful in establishing diagnosis. The EEG is not helpful in establishing the cause of the seizures, but in good hands may have prognostic value (Rose and Lombroso 1970, Torres and Blaw 1968). A normal interictal EEG is said to be associated with a good chance of normal development, whereas a periodic burst-suppression pattern is strongly correlated with severe cerebral disease and a poor prognosis. Proper interpretation of neonatal EEGs requires a highly trained, sophisticated encephalographer specifically attuned to the EEG patterns of the newborn and to their variation with gestational age and the state of arousal. When EEGs are not readily available or when electroencephalographers have not had considerable experience with the newborn, the interpretation should be used with caution. In general, the diagnostic evaluation and therapy should not be postponed while awaiting an EEG.

ANTICONVULSANT THERAPY

In older infants and children, prolonged convulsions may interfere with cerebral oxygenation and may result in brain damage. In the newborn infant, as has been indicated, convulsions are rarely generalized or repetitive. There is little evidence that the mild, subtle, neonatal seizures per se damage the brain. Therefore, I feel that unless seizures are frequent and severe or unless they are associated with apnea, there is little reason to use anticonvulsants. This opinion is not universally held (Volpe 1977). However, there is general agreement that *in the newborn* anticonvulsant medication is not the primary approach to control of seizures. Anticonvulsants should not be used until previous chemical evaluations and therapy have been completed.

Phenobarbital

Phenobarbital is the anticonvulsant drug of choice for the newborn. In addition to being an effective anticonvulsant, it may also decrease the cellular metabolism of damaged cells and may have an effect on cerebral circulation. It may thus protect cells damaged by anoxia and asphyxia. I recommend that phenobarbital be utilized *only* in severe or prolonged neonatal seizures (status) or where there are episodes of apnea that may produce further anoxic damage. Phenobarbital should be used to bring about prompt cessation of these states. When used, phenobarbital should be given in a leading dose of 15 to 20 mg/kg intravenously. It may be advisable to first give a dose of 10 mg/kg intravenously, followed 20 minutes later by a further dose of 5 mg, which may be repeated. However, if the seizures continue, the full 20 mg/kg may be given over 10–20 minutes. This leading dose should produce a therapeutic blood level of 15 to 20 μg/mL (Painter 1978).

Maintenance therapy after loading is another matter of individual bias. Because phenobarbital has a long half-life in the newborn (96+ hours) and because the effects of anoxia and the consequent cerebral edema (which causes the seizures) are transient, I do not use or recommend a maintenance dose of phenobarbital. Rather, I allow the loading dose to decay slowly over the first week of life. If seizures recur later, I reload the patient and continue the infant on a maintenance dose of 4–5 mg/kg/day orally. Others have differing views. Painter (1978) recommends an initial loading dose of phenobarbital and an oral, intravenous, or intramuscular maintenance dosage of 4–5 mg/kg/day for several weeks. Volpe (1977) recommends continuation of a similar maintenance dose until there is no evidence of neurologic disability. Blood levels must be measured because of the marked individual variability of newborns and because of changing metabolism with age. Blood level determinations will assure maintenance of a therapeutic level and will indicate possible toxic accumulation. Because of the long half-life, a maintenance dose of phenobarbital greater than 5 mg/kg in the newborn may cause increasing blood levels.

Phenytoin

Phenytoin (diphenylhydantoin) is used when phenobarbital is ineffective. Phenytoin must be given intravenously because its absorption after intramuscular administration is erratic, and phenytoin is poorly absorbed orally during the first months of life. An intravenous loading dose of 20 mg/kg will produce a therapeutic blood level. This loading dose should be given slowly with EKG monitoring and may be given in two parts separated by 20 minutes to an hour (Painter et al 1978). Maintenance, if used (see preceding discussion) requires 5 mg/kg given intravenously. Blood levels should be followed closely because signs of toxicity may be absent in the newborn.

Diazepam

Diazepam (Valium) is a poor choice as an anticonvulsant drug for the neonate. Its duration of action is short, and either phenobarbital or phenytoin will have to be used in addition for more prolonged seizure control. In addition, diazepam may interfere with bilirubin binding.

Sodium Valproate

Sodium valproate (Depakene) has not been approved for use in the neonate, nor have its efficacy and toxicity been adequately studied in neonatal seizures. There are suggestions that the hepatic toxicity is greater at younger ages. Therefore, this drug is not a primary choice at this time for treatment of neonatal seizures.

PROGNOSIS ASSOCIATED WITH NEONATAL SEIZURES

There is little evidence that the prognosis for infants with neonatal seizures is related to the seizures themselves. Rather, prognosis is related to their underlying cause. Long-term studies of the outcome of infants with neonatal seizures are few in number and difficult to intrepret because of the variability of selection factors in reported series. Some studies have excluded premature infants, whereas some have a high percentage of such infants and a high mortality rate (Seay and Bray 1977). In some studies, patients are those referred to 'a center, which increases the number of severely affected children included in the sample. Virtually no studies are unbiased. Mortality rates in published studies range from 10–40%. The variation results from selection factors and the duration of follow-up (Burke 1954, Craig 1960, Prichard 1964, Dennis 1978). The causes of death vary with the series and the age at death, but evidence of anoxia and intraventricular hemorrhage predominate, with infection and developmental anomalies being less common causes of mortality. The quality of survival is also affected by the previously mentioned biases and is compounded by variation and duration of follow-up and by accuracy of assessment. These factors have all made prognostication difficult. No reported studies followed children to school age to look for learning disorders (Gottfried 1973).

At least 60–80% of survivors of the reported series appear to be normal. Brown and co-workers (1972) found that mortality and morbidity were directly related to the day of onset of the seizure. He found that when seizures began on day 1, one-third of the infants died and 60% of the survivors were abnormal at 1 year. Infants whose seizures began on the second to the sixth day had a 97% change of surviving. One-half of those whose seizures started on the second day, 70% of those whose seizures began on the third day, and 90% of those whose seizures began on the fourth day were normal at follow-up.

Although serious attempts to correlate the neonatal neurologic examination with cause and prognosis have been made (Brown et al 1972, Ziegler et al 1976), the validity of neurologic examination on the newborn is open to serious question. Evidence of severe neurologic damage, such as lack of all primitive reflexes, and asymmetrical neurologic findings are associated with adverse sequellae (Ziegler et al 1976), but, except at the extremes, early prognostication is often wrong.

The National Collaborative Perinatal Project (NCPP) offered researchers an opportunity to evaluate the prognosis of children with neonatal seizures and to assess factors related to their long-term prognosis. This project, which was a prospective study of approximately 54,000 pregnancies whose products were followed to age 7, avoided the selection biases of previous reports and allowed the analysis of predictors of outcome. The results of these analyses have been reported (Holden et al 1981, Mellits et al 1981).

Two hundred seventy-seven infants were recognized to have seizures during the first 28 days of life. This gave an incidence of 0.5%. Other, subtle seizures may have gone unrecognized. Asphyxia manifested by a low Apgar score, meconium staining, and the need for prolonged resuscitation were common. The mean 5-minute Apgar score of the group was 6.8; and 19% of the group had an Apgar score of <7 at 15 minutes.

Forty-two percent of the infants began to seize during the first day of life, and more than one-half of those seizures began during the first 12 hours. Most seizures began during the first 3 days, and only 13% began after the first week of life.

Thirty-five percent of the infants died, two-third during the neonatal period. Death was associated with the 5-minute Apgar score, with the need for resuscitation after 5 minutes, and with low birth weight. Infants whose seizures began early, whose seizures lasted longer than 30 minutes, and whose seizures occurred on multiple days were all more likely to die.

Of the survivors, 70% did well. They had no evidence of mental retardation, cerebral palsy, or epilepsy. Six percent of the survivors had mental retardation alone, 2% had only cerebral palsy, and 9% had only epilepsy. Thirteen percent of the survivors had a combination of these neurologic sequellae.

Neonatal seizures were the major single perinatal factor related to later cerebral palsy. A child with neonatal seizures was 55–70 times more likely to have cerebral palsy than a child without neonatal seizures. A child with neonatal seizures was 5 times more likely to have mental retardation at age 7 than a child who had not had seizures. The child with neonatal seizures was also 18 times more likely to have epilepsy. Although neonatal seizures are a danger signal for later neurologic disability, it is important to emphasize that 70% of the survivors had *no* retardation, *no* cerebral palsy, and *no* epilepsy.

Using this same data and multiple regression analyses, my co-workers and I were able to identify factors that were significantly associated with specific outcomes and that would have predicted those outcomes in this population. These factors are shown in Table 11-3. It is noteworthy that the Apgar score, the need for resuscitation after 5 minutes of life, and a prolonged (>30 minutes) seizures were the most frequent variables associated with a poor outcome. A low birth weight was associated with death. There was little association of perinatal events and later epilepsy.

Table 11-3

Combinations of Variables Which Are Significantly Associated with Outcome and Which Might Be Utilized to Predict Outcome in Infants With Neonatal Seizures

Outcome	Variables
Death	Resuscitation after 5 minutes of age
	A seizure lasting more than 30 minutes
	Birth weight less than 2500 grams
Full scale 10 <70 at age 7	5-minute Apgar <7
	A seizure lasting more than 30 minutes
Cerebral palsy	Resuscitation after 5 minutes
Epilepsy	None
Any combination of MR, CP, epilepsy or death in infants surviving the neonatal period	5-minute Apgar score
	Onset time of seizures
	A seizure lasting more than 30 minutes

In view of the lack of correlation of mental retardation and cerebral palsy with the Apgar score, and the finding (Nelson et al 1981) that most children with a low Apgar at 15 minutes *and* seizures had cerebral palsy and mental retardation, one might speculate that seizures in the early neonatal period indicate the infant who had suffered a more severe or more prolonged period of intrauterine asphyxia. The Apgar score probably indicates asphyxia just prior to delivery. Perhaps when that asphyxia is sufficiently prolonged to damage the brain, that damage is manifested as neonatal seizures. The severity of that damage may be further demonstrated by the prolonged duration of a seizure or by the recurrent nature of the seizures over a number of days.

Thus, a child with a low 5-minute ro 10-minute Apgar score is at high risk for seizures; and, if the infant seizes, for an adverse outcome. Early identification using the Apgar score and seizures could provide an indication for intervention in the cycle of anoxia → edema → circulatory impairment → further anoxia proposed by Brann (1980). Methods to interrupt that cycle are needed. Studies of the use of osmotic agents to decrease edema, of the benefits and consequences of steroids, and of other agents to preserve damaged cells should be carried out. These studies are best done within an animal model, but the use of positron emission tomography may enable metabolic studies *in vivo* and evluation of the efficacy of intervention in the human newborn.

Now that we can identify the problem at a time when we could perhaps intervene and affect both the number of children who survive and the quality of their survival, studies of the best approaches to that intervention are urgently needed.

BIBLIOGRAPHY

Barnes R: In discussion to paper by WJ Little. *Obstetrical Transactions Society* (London) 1862;2:293–344.

Brann AW Jr: Effects of intrauterine asphyxia on the full-term brain, in *Neonatal Neurological Assessment and Outcome: Report of the 77th Ross Conference on Pediatric Research.* Columbus, OH, Ross Laboratories, 1980, pp 11-26.

Brann AW Jr, Dykes FD: The effects of intrauterine asphyxia on the full-term infant. *Clin Perinatol* 1977;4:149–161.

Brown JK, Cockburn F, Forfar JO: Clinical and chemical correlates in convulsions on the newborn. *Lancet* 1972;1:135–138.

Burke JB: The prognostic significance of neonatal convulsions. *Arch Dis Child* 1954;29: 342–345.

Craig WB: Convulsive movements in the first ten days of life. *Arch Dis Child* 1960;35:336–344.

Dennis J: Neonatal convulsions: Etiology, late neonatal status and long-term outcome. *Dev Med Child Neurol* 1978;20:143–158.

Dodson WE: Neonatal metabolic encephalopathies—Hypoglycemia, hypocalcemia, hypomagnesemia, and hypobilirubinemia. *Clin Perinatol* 1977;4:131–148.

Gilles FH: Lesions attributed to perinatal asphyxia in the human, in Gluck L (ed): *Intrauterine Asphyxia and the Developing Fetal Brain.* Chicago Year Book Medical Publishers, 1977, pp 99–107.

Gottfried AW: Intellectual consequences of perinatal anoxia. *Psychol Bull* 1973;80:231–242.

Herzlinger RA, Candall SR, Vaughn HG Jr: Neonatal seizures associated with narcotic withdrawal. *J Pediatr* 1977;91:638–641.

Holden KR, Mellits ED, Freeman JM: Neonatal seizures. I. Correlation of prenatal and perinatal events with outcomes. *Pediatrics* 1982;70:165–176.

Hopkins IJ: Seizures in the first week of life: A study of etiological factors. *Med J Aust* 1972; 2:647–651.

Keen JH: Significance of hypocalcaemia in neonatal convulsions. *Arch Dis Child* 1969;44: 356–361.

Lazzara A, Ahmann PA, Dykes FD, et al: Clinical predictability of intraventricular hemorrhage in preteam infants, abstracted. *Ann Neurol* 1978;4:187.

Little WJ: On the influence of abnormal parturition, difficult labours, premature birth, and asphyxia neonatorum, on the mental and physical condition of the child, especially in relation to deformities. *Obstetrical Transactions Society* (London) 1862;2:293–344.

Mellits ED, Holden KR, Freeman JM: Neonatal seizures. II. Multivariate analysis of factors associated with outcome. *Pediatrics* 1981;70:177–185.

Milner RDG: Neonatal hypoglycaemia—A critical reappraisal. *Arch Dis Child* 1972;47: 679–682.

Myers RE: Experimental models of perinatal brain damage: Relevance to human pathology, in Gluck L (ed): *Intrauterine Asphyxia and the Developing Fetal Brain.* Chicago, Year Book Medical Publishers, 1977, pp 37–97.

Nelson KB, Broman SH: Perinatal risk factors in children with serious motor and mental handicaps. *Ann Neurol* 1977;2:371–377.

Nelson KB, Ellenberg JH: Apgar scores as predictors of chronic neurologic disability. *Pediatrics* 1981;68:36–44.

Nyhan WL: Heritable metabolic disease and the differential diagnosis of asphyxia, in Gluck L (ed): *Intrauterine Asphyxia and the Developing Fetal Brain.* Chicago, Year Book Medical Publishers, 1977, pp 421–429.

Oh W, Vohr BR: The role of neonatal metabolic disorders on the neurological and developmental outcome of LBW infants, in Brann AW, Volpe JJ (eds): *Neonatal Neurologic Assessment and Outcome: Report of the 77th Ross Conference on Pediatric Research.* Columbus, OH, Ross Laboratories, 1980, pp 48–54.

Painter MJ, Pipinger C, McDonald H, et al: Phenobarbital and diphenylhyantoin levels in neonates with seizures. *J Pediatr* 1978;92:315–319.

Pildes RS, Cornblath M, Warren I, et al: A prospective controlled study of neonatal hypoglycemia. *Pediatrics* 1974;54:5–14.

Plum F, Howse DC, Duffy TE: Metabolic effects of seizures. *Res Publ Assoc Res Nerv Ment Dis* 1974;53:141–157.

Prichard JS: The character and significance of epileptic seizures in infancy, in Kellaway P, Peterson I (eds): *Neurological and Electroencephalographic Correlative Studies in Infancy.* New York, Grune & Stratton Inc, 1964.

Rose AL, Lombroso CT: Neonatal seizure states. A study of clinical, pathological, and electroencephalographic features in 137 full-term babies with a long-term follow-up. *Pediatrics* 1970;45:404–425.

Seay AR, Bray PE: Significance of seizures in infants weighing less than 2500 grams. *Arch Neurol* 1977;34:381–382.

Senior B: Neonatal hypoglycemia. *N Engl J Med* 1973;289:790–791.

Swaiman KF, Millstein TM: Pyridoxine-dependency and penicillin. *Neurology* 1970;20:78–81.

Torres F, Blaw ME: Longitudinal EEG—Clinical correlations in children from birth to 4 years of age. *Pediatrics* 1968;41:945–954.

Volpe JJ: Perinatal hypoxic—Ischemic brain injury. *Pediatr Clin North Am* 1976;23:383–397.

Volpe JJ: Neonatal seizures. *Clin Perinatol* 1977;4:43–63.

Wasterlain CG, Duffy TE: Neonatal status epilepticus: Decrease in brain glucose without decrease in blood glucose. *Neurology* 1975;25:365.

Wasterlain CG, Plum F: Vulnerability of developing rat brain to electro-convulsive seizures. *Arch Neurol* 1973;29:38–45.

Zelson C, Rubid E, Wasserman E: Neonatal narcotic addiction. *Pediatrics* 1971;48:178–189.

Ziegler AI, Calame A, Marchand C, et al: Cerebral distress in full-term newborns and its prognostic value. A follow-up study of 90 infants. *Helv Pediatr Acta* 1976;31:299–317.

CHAPTER 12

Febrile Seizures

Karin B. Nelson and Jonas H. Ellenberg

INTRODUCTION AND DEFINITION

Febrile seizures are a problem unique to young children. Beyond the age of approximately 5 years, humans usually do not have seizures with fever unless the illness causing the fever affects the brain directly, as in encephalitis or meningitis, or by other specific and readily recognizible mechanisms, eg, septic embolization or marked electrolyte shifts. In young children, in contrast, fever or its concomitants may be a sufficient precipitant of seizures. This age-related vulnerability to seizures with fever is common, appears to cluster in families, and was known in the time of Hippocrates to have a good prognosis.

Not every seizure with fever in a young child is a febrile seizure. Children sometimes suffer from meningitis or hypernatremic dehydration or toxic encephalopathy, and fever and seizures may be part of these disorders. Because these illnesses may damage the brain with or without seizures, it is important, when considering the natural history of febrile seizures, not to confuse the prognosis of meningitis, for example, with the prognosis of febrile seizures.

Most children who experience febrile seizures were previously normal; however, there is reason to think that neurologically abnormal children are somewhat more likely to have febrile seizures than normal children. Because children who were abnormal before a febrile seizure are likely to continue to be abnormal after it, it is important, when evaluating the prognosis of febrile seizures, to consider the intactness of the child before the occurrence of the seizure.

The definition of febrile seizures to be used in this discussion is taken, with minor modification, from the Consensus Development Meeting on Long-Term Management of Febrile Seizures (Consensus Development Panel 1980), which will be cited further elsewhere in this chapter.

> A febrile seizure is a seizure in infancy or childhood, usually occurring between 3 months and 5 years of age, associated with fever but without evidence of intracranial infection or recognized acute neurologic illness. Seizures with fever in children who have suffered a previous nonfebrile seizure are excluded. Febrile seizures are to be distinguished from epilepsy, which is characterized by recurrent nonfebrile seizures.

THE CLINICAL ENTITY

Febrile seizures occur most often in children between the ages of 6 months and 3 years, with a median age of occurrence 18 to 22 months. Such seizures are usually brief and self-limited and are most often generalized tonic-clonic convulsions. Other types of seizures, including focal seizures, multiple seizures, or prolonged seizures, may occur in some attacks, whether initial or subsequent (Table 12-1).

Table 12-1
Features of Febrile Seizures Observed in the NCPP

Features	First Seizure		Any Seizure	
	N	%	N	%
Pure	1391	81.6	1281	75.1
Complex*	314	18.4	425	24.9
Prolonged (>15 minutes)	96		129	
Multiple (>1 per 24 hours)	190		276	
Focal	56		69	

*Some of the complex seizures had multiple complex components and therefore the total number of complex seizures is less than the sum of its constituent parts.

The Illness Associated with Fever and Febrile Convulsions

Any illness or environmental factor that can elevate temperature in a young child can trigger febrile seizures. In fact, such illnesses are most often otitis media or respiratory infections, with the next most frequent being "flu" and gastroenteritis (Table 12-2). Viral agents can often be isolated (Lewis et al 1979, Stokes et al 1977). Syncopal mechanisms may underlie some febrile seizures (Stephenson 1978).

Table 12-2
Associated Conditions in Children with Febrile Seizures

Condition	Frequency	
	N	Percentage
Otitis media	289	16.9
Other URI	475	27.8
Pneumonia	183	10.7
Flu	18	1.1
Gastroenteritis	82	4.8
Roseola	59	3.5
No condition	55	3.2
Other	152	8.9
Unknown	393	23.0
Total	1706	99.0

Fever and seizures may follow immunization procedures. Several workers have suggested that some of these may be febrile seizures, precipitated by the fever the immunizations often provoke. This possibility is reinforced by observation in the NCPP that children who had seizures after shots were almost always febrile—often highly febrile—and that more than one-half of children who had seizures after immunization procedures had a personal history of other febrile seizures or a history of febrile seizures in a sibling or parent (DG Hirtz, KB Nelson, JH Ellenberg, unpublished data, 1982). The outcome of these seizures was good in children whose immunization-associated seizure lasted less than an hour. Thus, some, and perhaps many, of the seizures following immunization may have the same mechanism as febrile seizures.

Other factors may contribute to susceptibility to febrile seizures, including genetic predisposition, specific toxic constituents in some infectious diseases such as shigellosis, and iatrogenic factors such as overhydration, tap water enemas (which may induce hyponatremia), or medications that may lower the convulsive threshold. With respect to the last-mentioned consideration, Nealis and co-workers (Nealis et al 1976) have observed experimentally that diphenhydramine (Benadryl) potentiates fever-induced seizures in younr animals. Whether antihistamines or decongestants with central excitatory capabilities can increase vulnerability to seizures in children with fever has apparently not been investigated.

Fever and Febrile Seizures

Febrile seizures usually occur during the first day and often in the earliest hours of acute infectious illness. The seizure may be the initial sign of illness to be recognized by the parent. Except when there is a sharp secondary increase in body temperature (as may happen when acute otitis media supervenes upon an upper respiratory infection), a seizure occurring after the first day of illness should lead the clinician to seriously consider other diagnostic possibilities.

Children with high fevers are more likely to experience seizures than those with less extreme elevations of temperature. Whether it is the rate of rise of fever, the height of body temperature attained, or associated factors that trigger the seizure is unknown. As Lennox-Buchthal (1973) observed, a seizure may occur well before the temperature reaches its peak or after the temperature has dropped; and usually a child who has had a febrile seizure will later tolerate a higher fever without a seizure.

Intuition suggests that children who seize at relatively low levels of fever may have relatively low seizure thresholds and therefore be at greater risk of later spontaneous seizures. There are few data to test this hypothesis, but the child who has a seizure with only mild elevation of body temperature should be observed with care and the diagnosis of febrile seizure considered to be somewhat tentative.

In general, reliable information on the child's temperature at the time of the seizure, or just before it, is seldom available. The temperature recorded is usually that noted some time after the seizure, when the child reaches medical attention and the seizure has terminated.

Differential Diagnosis

The usual medical workup for seizures with fever (see Management, following) is designed to identify common entities that demand specific treatment. Most of these, like meningitis and hypernatremic dehydration, are excluded by definition from "febrile seizures" as the term is used here. However, the number of conditions that can present with fever and convulsions in young children is large, and some of these conditions do involve the brain directly and have implications for prognosis quite different from the others; however, they may not be identified by the usual medical investigation. Some uncommon metabolic conditions, such as ketotic hypoglycemia (Cordelli and Banaudi 1980) and ornithine carbamoyltransferase deficiency (Tsuboi 1976) can present with seizures and fever in young children and might elude the standard workup. Some conditions of uncertain frequency and unclear relationship with seizures and outcome, such as serologically diagnosed *Toxocara* infestation, may also present with seizure and fever (Glickman et al 1979).

It appears likely that future progress in understanding febrile seizures will include identification of subsyndromes with specific pathogenetic mechanisms and specific natural histories. A possible example of the identification of such a subgroup is the recent observation that cytomegalovirus was found in the urine of children who developed nonfebrile seizures after febrile seizures twice as often as in children who did not develop nonfebrile seizures (Iannetti et al, 1982). If confirmed, this study indicates a new direction for diagnostic efforts. We can hope for further recognition, within the probably heterogeneous entity "febrile seizures," of specific diagnostic categories.

Genetic Factors

The families of children with febrile seizures contain more members with seizure disorders, febrile and perhaps nonfebrile, than the families of unaffected children. As many as 60% of children with febrile seizures have relatives who have had at least one seizure. Seizures have been reported in 7% to 10% (Annegers et al 1982, van den Berg 1974) of siblings of children with febrile seizures in several series, and 20% in one (Tsuboi 1976). Two percent to 10% of parents are similarly involved.

The excess of affected parents and a risk to siblings well below 25% in most studies suggest that an autosomal recessive mode of inheritance is unlikely. Although the frequency of febrile seizures in males has exceeded that in females in most series, the difference is too slight to be compatible with a sex-linked form of transmission. A dominant mode of inheritance with reduced penetrance (Frantzen et al 1970, Lennox-Buchthal 1971) or polygenic inheritance appears likely, with current opinion favoring the latter (Kagawa 1975); and nongenetic factors shared by families may be relevant (Schiottz-Christensen 1972).

Assuming that vulnerability to febrile seizures is at least in part genetically determined, what is it that is inherited? Is it a specific tendency to seizure with fever when immature, or is it a more general lowering of convulsive threshold (Diaz and Shields 1981)? Or is there a subgroup among children with febrile seizures who later develop specific types of epilepsy?

Whether nonfebrile seizures are more common in the families of individuals with febrile seizures is not entirely clear. Nonfebrile seizure disorders appeared to be more frequent in the siblings of children with febrile seizures than in the general population in some studies (Millichap 1968, Ounsted et al 1966) but not in another (Frantzen et al 1970). Present evidence does not permit a firm conclusion as to whether the trait inherited is specific to febrile seizures or includes a more general vulnerability to seizures. However, there is more data to support the latter hypothesis.

As will be discussed further, a family history of nonfebrile seizures is a risk factor for the development of nonfebrile seizures after febrile seizures (Nelson and Ellenberg 1981). However, that increase was not marked unless one or more other risk factors were also present.

PREVALENCE

Febrile seizure is the most common seizure disorder in any age group, occurring in

2–5% of young children (Annegers et al 1982, Nelson and Ellenberg 1978, Wallace 1981). Two-thirds of all children with seizures in early childhood have febrile seizures only. In most series, boys outnumber girls; and black children have febrile seizures with slightly higher frequency than white children. Febrile seizures are reported to be approximately twice as common in certain Asian countries as in western communities, and once there has been one febrile seizure, the recurrence rate is reported to be as high as 80%, a much higher rate than in Western studies (Hauser 1981). A variation of frequency of febrile seizures by geographic region is not surprising for a characteristic that might be related to genetic drift in different locations. Common feverish illnesses will also be different by region. As an extreme example, in areas in which malaria is endemic, as many as one-half the seizures with fever are malarial convulsions. The reported prognosis may also be different, both because some of these children will have cerebral malaria, a brain-damaging disease, and because the local remedies are often neurotoxic (Asirifi 1972).

We are dependent for knowledge of the occurrence of seizures upon history: ascertainment requires that someone has observed the attack or attacks and that the informant be willing to tell us about it. Hauser (1981) remarks that in addition to possible real differences in seizure frequencies in different geographic areas, there may be some difference in ascertainment because a high proportion of febrile seizures occur during sleep (Leviton and Cowan 1981); and in general more people sleep in one room in some of the countries reporting high febrile seizure rates. High housing density, with its possibility greater opportunity for observation of the sleeping child, as well as a greater opportunity for contracting infectious illnesses, could also underlie the observation that the prevalence of febrile seizures is inversely related to socioeconomic status, with poorer families reporting considerably higher frequencies of febrile seizures than the more affluent.

It is intriguing to consider that one child may have a febrile seizure while someone is looking, be whisked to an emergency room by terrified parents, undergo an extensive workup, be placed on chronic treatment, have side effects and blood levels of medication monitored for several years, have his parents view him as changed and vulnerable, and so on; all this while the child in the next apartment has a febrile seizure in the bedroom alone at night, and occasions no drama at all.

PROGNOSIS

Death

A child rarely dies during a febrile seizure. Early studies of hospitalized series reported death rates up to 10%, but included cases of meningitis, severe preexisting neurologic handicap, and major electrolyte disturbances. The one child who died in a Danish series was a severely retarded youngster whose seizure lasted 5 hours (Frantzen et al 1968). Subsequent large cohort studies have not reported deaths (Hauser and Kurland 1975, Nelson and Ellenberg 1978).

Motor Handicap

Although early studies reported that severe handicap could be observed following febrile seizures, these reports did not distinguish children with meningitis, preexisting abnormalities, or specific neurologic diseases from those who meet the definition of febrile seizures employed here. In prospective studies of defined populations using the current definition, no new persisting hemipareses or other motor deficits have appeared with febrile seizures (Hauser and Kurland 1975, Nelson and Ellenberg 1978). However, transient unilateral weakness (Todd's paresis) occurred in approximately 0.5% of the population with febrile seizures.

Mental Retardation

Mental retardation has been found in higher frequency in selected populations of children who have had febrile seizures, but earlier studies were subject to the same limitations already noted regarding condition prior to the seizure, the acute illness, and selective sampling of the sample studied.

In a unique Danish study, 14 monozygous twin pairs, one of whom in each pair had had a febrile seizure, were compared on psychometric measures (Schmidley and Simon 1981). A mean difference of five IQ points was noted, the seizure-free twin averaging higher. These twins were not examined prior to the occurrence of the seizures. In the NCPP, among 431 pairs of siblings of whom one had had one or more febrile seizures (but none without fever) while the other was seizure-free, the mean IQ of children with febrile seizures was the same as the mean IQ of their brothers and sisters who had had no seizures (Ellenberg and Nelson 1978).

Smith and Wallace (1982) have reported that developmental quotients were lower in children with febrile seizures who experienced recurrences than in children who had no further attacks; however, in that series the treatment groups were not comparable with regard to expectation for intellectual outcome prior to the initiation of therapy. Rossiter et al (1977) did not find a change in developmental quotient associated with seizures.

School Progress

At the age of 11 years, children in the British National Child Development Study who had had febrile seizures (none without fever), were similar to those who had never had a seizure in performance on tests of general ability, reading comprehension, and arithmetic (Rossiter et al 1977). Among siblings of normal intelligence in the NCPP, one of whom had had one or more febrile seizures, there was no difference in the frequency of poor early academic achievement as judged by the Wide Range Achievement Test administration when the children were 7 years old (Ellenberg and Nelson 1978).

Epilepsy

All studies that have examined the question have found recurrent nonfebrile seizures to develop more often in persons who have experienced febrile seizures than in those who have not. Studies from referral centers and specialty clinics, studies of samples of hospitalized children and retrospective studies of individuals who have presented themselves later in life for care of serious handicaps have all been used in the past to judge the magnitude of the increase in risk of nonfebrile seizures after febrile seizures; none of these study types provides an appropriate basis for an investigation of natural history. Some of the estimates of risk of epilepsy have been enormously high in such studies, but at least as impressive has been the great variability observed in these highly selected samples (Figure 12-1) (Ellenberg and Nelson 1980).

The importance of selective factors in relation to outcome is illustrated by an

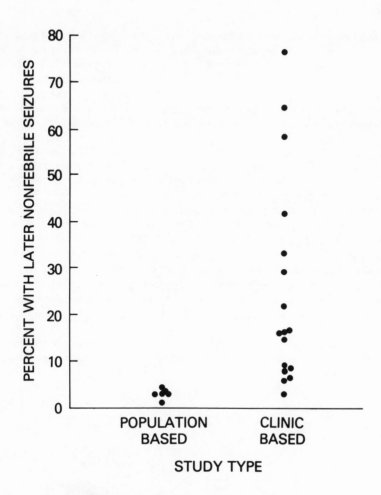

Figure 12-1 Percentage of children who experience nonfebrile seizures after one or more febrile seizures, in population-based (left) and clinic-based (right) studies. From Ellenberg and Nelson, 1980. Reproduced with permission from American Medical Association.

observation from the National Child Development Study (Ross et al 1980). More than one-half the children with febrile seizures were treated exclusively by their general practitioners, and only 0.5% of these later had seizures without fever. The remainder were admitted to the hospital overnight or longer, and 12% of the hospitalized group developed nonfebrile seizures.

With the advent of cohort studies, a fairly consistent answer has emerged: overall, nonfebrile seizures develop in 2% to 6% of children who have had febrile seizures (Annegers et al 1979, Nelson and Ellenberg 1976, van den Berg and Yerushalmy 1969) (Figure 12-1). Because approximately 0.9% of the general population has at least one nonfebrile seizure, the risk in those with febrile seizures is clearly raised. The absolute level of risk is not high, however.

There have been a number of efforts to discover whether particular subgroups face a special degree of risk of epilepsy after febrile seizures. It is generally agreed that a history of seizures without fever in the immediate family and neurologic abnormality (including developmental delay) constitute such risk factors. Characteristics of the initial febrile seizure, chiefly a duration of the seizure in excess of 10 to 15 minutes, focal convulsion, and multiple seizures in a single day are also relevant: a child whose first febrile seizure had one or more of these features is more likely to develop subsequent nonfebrile attacks. In the NCPP, we examined the frequency of these characteristics and their impact on outcome (Nelson and Ellenberg 1978). Sixty percent of children were normal prior to the first seizure, had a negative family history of nonfebrile seizures, and had an uncomplicated initial seizure. The frequency of nonfebrile seizures in such children was 2%, which is only 1% higher than in children who had never had a febrile seizure—a difference that, despite large sample size, was not statistically significant. Children with one risk factor constituted a third of all children with febrile seizures in the NCPP (Figure 12-2); 3% of them had a nonfebrile seizure by the age of 7, a risk that exceeds the 1% risk in the general population but remains relatively low. A small subgroup (6% of those with febrile seizures) had two or more risk factors. In this small subgroup, the risk of nonfebrile seizures was 13%, thirteen times greater than that of the general population. Yet even in this highest risk group, a large majority (87%) did not develop nonfebrile seizures.

After the age of 1 year, age at onset of febrile seizures was not related to the likelihood of subsequent epilepsy (Nelson and Ellenberg 1976); however, onset in the

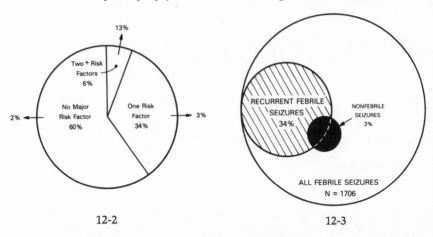

12-2   12-3

Figure 12-2 Nonfebrile seizures by age 7 in children with febrile seizures, based on results from the Collaborative Perinatal Project on the outcome of 1706 children. The risk factors evaluated were history of nonfebrile seizures in the immediate family, suspect or abnormal status in the child prior to first febrile seizure, and complex first febrile seizure. From Ellenberg and Nelson (1981). Reproduced with permission from Raven Press.

Figure 12-3 Among all children with febrile seizures (outer circle), a third had recurrences (hatched circle). Children with subsequent nonfebrile seizures (solid circle) came almost equally from among those who did and those who did not have at least one recurrence. From Nelson and Ellenberg (1981). Reproduced with permission from Raven Press.

181

first year, and especially in the first 6 months of life, was associated with higher risk of epilepsy. In multivariate analysis, once the major risk factors cited earlier were entered, age of onset did not add significant additional predictive power (Nelson and Ellenberg 1978).

The number of febrile seizures experienced has been reported by some workers as a predictor of epilepsy (Millichap 1968). One-half of the children in the NCPP who had at least one nonfebrile seizure after febrile seizures never had a second febrile seizure; the first seizure of their lives was febrile, the second nonfebrile (Figure 12-3) (Nelson and Ellenberg 1981). Clearly recurrence is not a necessary step on the road some patients follow from febrile seizures to epilepsy. Overall, the frequency of nonfebrile seizures was twice as high among children who had recurrences as among those who did not (Figure 12-4). That doubling of risk came with the second febrile seizure, and there was no further increase with a greater number of febrile seizures (Nelson and Ellenberg 1981). The absolute level of risk remained below 5% in the presence of one or more recurrences. When the population was subdivided according to the risk factors already cited for epilepsy after febrile seizures (prior neurologic or developmental abnormality, family history of nonfebrile seizures, and an initial seizure that was prolonged, focal, or multiple in the first day), it was observed that the low-risk group remained at low risk, however many recurrences they experienced, and the at-risk groups showed a possible irregular trend toward increase in risk that was not statistically significant. Data from the Rochester, Minnesota, study (Annegers et al 1979) was very similar and showed no increase in risk with increasing number of febrile seizures experienced and no statistically significant increase in risk with recurrences within the higher risk group (Figure 12-5).

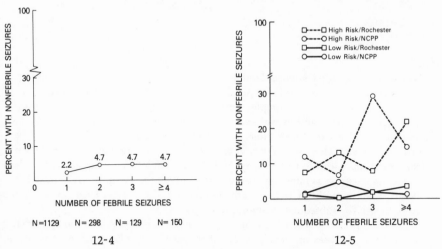

Figure 12-4 The rate of later nonfebrile seizures associated with a first recurrence was twice the rate in children with no recurrence. There was no further observed increase in the rate of nonfebrile seizures associated with recurrence after the first. From Nelson and Ellenberg (1981). Reproduced with permission from Raven Press.

Figure 12-5 Data from the Rochester, Minnesota, study and from the NCPP showing rate of later nonfebrile seizures experienced in high- and low-risk groups of these two studies.

Multivariate analysis confirmed, within the NCPP sample, that once the major risk factors were considered, seizure number did not add significant additional predictive power. In summary, number of febrile seizures experienced did not appear to be a major determinant of later nonfebrile seizures.

A number of factors do *not* alter the risk of epilepsy in persons who have had febrile seizures: race, sex, low Apgar scores, and low birth weight were not risk factors (Nelson and Ellenberg 1976).

Although only a small proportion of children with febrile seizures became epileptic, 13% of children who were epileptic by the age of 7 years began their seizure histories with one or more febrile seizures. When nonfebrile seizures developed, they usually had their onset relatively soon, approximately three-quarters beginning within the first 3 years after the initial febrile seizure (Table 12-3) (Aicardi and Chevrie 1976, Nelson and Ellenberg 1976).

Table 12-3
Interval from First Febrile to First Nonfebrile Seizure

| Time from First Febrile to First Nonfebrile Seizure (months) | Frequency | |
	N	Cumulative Percentage
0–12	22	42.3
13–24	10	61.5
37–48	6	86.5
49–60	5	96.2
61–84	2	100.0
Total	52	

Febrile Seizures and Temporal Lobe Epilepsy

Studies with patients with temporal lobe epilepsy (psychomotor epilepsy, or in more recent terminology, complex partial seizures)—notably the medical series of Ounsted et al (1966) and the surgical series of Falconer et al (1964)—have indicated that these patients relatively often had a history of prolonged seizures in infancy, often with fever. These workers have suggested that lengthy febrile seizures in early childhood "may lead to those lesions in the temporal lobe and amygdaloid nucleus which are regarded as important precursors of psychomotor epilepsy (Ounsted et al 1966). Their hypothesis is that early febrile seizures can produce the anatomic groundwork for subsequent temporal lobe epilepsy.

The definition of febrile seizures used by Ounsted and co-workers and by Falconer did not exclude cases of meningitis or other specific encephalopathies. The febrile seizures were retrospectively identified in older children or adults who had serious and multifaceted seizure disorders, and the selection factors involved make generalization from these series uncertain.

Leviton and Cowan (1981) have reviewed this topic. They pointed out that three studies have noted an increase in complex partial seizures in persons who earlier had febrile seizures, but no greater an increase for complex partial than for other types of epilepsy. They estimated that febrile seizures could not account for more than approximately 10% of temporal lobe epilepsy; they proposed alternative and non-causal models of the association between the disorders.

A population study, "Temporal lobe epilepsy—not a consequence of childhood febrile convulsions in Denmark," does not confirm the hypothesis that febrile seizures cause subsequent chronic temporal lobe epilepsy (Lee at al 1981).

Recurrences

Overall, one-third of children who have a febrile seizure experience at least one recurrence; and of those who have a recurrence, one-half have at least one further febrile seizure. Nine percent have three or more attacks. The earlier the first seizure, the greater the chance of recurrence: one-half the children whose first febrile seizure occurs before the first birthday have at least one recurrence, whereas only one-fifth the children whose first attack is after 36 months have a subsequent febrile seizure.

Almost one-half of second attacks occur within 6 months of the first seizure, and almost three-quarters occur within 12 months following the first (Nelson and Ellenberg 1978) (Table 12-4). Children with prolonged, focal, or multiple first seizures were not more likely to experience recurrences than children whose first febrile seizure was uncomplicated (Nelson and Ellenberg 1978). Most prolonged, focal, or multiple seizures are the first seizure of the child's life (Table 12-1) and have already occurred when the child is first brought to medical attention for febrile seizures.

Table 12-4
Interval to Recurrence of Febrile Seizures

Time from First to Second Seizure (months)	Frequency	
	N	Cumulative Percentage
0–2	114	22
3–6	136	47
7–12	135	73
13–24	79	88
25–48	54	98
49–84	10	100
Total	528	

Of the variety of factors examined as possible predictors of recurrence, the only consistently identified characteristic is age at which the initial seizure occurred. In general, factors that predict epilepsy after febrile seizure are not the same characteristics that predict recurrences.

The predictors of *favorable* prognosis in febrile seizures can be stated in *positive* terms as: normal neurologic development, family history free of nonfebrile seizure disorders, and all seizures experienced to be simple or pure febrile seizures. These factors are reminiscent of the characteristics cited by Sato and co-workers (1976) as favorable prognostic factors in absence (petit mal) epilepsy: normal intelligence, negative family history of seizure disorders, no seizures other than characteristic absence attacks, and normal background on the EEG. (The EEG as a predictor in febrile seizures is discussed later.) Other investigators have found rather similar factors to indicate favorable prognoses in other seizure disorders.

The Electroencephalogram as a Predictor in Febrile Seizures

The EEG has proved its utility in many clinical situations. It is a standard tool in diagnosis and prognosis of absence seizures, for example. In adults who have had a single seizure, the EEG is an important aid in judging the likelihood of subsequent recurrences (Hauser 1981). However, with respect to febrile seizures, the role of the EEG is far less clear.

In the period immediately following a febrile seizure, the EEG is likely to demonstrate unilateral or bilateral posterior slowing. Fever alone can produce such a record, and there is no known predictive significance. Paroxysmal abnormalities may appear at a later date in children who have had febrile seizures. Spike-wave tracings are found in an astonishing proportion—up to 40% or more—of children with past febrile seizures, if follow-up is continued for several years (Hauser 1981). Rolandic discharges have also been described in children who have had febrile seizures in the past and in their siblings (Kajitani et al 1981). As a marker for some influence, very possibly genetic, these electroencephalographic observations are of interest and warrant further research. At present for the clinician, however, it may be of little or no help to know the evolving electroencephalographic characteristics of individual children; and, indeed, these may be a possible source of confusion because the majority of studies do not find that even paroxysmal or epileptiform abnormalities predict either recurrences of febrile seizures or the development of subsequent epilepsy.

The major role of EEG in the management of children with febrile seizures at present is to help to rule out underlying structural pathology in the child who has experienced a focal seizure or a lengthy seizure.

MANAGEMENT

Management of children with febrile seizures should focus on the rapid termination of any seizure, on establishing the diagnosis by exclusion of other illnesses that require specific interventions, and on helping the family understand the disorder. Decisions concerning chronic therapy are of considerably less importance than are these primary considerations.

Acute Care

During the acute episode, the airway must be kept clear and aspiration prevented. The child should be protected from physical trauma; clothing and blankets should be removed; and sponging and rectal antipyretics should be used to reduce fever. If a well-equipped medical facility is some distance away or if the seizure has already lasted for some time, transport should be swiftly arranged; most seizures are self-limited, but it is better to err on the side of safety.

If the child is seen while the seizure is still in progress, the convulsion should be brought under control as quickly as can safely be accomplished. The specific approach will depend upon the circumstances and the facilities available and the agents with which the medical attendant is most familiar (see Chapter 14). Diazepam (Valium) may be administered, 0.3 mg/kg by IM injection or slowly by IV. If necessary this dose may be repeated in 10 minutes. Careful attention should be given to cardiac and respiratory rate and blood pressure, especially if barbiturates have previously been administered. Diazepam intravenously may be used, but special care must be taken if other anticonvulsants have already been administered. The protective action of diazepam is brief. Many clinicians administer an intramuscular dose of phenobarbital, but it is uncertain whether, given the pharmacokinetics, this is an effective measure.

Paraldehyde may be administered rectally (1 mL per year of age; not to exceed 5 mL regardless of age). Where respiratory support is available, a lengthy seizure can be treated with intravenous phenobarbital or with paraldehyde by intravenous drip (10 mg in 100 mL of solution, slowly over 10 to 20 minutes). In rare instances, short-acting barbiturates or volatile anesthetics may be required and are best administered by an anesthesiologist.

As soon as the seizure is controlled and the child's condition stable, a search for the cause of the fever should be undertaken.

The Workup

If the convulsion was brief, nonrepetitive, and nonfocal, if it occurred early in an infectious illness and with high fever, and if the child awakens alert and free of fresh neurologic findings after the seizure, then a simple workup and further observation is usually all that is required (Gerber and Berliner 1981, Heijbel et al 1980, Jaffe et al 1981, Wolf 1978). In that situation, the investigation can focus on finding a cause for the fever, rather than finding a cause for the seizure. The need for a blood count and urinalysis can be judged on the basis of their utility in diagnosing the cause of the fever. Even if these conditions are met, if the child is less than 1 year old or if close and intelligent observation cannot be confidently expected, many clinicians will choose to perform a lumbar puncture to exclude the possibility of meningitis. Other investigations have an extremely low yield, and skull x-rays virtually none (Nealis et al 1977) in this situation.

If the clinical circumstances of the seizure are different from those cited, it is necessary to rule out any condition that might require prompt and specific treatment. The most immediate concern is to rule out bacterial meningitis or other intracranial infection. Even a child with a history of previous febrile seizures must be reevaluated at any new episodes for possible meningitis. Electrolyte disturbances, intoxication, trauma, and a host of infrequent but serious disorders such as the hemolytic-uremic syndrome, septic embolization, lead intoxication, and so on, also require consideration. In more complex clinical situations, the investigation must obviously be tailored to the individual case.

A lumbar puncture will usually be appropriate when the history and physical examination depart from the reassuring situation outlined previously, especially if the child is younger than 1 year. Lumbar puncture is always indicated, whether or not there has been a seizure, if any clinical sign suggestive of meningitis is present. Performed on a well-immobilized child free from increased intracranial pressure, lumbar puncture is in general a safe procedure. However, in the bacteremic infant, lumbar puncture can in a small proportion of cases introduce bacteria into the spinal fluid and *produce* meningitis (Teele et al 1981). Repeated convulsions may be capable of producing some spinal fluid pleocytosis even in the absence of infection (Schmidley and Simon 1981). In addition, early in the course of meningitis, an infected spinal fluid may not yet exhibit pleocytosis or changes in protein or glucose content, so that false reassurance can be derived from a lumbar puncture performed early in the course (Lorber and Sunderland 1980). Therefore performance of a lumbar puncture in a highly febrile young infant does not eliminate the need for careful follow-up.

If the seizure was focal and especially if new neurologic signs should be present, EEG and skull radiography or scanning may be helpful in ruling out underlying structural pathology. Electroencephalography must be delayed for 7 to 10 days following the seizure and resolution of the fever, or false localization, usually to an occipital area, is possible.

The examination most helpful in deciding whether serious disease is present after a febrile seizure is the *second clinical evaluation*, performed 1 to 4 hours following the initial examination. An observation area in the office or clinic, or an overnight observation unit in the hospital, is invaluable as a place for the child to be watched until his clinical status can be confidently evaluated, where his parents can calm down from the distress of the events surrounding the convulsion, and where the initial discussion with the parents can take place. Because febrile seizures are the most common cause of seizures with fever in young children and because the outcome of these is usually benign, well-grounded reassurance will usually be possible at the time of discharge from such a unit, despite what is often a stormy and anxiety-provoking circumstance on admission some hours earlier. Parents not familiar with febrile seizures often think during the seizure and the postictal period that their child is dying (Baumer et al 1981). Observation for a time for the child in an observation unit allowing the physician an opportunity to watch the child rouse and giving an opportunity also for the initial discussion with the medical attendant can be very important to the parents. Admission to the hospital, on the other hand, should be reserved for children suspected of having a serious underlying illness, because children with febrile seizures usually have viral illnesses that are a potential source of infection for other patients and because hospitalization increases the likelihood of unnecessary testing (Surpure 1980).

PROPHYLACTIC TREATMENT

Once the acute illness is over, it is necessary to decide whether or not to undertake prophylactic treatment for febrile seizures, either intermittent (at the time of febrile illness) or chronic. As will be discussed, chronic treatment with anticonvulsant medications can produce undesirable side effects in young children. Ideally it would be preferable in at least some regards to limit drug exposure to the period during which children are actually at risk for recurrences of febrile seizures, which is in the early hours of acute febrile illness.

Agents to Reduce Fever

It is reasonable to ask whether, if an abrupt rise in body temperature could be prevented, the seizure could be prevented. Two studies have evaluated the effectiveness of such antipyretic measures as tepid sponging and aspirin administration in the prevention of recurrences of febrile seizures. Antipyretic agents given alone (Camfield et al 1980) or with 30 mg phenobarbital (Masala et al 1980) as soon as fever was noted did not appear to protect against the recurrence of febrile seizures. These observations suggest that antipyretic measures cannot be relied on to prevent febrile seizures, but it remains prudent to counsel parents against overdressing (the common practice of bundling) the small child who is becoming ill in excessively warm garments or blankets. Beyond that, the clinician will probably want to control a fever below some upper limit. Two questions arise. What antipyretic agents should be used? What degree of temperature control should be sought?

Aspirin and acetaminophen are roughly comparable in antipyretic efficacy, although they differ somewhat in pharmacokinetics. Wilson (1981) has discussed the theoretical trade-off of the use of these agents, but for the present there is little definite evidence that one is better than the other for general use in control of fever in young children. No strong recommendation can be made that fever should be permitted to rise to any specifiable level but not higher. However, most clinicians seek to keep the body temperature below 102 °F. Fever serves a biological function in the control of at least some infectious illnesses (Kluger 1980), and the goal should probably be to limit, but not eliminate, hyperpyrexia.

Anticonvulsant Medications for Intermittent Prophylaxis

Administration of phenobarbital in the usual 3–5 mg/kg doses at the time of acute feverish illness does not prevent febrile seizures because considerable time is required to achieve a stable therapeutic blood level. Pharmacokinetic considerations (Porter 1981) make this conclusion apparent, and clinical studies provide empirical substantiation (Wolf et al 1977). Although many physicians still recommend oral phenobarbital at times of illness, this approach may be more useful in reassuring parents and physicians than in preventing recurrences.

Phenobarbital could be used in a loading dosage, but it is difficult to be enthusiastic about that approach because of the potential danger of oversedation and respiratory depression in ill children.

The rapidly absorbed anticonvulsant medication diazepam does produce therapeutic levels of anticonvulsant medication within minutes (Dulac et al 1978, Keinanen-Kiukaanniemi et al 1979, Munthe-Kaas 1980). There is individual variation in the absorption of diazepam per rectum, although clinical effect was not clearly related to blood drug level (Kanto et al 1980). Knudsen (1979) admitted to the hospital 317 children who had febrile seizures and returned with a new episode of fever (38.5 °C) and treated them with rectal diazepam. No case of sigificant respiratory depression or other serious side effects was observed, even after repeated doses of diazepam. However, sedation was common, and for one of the three children who developed meningitis in this illness, "the possibility cannot be excluded that establishment of the diagnosis was delayed a few hours" (Knudsen 1979). Knudsen stressed the need for very careful instruction of the parents if diazepam is administered in the home, especially if the child is under concurrent treatment with phenobarbital.

Hoppu and Santavuori (1981) evaluated home therapy with diazeam rectal solution, in epileptic children subject to prolonged seizures. Presumably most or all of these children were on regular daily anticonvulsant medication as well. In 65 usages in 17 children, there was one episode of "temporary difficulty in breathing," and in another case there was "brief, respiratory arrest necessitating assisted ventilation for a few minutes." The doses in these cases were not large (0.5–0.6 mg/kg).

Thorn (1981) compared rectal administration of diazepam at the onset of illness with continuous treatment with phenobarbital in the prevention of recurrent febrile seizures. Both approaches did reduce recurrent attacks. With the intermittent treatment, parents sometimes did not recognize that illness was present until the seizure occurred. However, overall, more recurrences took place in children on continuous phenobarbital therapy because compliance failure was so common with the latter approach. Empirically, then, the intermittent approach with diazepam was associated with fewer recurrences than chronic treatment with phenobarbital; failure to recognize illness early, although it did occur, was less often a problem than compliance failure.

Another European investigator has suggested that diazepam, given by mouth at the onset of feverish illnesses can prevent febrile seizures (Dianese 1979 and 1980).

Intermittent prophylaxis with oral or rectal valproate (Depakene syrup) might also be feasible because valproate is rapidly absrobed. Because dilution of the syrup to reach the dosage appropriate for very young children has been associated with errors in mixing and dosing (Wallace 1981), valproate might best be administered in a preparation better suited to this age group, such as a lower dosage syrup or a rectal suppository. The availability of a safe and convenient dispenser capable of delivering a measured rectal dose, or a rectal suppository, would facilitate testing of rectal administration of diazepam and valproate for this purpose in an American population.

The rectal route to intermittent prophylaxis may have some advantages in acutely ill children because feverish babies often vomit, and absorption by the rectal route may be more reliable. However, as Addy (1981) remarks, "the prospect of a family being ruled by the thermometer and of children being subjected to rectal injection whenever the mercury passes a particular mark cannot be viewed entirely with equanimity."

Further evaluation of the safety and efficacy of intermittent home treatment, orally or rectally, with diazepam or valproate is required before this approach can be recommended for general use.

Termination of a Seizure Once It Has Begun, or Prevention of Immediate Recurrence

If, as is generally accepted, seizure duration beyond some still incompletely defined limit is associated with risks to the child, then optimal means for the safe termination of seizures is important in secondary prevention. Lengthy seizures seen in a hospital or clinic setting are treated as status epilepticus, by means that require the presence of special facilities and personnel. If rapidly absorbed and safe agents can be shown to be safe and effective for terminating ongoing seizures at home, they might be used once a seizure begins, or they might also be used after even a brief and self-limited seizure, to ensure against immediate recurrence.

It is now fairly common for British and European journals to recommend the prescription of rectal diazepam for administration by parents in the home, using the regular parental solution administered with disposable syringes (Bacon et al 1981a, van der Berg 1974) or, in some countries, specially packaged rectal suppositories of diazepam (Thorn 1981).

Both valproate and diazepam have been used in small series for the termination of ongoing seizures. Knudsen (1979) found rectal diazepam, administered in solution, to be effective if the seizure had been in process 15 minutes or less, and less effective if seizures were more prolonged before treatment was begun. Rectal valproate or valproic acid have been found in very small series to produce serum levels comparable to those following oral administration (Cloyd and Kriel 1981) and to be effective in controlling status epilepticus (Thorpy 1980, Vajda 1978).

Further development and testing of rapidly absorbable agents safe enough for administration at home might enable some families to treat any seizure that occurs near the time of its onset and to forestall lengthy or repetitive convulsions.

Anticonvulsant Agents for Chronic Prophylaxis

There has been considerable controversy concerning the optimal approach to the chronic management of children who have had one or more febrile seizures. Two of the most popular standard textbooks of pediatrics give opposite advice, one counseling daily anticonvulsant therapy for all such children, one recommending treatment only if nonfebrile seizures supervene. The advent of cohort studies, with the reassurance these have provided as to the relative benignity of febrile seizures, has permitted many clinicians to conclude that many or most children may not require treatment. However, there is not yet general agreement as to just whom, if anyone, to treat. Part of the remaining problem is the fact that predictors of recurrence of febrile seizures are, in the main, different characteristics than factors predictive of eventual epilepsy. Because it has never been demonstrated that chronic prophylaxis can prevent eventual epilepsy, some clinicians might conclude that treatment, if prescribed, should be aimed chiefly at the prevention of recurrences. If this is the approach chosen, then the most rational course might be treatment only of children whose initial seizure occurred at an early age, as early age of onset is the only well-established predictor of recurrence.

However, it has not been demonstrated that chronic prophylaxis *cannot* lessen the likelihood of eventual epilepsy; and almost all the recent recommendations for treatment have included advice to treat children with the risk factors for epilepsy. It would obviously be desirable to know that an often-troublesome treatment (see later), if prescribed, is capable of achieving the intended goal. The wait for such data may be long indeed, however, as the sample size and duration of follow-up that would be required for a clinical trial addressing this question would make such an undertaking extremely expensive (Ellenberg and Nelson 1981). We know of no such trial on the horizon.

TREATMENT REGIMENS FOR PREVENTION OF RECURRENCES

This section concerns medical treatment regimens that have been evaluated for their efficacy and safety in the prevention of recurrences of febrile seizures. Efficacy will be discussed first, and complications of treatment will follow.

Efficacy in the Prevention of Recurrences

A number of studies attest the effectiveness of daily administration of phenobarbital in reducing the risk of recurrent febrile seizures (Camfield et al 1980, Faerø et al 1972, Knudsen and Vestermark 1978, Monaco et al 1980, Ngwane and Bower 1980, Pilgaard et al 1981, Thorn 1975, Wolf et al 1977). In children with adequate blood levels, the rate of recurrences has been halved or even further reduced. The reduced risk of recurrences has been noted whether the initial seizure was simple or lengthy or focal. A dose of 3 to 5 mg/kg is usually employed, in a once or twice per day regimen. A blood level of 15–16 μg/mL is the goal (although that goal is often not reached, as will be discussed later). Only a small proportion of children have recurrences with phenobarbital levels above 20 μg/mL.

Primidone, in a dosage of 15–20 mg/kg per day in two divided doses, has been reported to be similar to phenobarbital in control of recurrent febrile seizures (Minagawa et al 1980). Phenytoin is apparently ineffective in the usual dosages (Bacon et al 1981b, Millichap 1968, Monaco et al 1980).

Carbamazepine, 20 mg/kg (Monaco et al 1980) or at a blood level of 0.4 to 0.7 mg/dL (Camfield et al 1981) has not prevented recurrences of febrile seizures.

Several groups have reported that valproate is effective in febrile seizures (Minagawa and Miura 1981, Ngwane and Bower 1980, Wallace and Smith 1980, Williams et al 1979), with a suggestion that a three-a-day dose schedule is more useful than bid. Dosages of 20–25 and 30–60 mg/kg/day have been employed.

Although valproate and primidone are alternatives to phenobarbital, experience with phenobarbital is larger than with any other agent in the therapy of febrile seizures.

Medical Complications of Anticonvulsant Therapy

Wilson (1981b) has summarized the major adverse somatic effects of phenobarbital and valproate, the two agents most likely to be considered in the treatment of febrile seizures.

Skin rashes that can progress to exfoliative dermatitis and interference, via enzyme induction, with the action of hormone medications are occasional problems with phenobarbital. In a controversial paper (Gold et al 1978), phenobarbital has been implicated in the development of brain tumors in children. In experimental work of unknown clinical relevance, phenobarbital is a promotor of chemically induced cancer (Wilson 1981b), and early exposure to phenobarbital apparently causes long-term (possibly permanent) alterations in metabolism of carcinogenic substances (Faris and Campbell 1981).

Early exposure to phenobarbital has produced permanent alterations in hormone production and permanent reproductive dysfunction in rats, both male and female (Gupta et al 1980ab). In humans, boys aged 15 to 24 months treated with 5 mg/kg of phenobarbital for febrile seizures showed alteration of basal and stimulated secretion of gonadotrophin and prolactin, apparently due to alteration of pituitary responsiveness to gonadotrophin-releasing hormone (Masala et al 1980). Eventual reproductive function in humans exposed early in life to phenobarbital has not, to our knowledge, been investigated.

Anticonvulsant doses of phenobarbital in rats is associated with reduction in total brain weight (Diaz and Schain 1978) and, in tissue culture, reduces enzyme markers of neuronal development (Bergey et al 1981).

Valproate has been associated with fulminant, and sometimes fatal, hepatic failure and acute pancreatitis (Bergey et al 1981, Browne 1980). Lesser complications include hair loss, weight gain, gastrointestinal discomfort, and platelet dysfunction. Given to young experimental animals, valproate has been reported to inhibit brain growth (Diaz and Shields 1981).

In summary, clinically recognized medical problems with phenobarbital are uncommon. Whether the experimental observations of long-term alterations in sexual function or tumor susceptibility can be documented in human populations is a question for future research. Most of the problems with valproate are minor, but the low level risk of catastrophe, and the fact that the drug is new enough to some of its side effects to be still unknown, must give pause to the practitioner who is considering use of this drug in young children with a usually benign disorder.

Psychological Side Effects

Anecdotal reports of behavioral alterations in children treated with phenobarbital are very familiar to clinicians. Objective study of such alterations has presented difficulties related, in part, to the absence of a testing instrument that spans the spectrum of ages at which children are treated for febrile seizures. Two or three years, while not a long time in adult terms, covers a huge range of changes in normal learning and behavior in young children. Reviews on psychological effects, chiefly of anticonvulsants, are available (Hirtz 1981, Stores 1981, Trimble and Corbett 1980, Trimble and Reynolds 1976). Most studies of behavioral changes with phenobarbital have shown alterations in activity, irritability, and sleep pattern in young children, with a frequency of hyperactivity as high as 40% (Wolf and Forsythe 1978). There is a peculiar quality of behavioral change in some children, poorly captured by most descriptions in print, that can perhaps best be characterized as "meanness," or as a dysinhibition of some behavior that is easier for the unmedicated child to restrain. Some of the effect is transient, resolving if parents tolerate continuation of treatment or if the dose is decreased and thereafter gradually returned to its previous level (Bacon et al 1981ab, Hellstrom and Barlach-Christoffersen 1980). However, there are probably persisting changes in at least some children who continue to take phenobarbital. Valproate is probably associated with less disturbance of behavior but is even less well studied in this regard.

Whether there are cognitive alterations with phenobarbital has been controversial, and their study has been compounded by methodological problems (Camfield et al 1980, Wolf et al 1981). In adults, there is a dose-related reduction in intellectual efficiency within the clinical dosage range with phenobarbital (Hutt et al 1968, Trimble and Reynolds 1976). Studies in children are not yet conclusive, and effects, if any, must be fairly subtle. However, *if* subtle effects can be shown to be present, they must be taken very seriously, because they could easily be cumulative (Stores 1981).

Studies to describe the nature and time course of behavioral and cognitive alterations with anticonvulsant agents are underway at a number of centers, and information on this subject is likely to increase.

Practical Problems

Although daily treatment with phenobarbital or valproate can reduce the frequency of recurrences if either is given regularly, it is general experience that often it is not administered reliably in long-term use.

Prior to the initiation of strong efforts to encourage the regular administration of medication, Wolf and co-workers (1977) found only 13% of the children to have a blood level of phenobarbital above 15 μg/mL; and 3 weeks after the initiation of treatment, Wallace (1981) found fewer than one-half to be still taking the original treatment. Even in a study that aimed for a level of 10 μg/mL of phenobarbital, Camfield and co-workers (1980) found that, despite their careful follow-up efforts, 30% of the children were below that level. Wolf (1977) stated that to achieve good cooperation required "intense persuasion, close follow-up, repeated testing, and many evening and weekend calls." With lesser input of physician energy, lower rates of compliance follow. One reason for the poor cooperation by parents is probably the fact that many stop worrying about the child once, after the seizure, they find the youngster looking well again. Some parents express anxiety about the possibility of addiction to barbiturate. Some forget, and some are probably troubled by the inconvenience and expense of medical follow-up and blood testing. A substantial share of the poor compliance is apparently related to the changes in behavior the child may exhibit while on phenobarbital, such as irritability and sleep disturbance.

Treatment with valproate is expensive (Goldberg 1981), and was in one study less often accepted by parents than phenobarbital despite the lesser rate of behavioral side effects (Wallace 1981).

Thus, the clinician who seeks to maintain compliance must devote considerable energy to monitoring blood levels and to persuading parents to continue treatment despite the child's apparent well-being without treatment and often in the presence of troubling side effects when on medication.

Consensus Meeting on Management
of Children with Febrile Seizures

A Consensus Development Conference on Febrile Seizures was held at the National Institutes of Health on May 19–21, 1980. The purpose of the Conference was to bring together practicing physicians, research scientists, consumers, and others in an effort to reach general agreement on the risks of sequelae in children with febrile seizures and to compare them with the potenital risks and benefits of prophylaxis with anticonvulsants.

The members of the Consensus Development Panel represented the disciplines involved with treatment and evaluation of management of children with febrile seizures. The physicians were nominated for their role on the panel by four speciality medical associations: the American Academy of Pediatrics, the American Academy of Neurology, the American Academy of Family Physicians, and the Child Neurology Society. The panel met following the formal presentations and discussions to examine and debate the issues based on the evidence presented. A summary was prepared as the result of these deliberations. A portion of the summary was as follows:

> A rational approach to the management of febrile seizures should take into account that the long-term prognosis is excellent, that prophylaxis reduces the risk of subsequent febrile seizures, and that there is no evidence that prophylaxis reduces the risk of subsequent nonfebrile seizures.

> An initial workup of febrile seizures should include a complete history and complete pediatric and neurological examination, including characterization of the febrile illness, degree of temperature elevation, and complete description of the febrile seizure. If a CNS infection is suspected, a lumbar puncture is indicated.

> The role of the electroencephalogram (EEG) in the workup of febrile seizures remains controversial. Abnormal EEGs do not reliably predict the development of epilepsy in patients with febrile convulsions.

> Other studies, such as a complete blood count, measurement of levels of serum electrolytes, calcium, and glucose in the blood, and skull x-rays or computerized (CT) scanning of the brain are rarely useful in the uncomplicated febrile seizure.

Febrile convulsions rarely presage complex partial seizures or other forms of epilepsy and are generally benign and self-limited.

Anticonvulsant prophylaxis in therapeutic levels may be considered under any of the following conditions:
a) In the presence of abnormal neurological development (eg, cerebral palsy syndromes, mental retardation, microcephaly).
b) When a febrile seizure is:
   1. longer than 15 minutes; or
   2. focal; or
   3. followed by transient or persistent neurological abnormalities.
c) History of nonfebrile seizures of genetic origin in a parent or sibling.

The physician occasionally may elect, in certain selected cases, to provide an anticonvulsant treatment when a patient has multiple febrile seizures or when seizures occur in an infant under the age of 12 months.

When anticonvulsant prophylaxis is instituted, it is usually continued for at least 2 years or 1 year after the last seizure, whichever is the longer period of time. Discontinuation of therapy should be done slowly over a 1- to 2-month period.

Parents and others who are responsible in the care of young children play a key role in the prevention and management of febrile seizures. Family education and counseling should address:

• the relatively benign nature of febrile seizures;
• the recognition of and management of fever;
• the use of antipyretic agents;
• medication and compliance;
• side effects of medication;
• first aid for a seizure; and
• when and how to seek emergency assistance, if needed.

Educational materials may be an effective means to complement the physician's efforts toward family education.

Since nurses and allied health professionals, health educators, and social workers are important in family education and counseling, they should receive adequate information in the management of febrile seizures.

Efforts should also be directed to disseminating this knowledge to the public, including day care centers, through mass media and other means.

CONCLUSIONS

Febrile seizures are common, and the majority of children who experience them do well, whether or not they have recurrences. Subgroups whose prognosis differ from the overall group have been recognized, based upon family seizure history, neurologic well-being before the first seizure, and characteristics of the first seizure. Further delineation of subgroups with different outlooks may in the future improve our ability to offer more accurate prognoses.

Most febrile seizures are brief, and most are due to infectious illnesses that are readily recognized. Management of the child with febrile seizures involves safe and rapid termination of the seizure or seizures. For the child whose underlying illness poses a direct or indirect threat to his/her neurologic integrity (via infectious,

194

metabolic, or toxic means), diagnostic and therapeutic measures must be mobilized promptly and intelligently. Following the initial febrile seizure, there must be a discussion with the parents concerning what has happened, and its implications (if any) for the future. Parents and other caretakers should be informed of what to do in the event of a seizure in this child or his sibling, and how to reach competent medical attention quickly.

In deciding whether or not to prescribe long-term anticonvulsant medication, clinicians should recognize that the majority of parents, even if they initiate treatment, will not continue it at therapeutic levels without energetic and continuing urging from the physician. The balance of risks and benefits from daily administration of anticonvulsant agents is not known, and the only benefit established is a lowering of the risk of recurrent febrile seizures. It is not known whether treatment can alter the already low risk of later epilepsy. Given the uncertainties of long-term benefit and some possibility, in young children, of long-term risk from medication, there is wisdom in Addy's (1981) advice: "Epilepsy should not be treated until it occurs."

BIBLIOGRAPHY

Addy DP: Prophylaxis and febrile convulsions. *Arch Dis Child* 1981;56:81–83.

Aicardi J, Chevrie JJ: Febrile convulsions: Neurological sequelae and mental retardation, in Brazier MAB, Coceani F (eds): *Brain Dysfunction in Infantile Febrile Convulsions*. New York, Raven Press, 1976, pp 247–257.

Annegers JF, Hauser WA, Anderson VE, et al: The risks of seizure disorders among relatives of patients with childhood onset epilepsy. *Neurology* 1982;32:174–179.

Annegers JF, Hauser WA, Elveback LR, et al: The risk of epilepsy following febrile convulsions. *Neurology* 1979;29:297–303.

Asirifi Y: Aetiology of cerebral palsy in developing countries. *Dev Med Child Neurol* 1972; 14:230–232.

Bacon CJ, Cranage JD, Hierons AM, et al: Behavioural effects of phenobarbitone and phenytoin in small children. *Arch Dis Child* 1981a;56:836–840.

Bacon CJ, Mucklow JC, Rawlins MD, et al: Placebo-controlled study of phenobarbitone and phenytoin in the prophylaxis of febrile convulsions. *Lancet* September 19, 1981;2: 600–604.

Baumer JH, David TJ, Valentine SJ, et al: Many parents think their child is dying when having a first febrile convulsion. *Dev Med Child Neurol* 1981;23:462–464.

Bergey GK, Swaiman KF, Schrier BK, et al: Adverse effects of phenobarbital on morphological and biochemical development of fetal mouse spinal cord neurons in culture. *Ann Neurol* 1981;9:584–589.

Browne TR: Valproic acid. *N Engl J Med* 1980;302:661–666.

Camfield PR, Camfield CS, Tibbles JAR: Ineffectiveness of carbamazepine for febrile seizure patients requiring prophylaxis but intolerant to or uncontrolled by phenobarbital, presented at the annual meeting of the Child Neurology Society, Halifax, Nova Scotia, 1981.

Camfield CS, Chaplin S, Doyle A-B, et al: Side effects of phenobarbital in toddlers: Behavioral and cognitive aspects. *J Pediatrics* 1980;95:361–365.

Camfield PR, Camfield CS, Shapiro SH, et al: The first febrile seizure-antipyretic instruction plus either phenobarbital or placebo to prevent recurrence. *J Pediatrics* 1980;97:16–21.

Cloyd JC, Kriel RL: Bioavailability of rectally administered valproic acid syrup. *Neurology* 1981;31:1348–1352.

Consenusus Development Panel: Febrile seizures: Long-term management of children with fever-associated seizures. *Pediatrics* 1980;66:1009–1012.

Cordelli F, Banaudi P: Febrile seizures and ketotic hypoglycemia-possible relationships (Italian). *Pediatr Med Chir* 1980;4:505–511.

Dianese G: Prophylactic diazepam in febrile convulsions. *Arch Dis Child* 1979;54:244–245.

Dianese G: Treatment of the febrile seizures. *J Pediatrics* 1980;96:516–517.

Diaz J, Schain RJ: Phenobarbital—Effects of long-term administration on behavior and brain of artificially reared rats. *Science* 1978;199:90–91.

Diaz J, Shields D: Effects of dipropylacetate on brain development. *Ann Neurol* 1981;10: 465–468.

Dulac O, Aicardi J, Rey E, et al: Blood levels of diazepam after single rectal administration in infants and children. *J Pediatrics* 1978;93:1039–1041.

Ellenberg JH, Nelson KB: Febrile seizures and later intellectual performance. *Arch Neurol* 1978;35:17–21.

Ellenberg JH, Nelson KB: Sample selection and the natural history of disease. *JAMA* 1980; 243:1337–1340.

Ellenberg JH, Nelson KB: Long-term clinical trials on the use of prophylaxis for prevention of recurrences of febrile seizures and epilepsy, in Nelson KB, Ellenberg JH (eds): *Febrile Seizures.* New York, Raven Press, 1981, pp 267–278.

Faerø O, Kastrup K, Nielson E, et al: Successful prophylaxis of febrile convulsions with phenobarbital. *Epilepsia* 1972;13:279–285.

Falconer MA, Serafetinides EA, Corsellis JA: Etiology and pathogenesis of temporal lobe epilepsy. *Arch Neurol* 1964;10:233–243.

Faris RA, Campbell, TC: Exposure of newborn rats to pharmacologically active compounds may permanently alter carcinogen metabolism. *Science* 1981;211:719–721.

Frantzen E, Lennox-Buchthal M, Nygaard A: Longitudinal EEG and clinical study of children with febrile convulsions. *Electroencephalogr Clin Neurophysiol* 1968;24:197–212.

Frantzen E, Lennox-Buchthal M, Nygaard A, et al: A genetic study of febrile convulsions. *Neurology* 1970;20:909–917.

Gerber MA, Berliner BC: The child with a "simple" febrile seizure; appropriate diagnostic evaluation. *Am J Dis Child* 1981;135:431–433.

Glickman LT, Cypess RH, Crumrine PK, et al: *Toxocara* infection and epilepsy in children. *J Pediatrics* 1979;94:75–78.

Gold E, Gordis L, Tonascia J, et al: Increased risk of brain tumors in children exposed to barbiturates. *J Natl Cancer Inst* 1978;61:1031–1034.

Goldberg MA: Costs of anticonvulsant therapy. *Ann Neurol* 1981;9:95.

Gupta C, Shapiro BH, Yaffe SJ: Reproductive dysfunction in male rats following prenatal exposure to phenobarbital. *Pediatr Pharmacol* 1980a;1:55–62.

Gupta C, Sonawane BR, Yaffe SJ, et al: Phenobarbital exposure in utero: Alterations in female reproductive function in rats. *Science* 1980b;208:508–510.

Hauser WA: The natural history of febrile seizures, in Nelson KB, Ellenberg JH (eds): *Febrile Seizures.* New York, Raven Press, 1981, pp 5–17.

Hauser WA, Kurland LT: The epidemiology of epilepsy in Rochester, Minnesota, 1935 through 1967. *Epilepsia* 1975;16:1–66.

Heijbel J, Blom S, Bergfors PG: Simple febrile convulsions. A prospective incidence study and an evaluation of investigations initially needed. *Neuropaediatrie* 1980;11:45–56.

Hellstrom B, Barlach-Christoffersen M: Influence of phenobarbital on the psychomotor development and behavior in preschool children with convulsions. *Neuropaediatrie* 1980; 11:151–160.

Hirtz DG: Effects of treatment for prevention of febrile seizure recurrence on behavioral and cognitive function, in Nelson KB, Ellenberg JH (eds): *Febrile Seizures.* New York, Raven Press, 1981, pp 193–202.

Hoppu K, Santavuori P: Diazepam rectal solution for home treatment of acute seizures in children. *Acta Paediatr Scand* 1981;70:369–372.

Hutt SJ, Jackson PM, Belsham A, et al: Perceptual-motor behaviour in relation to blood phenobarbitone level: A preliminary report. *Dev Med Child Neurol* 1968;10:626–632.

Iannetti P, Fiorilli M, Sirianni MC, et al: Nonfebrile seizures after febrile convulsions: Possible role of chronic cytomegalovirus infection. *J Pediatrics* 1982;101:27–31.

Jaffe M, Bar-Joseph G, Tirosh E: Fever and convulsions—Indications for laboratory investigations. *Pediatrics* 1981;67:729–731.

Kagawa K: A genetic study of febrile convulsions (Japanese), translated in *Epilepsy Abstracts*. *Brain Dev* 1975;5:369–384.

Kajitani T, Ueoka K, Nakamura M, et al: Febrile convulsions and rolandic discharges. *Brain Dev* 1981;3:351–359.

Kanto J, Iisalo E, Kangas L, et al: A comparative study on the clinical effects of rectal diazepam and pentobarbital on small children. Relationship between plasma level and effect. *Int J Clin Pharmacol Therapy Toxicol* 1980;18:348–351.

Keinanen-Kiukaanniemi S, Simila S, Luoma P, et al: Antipyretic effect and plasma concentrations of rectal acetaminophen and diazepam in children. *Epilepsia* 1979;20:607–612.

Kluger MJ: Fever. *Pediatrics* 1980;66:720–724.

Knudsen FU: Rectal administration of diazepam in solution in the acute treatment of convulsions in infants and children. Anticonvulsant effect and side effects. *Arch Dis Child* 1979;54:855–857.

Knudsen FU, Vestermark S: Prophylactic diazepam or phenobarbitone in febrile convulsions: A prospective, controlled study. *Arch Dis Child* 1978;53:660–663.

Lee K, Diaz M, Melchior JC: Temporal lobe epilepsy—Not a consequence of childhood febrile convulsions in Denmark. *Acta Neurol Scand* 1981;63:231–236.

Lennox-Buchthal M: Febrile and nocturnal convulsions in monozygotic twins. *Epilepsia* 1971; 12:147–156.

Lennox-Buchthal MA: Febrile convulsions: A reappraisal. *Electroencephalogr Clin Neurophysiol* 1973;32(suppl):1–138.

Leviton A, Cowan LD: Do febrile seizures increase the risk of complex partial seizures? An epidemiologic assessment, in Nelson KB, Ellenberg JH (eds): *Febrile Seizures*. New York, Raven Press, 1981, pp 65–74.

Lewis HM, Parry JV, Parry RP, et al: Role of viruses in febrile convulsions. *Arch Dis Child* 1979;54:869–876.

Lorber J, Sunderland R: Lumbar puncture in children with convulsions associated with fever. *Lancet* 1980;1:785–786.

Masala A, Meloni T, Alagna S, et al: Pituitary responsiveness to gonadotrophin-releasing and thyrotrophin-releasing hormones in children receiving phenobarbitone. *Br Med J* 1980;281:1175–1177.

Millichap JG: *Febrile Convulsions*. New York, Macmillan Company, 1968.

Minagawa K, Miura H: Phenobarbital, primidone and sodium valproate in the prophylaxis of febrile convulsions. *Brain Dev* 1981;3:385–393.

Minagawa K, Miura H, Kaneko T, et al: Effectiveness of daily primidone for the prevention of febrile convulsions: A further study (Japanese). *Brain Dev* 1980;4:287–296.

Monaco F, Sechi GP, Mutani R, et al: Lack of efficacy of carbamazepine in preventing the recurrence of febrile convulsions, in Johannessen SI, Morselli PL, Pippenger CE, et al: *Antiepileptic Therapy: Advances in Drug Monitoring*. New York, Raven Press, 1980, pp 75–79.

Munthe-Kaas AW: Rectal administration of diazepam: Theoretical basis and clinical experience, in Johannessen SI, Morselli PL, Pippenger CE, et al: *Antiepileptic Therapy: Advances in Drug Monitoring*. New York, Raven Press, 1980, pp 381–389.

Nealis JGT, Depiero TJ, Rosman NP: The effect of diphenhydramine (Benadryl) and phenobarbital on experimental febrile convulsions. *Neurology* 1976;26:393–394.

Nealis JGT, McFadden SW, Asnes RA, et al: Routine skull roentgenograms in the management of simple febrile seizures. *J Pediatr* 1977;90:595–596.

Nelson KB, Ellenberg JH: Predictors of epilepsy in children who have experienced febrile seizures. *N Engl J Med* 1976;295:1029–1033.

Nelson KB, Ellenberg JH: Prognosis in children with febrile seizures. *Pediatrics* 1978;61:720–727.

Nelson KB, Ellenberg JH: The role of recurrences in determining outcome in children with febrile seizures, in Nelson KB, Ellenberg JH (eds): *Febrile Seizures*. New York, Raven Press, 1981, pp 19–25.

Ngwane E, Bower B: Continuous sodium valproate or phenobarbitone in the prevention of "simple" febrile convulsions. *Arch Dis Child* 1980;55:171–174.

Ounsted C, Lindsay J, Norman R: *Biological Factors in Temporal Lobe Epilepsy*. Suffolk, England, The Lavenham Press Ltd, 1966.

Pilgaard S, Hansen FJ, Paerregaard P: Prophylaxis against febrile convulsions with phenobarbital. A 3-year prospective investigation. *Acta Paediatr Scand* 1981;70:67–71.

Porter RJ: Pharmacokinetic basis of intermittent and chronic anticonvulsant drug therapy, in Nelson KB, Ellenberg JH (eds): *Febrile Seizures*. New York, Raven Press, 1981, pp 107–118.

Ross EM, Peckham CS, West PB, et al: Epilepsy in childhood: Findings from the National Child Development Study. *Br Med J* 1980;281:207–210.

Rossiter EJR, Hallowes R, Pearson RD: Developmental assessment of children who had one or more convulsive episodes. *Aust Paediatr J* 1977;13:182–186.

Sato S, Dreifuss FE, Penry JK: Prognostic factors in absence seizures. *Neurology* 1976;26:788–796.

Schiottz-Christensen E: Genetic factors in febrile convulsions. An investigation of 64 same-sexed twin pairs. *Acta Neurol Scand* 1972;48:538–546.

Schmidley JW, Simon RP: Postictal pleocytosis. *Ann Neurol* 1981;9:81–84.

Smith JA, Wallace SJ: Febrile convulsions: Intellectual progress in relation to anticonvulsant therapy and to recurrence of fits. *Arch Dis Child* 1982;57:104–107.

Stephenson JBP: Two types of febrile seizure: Anoxic (syncopal) and epileptic mechanisms differentiated by oculocardiac reflex. *Br Med J* 1978;2:726–728.

Stokes MJ, Downham MAPS, Webb JKG, et al: Viruses and febrile convulsions. *Arch Dis Child* 1977;52:129–133.

Stores G: Behavioral effects of antiepileptic drugs, in Nelson KB, Ellenberg JH (eds): *Febrile Seizures*. New York, Raven Press, 1981, pp 185–192.

Surpure JS: Febrile convulsions. *Clin Pediatr (Phila)* 1980;19:361–362.

Teele DW, Dashefsky B, Rakusan T, et al: Meningitis after lumbar puncture in children with bacteremia. *N Engl J Med* 1981;305:1079–1081.

Thorn I: A controlled study of prophylactic long-term treatment of febrile convulsions with phenobarbital. *Acta Neurol Scand* 1975;(suppl)60:67–73.

Thorn I: Prevention of recurrent febrile seizures: Intermittent prophylaxis with diazepam compared with continuous treatment with phenobarbital, in Nelson KB, Ellenberg JH (eds): *Febrile Seizures*. New York, Raven Press, 1981, pp 119–126.

Thorpy MJ: Rectal valproate syrup and status epilepticus. *Neurology* 1980;30:1113–1114.

Trimble M, Corbett J: Anticonvulsant drugs and cognitive function, in Wada JA, Penry JK (eds) *Advances in Epileptology: The Tenth Epilepsy International Symposium*. New York, Raven Press, 1980, pp 113–120.

Trimble MR, Reynolds EH: Anticonvulsant drugs and mental symptoms: A review. *Psychol Med* 1976;6:169–178.

Tsuboi T: Polygenic inheritance of epilepsy and febrile convulsions: Analysis based on a computational model. *Br J Psychiatry* 1976;129:239–242.

Vajda FJE, Mihaly GW, Miles JL, et al: Rectal administration of sodium valproate in status epilepticus. *Neurology* 1978;28:897–899.

Valman HB: Convulsions in the older infant. *Br Med J* 1980;281:1113–1114.

van den Berg BJ: Studies on convulsive disorders in young children. IV. Incidence of convulsions among siblings. *Dev Med Child Neurol* 1974;16:457–464.

van den Berg BJ, Yerushalmy J: Studies on convulsive disorders in young children. I. Incidence of febrile and nonfebrile convulsions by age and other factors. *Pediatr Res* 1969;3:298–304.

Wallace SJ: Prevention of recurrent febrile seizures using continuous prophylaxis: Sodium valproate compared with phenobarbital, in Nelson KB, Ellenberg JH (eds): *Febrile Seizures.* New York, Raven Press, 1981, pp 135–142.

Wallace SJ, Smith JA: Successful prophylaxis against febrile convulsions with valproic acid or phenobarbitone. *Br Med J* 1980;281:353–354.

Wilson JT: Observed and potential risks of anticonvulsant medications in children, in Nelson KB, Ellenberg JH (eds): *Febrile Seizures.* New York, Raven Press, 1981, pp 153–167.

Williams AJ, Evans-Jones LG, Kindley AD, et al: Sodium valproate in the prophylaxis of simple febrile convulsions. *Clin Pediatr* 1979;18:426–430.

Wolf SM: Laboratory evaluation of the child with a febrile convulsion. *Pediatrics* 1978;62:1074–1076.

Wolf SM, Carr A, Davis DC, et al: The value of phenobarbital in the child who has had a single febrile seizure: A controlled prospective study. *Pediatrics* 1977;59:378–385.

Wolf SM, Forsythe A: Behavior disturbance, phenobarbital and febrile seizures. *Pediatrics* 1978;61:728–731.

Wolf SM, Forsythe A, Stunden AA, et al: Long-term effect of phenobarbital on cognitive function in children with febrile convulsions. *Pediatrics* 1981;68:820–823.

CHAPTER **13**

Sensory Evoked Seizures

Michael E. Newmark

Sensory evoked seizures—seizures that are evoked by a specific sensory stimulus —form a small but important set of seizure disorders. Although the relevant stimuli may vary widely, patients with sensory evoked seizures (often entitled "reflex epilepsy") may be broadly classed into two subgroups. The first group consists of patients who may have attacks that are almost always evoked by a specific sensory stimulus. An example is the photic induced seizure patient, who may have attacks provoked by flickering light within a range of flash frequencies. Photosensitive individuals have reproducible seizures that are induced by a flicker stimulus and that produce well-defined electroencephalographic abnormalities (the photoparyoxysmal response). Other related, visually evoked seizures, including pattern-induced seizures, television epilepsy, and reading epilepsy are also provoked by specific sensory stimulation.

In the second group of patients with sensory evoked seizures, the sensory stimulation is not so specific. The induced seizures may be variable or may be inconstantly produced by the sensory stimulus, and seizures may occur spontaneously. Because as many as 5% to 6% of epileptic patients report that a sensory stimulus may exacerbate a seizure disorder (Servit et al 1962), this second type of sensory evoked seizure is relatively common. Before a seizure is attributed to a sensory stimulus, the following characteristics must be determined:

1. Does the seizure evoked by the stimulus have repetitive, stereotyped, clinical symptoms, or do the symptoms of the evoked seizures vary among attacks?
2. Are there consistent, diagnostic EEG patterns associated with the stimulus?
3. Do the seizures occur spontaneously?
4. Can the seizures be evoked under laboratory conditions?

If the seizure is defined using these parameters, the relationship between the sensory stimulation and the evoked seizure is best established.

In the following discussion, several sensory evoked seizures are described (Table 13-1). The visually evoked seizures, especially the photic induced attacks, will be emphasized, because the greatest amount of clinical and experimental data have been collected for these disorders. As they are the best documented, the visually evoked seizures may serve as a model for the entire group of sensory evoked seizures.

Table 13-1
Sensory Evoked Seizures

Seizure Type	Stimulus
Visually evoked	Flicker
	Television
	Pattern
	Eye closure
	Eye movement
	Reading
	Self-induced
Language-induced	Speech
	Writing
Auditory evoked	Pure sound
	Music
Startle-induced	
Movement-induced	Dystonia
	Paroxysmal choreoathetosis
	Movement-induced seizures
	Jumping Frenchmen of Maine
Miscellaneous	Vestibular
	Eating
	Decision-making
	Sex

VISUALLY EVOKED SEIZURES

Visually evoked seizures may be evoked by the following stimuli: flicker, television, pattern, reading, and eye closure. Several of the visually evoked seizures may be self-evoked, particularly by hand-waving or by watching television.

Photosensitivity

Photosensitivity may be defined as an abnormal electroencephalographic or clinical response to flickering light (Newmark and Penry 1979). The clinical manifestation of photosensitivity, the photic induced seizure, consists almost exclusively of generalized tonic-clonic, absence, or myoclonic seizures. The photomyogenic response, a specific photic induced clinical response, is not included in this definition of photosensitivity and is present primarily in nonepileptic individuals. Photosensitivity has been noted since the third century BC, when Apuleius observed that the rotations of a potter's wheel before the eyes of an epileptic person might cause a seizure (Temkin 1971). However, not until the 20th century were photic induced seizures specifically described (Goodkind 1936), and electroenceaphalographic responses to flickering light were first described in 1934 (Adrian and Matthews 1934).

Seizures produced by flicker stimulation may occur after environmental photic stimulation; they may occur after stroboscopic testing in the laboratory, or patients may merely have an electroencephalographic abnormality without a clinical response. Some patients may have a seizure only when exposed to a laboratory stroboscope under the special conditions of the laboratory. These patients form a separate group and have an excellent prognosis (Doose and Gerken, 1973).

The prevalence of photosensitivity in the general population is not known. In a retrospective study by Wadlington and Riley (1965), only 25 patients had photic induced seizures in an EEG population of 20,000. Two hundred twenty-five more individuals had photic induced electrical abnormalities without clinical seizures. Other investigators have found a higher seizure rate. Jeavons and Harding (1975) were able to obtain a series of 460 photosensitive patients of whom 332 had seizures produced by environmental, photic stimuli.

Numerous environmental stimuli have precipitated visually evoked seizures (Table 13-2). Common to these stimuli has been the sudden appearance of a bright flickering light or a brightly lit pattern. Occasionally, other seizure-inducing stimuli are present, as, for example, thunder in patients susceptible to lightning or surprise in the patients susceptible to a sudden appearance of sunlight.

Table 13-2
Visual Stimuli that Have Evoked Seizures

Stimuli	Reference
Lightning	Hishakawa et al (1967)
Headlights of cars	Hishakawa et al (1967)
Riding as a passenger in an automobile	Cobb (1947); Daly and Bickford (1951)
Driving an automobile	Livingston (1972)
Patterns of sunlight	Whitty (1960)
Red- and white-checked tablecloths	Whitty (1960)
Nonspecific quadrille patterns	Ernst (1969)
Sudden appearance of the sun or bright light	Goodkind (1936) Davidson and Watson (1956)
Flickering light or sunlight	Herrlin (1960)
The beating blades of a helicopter	Foster (1975)
Riding a bicycle in bright sunlight	Kutt et al (1963)
Walking by a picket fence	Forster and Campos (1964)
Reflections from water while swimming	Jeavons and Harding (1975)
Sunlight reflected from snow	Jeavons and Harding (1975)
Flickering artificial light	Jeavons and Harding (1975)

Environmental, photic stimuli usually cause generalized tonic-clonic seizures (Jeavons and Harding 1975, Wadlington and Riley 1965). An aura is often not present but fixed gaze or crying out (Bickford et al 1953, Wadlington and Riley 1965), a funny feeling in the eyes (Keith et al 1953), or an intense discomfort (Forster and Campos 1964) have been described. Absence seizures have also been reported and may appear abruptly or repetitively, as in a 17-year-old girl who was left dazed from her absence seizures after riding up a long avenue flanked by trees (Cobb 1947). The attacks may consist of a blank response for a few seconds (Whitty 1960), spells of eye-blinking and fogginess in thought (Davidson and Watson 1956), loss of awareness, rolling of eyes and cessation of activity without loss of posture (Brausch and Ferguson 1965), or feelings of light-headedness and blinking associated with extension of the head and neck (Brausch and Ferguson 1965). The absence seizures induced by flickering light may have prominent myoclonic components (Bertha and Lechner 1956) or may terminate with a generalized tonic-clonic seizure (Chao 1962).

Myoclonic seizures have been reported (Rao and Prichard 1955), and the myoclonus may involve the arms and legs without loss of consciousness (Jeavons 1977) or it may be severe enough to throw the patient down (Rao and Prichard 1955). It may last for several minutes with involvement of limbs, axial and facial muscles, and eyelids (Goodkind 1936). The myoclonus may be associated with changes in consciousness and begin to resemble absence attacks (Daly and Bickford 1951). As with absence seizures, the myoclonic attacks occasionally develop into generalized tonic-clonic seizures (Bickford et al 1953). Partial seizures, both elementary and complex, are rarely induced by environmental, photic stimuli. For example, only 5 of the 181 patients described by Jeavons and Harding 1975) with seizures occurring after exposure to environmental stimuli had partial seizures. The few complex partial seizures have usually consisted of visual hallucinations or nonspecific diminution of alertness.

In contrast to seizures produced by environmental stimuli, the seizures produced by laboratory stroboscopic stimuli have usually been myoclonic or, rarely, generalized tonic-clonic or absence. A photoparoxysmal response may also occur without a clinical accompaniment (Herrlin 1954), but this phenomenon may be explained by the practical technique of discontinuing photic stimulation after the beginning of an abnormal EEG response. The myoclonic seizure produced by photic stimulation must be differentiated from the clinical photomyogenic response. The photic induced myoclonic seizure has the typical photoparoxysmal EEG changes, and the myoclonus is clinically more variable and has longer latency (Bickford and Klass 1969) than the myoclonus associated with the photomyogenic response. Photic induced myoclonic seizures often involve a change in mental status and may progress to generalized tonic-clonic seizures, unlike the photomyogenic response.

Generalized tonic-clonic seizures are rarely produced by stroboscopic stimulation, primarily because of the cautious technique of most investigators. Photic induced absence seizures are frequent and have been reported in approximately one-quarter of the patients with spontaneous absence (Penry et al 1975). Although the photic induced absence may not be accompanied by motor changes, it is often accompanied by myoclonus (Bickford et al 1953), and occasional attacks may last 1 minute (Jeavons and Harding 1975). In the prolonged attacks, automatisms may appear, which may be confused with the deliberate hand movements of self-induced seizures.

The method of stroboscopic examination is quite variable. Important features of photic stimulation include the light intensity of the stroboscope, the level of background illumination, the flicker frequency, the color of the flicker stimulus, the position of the eyelids, the state of alertness of the individual, and the inclusion of pattern with the flicker stimulation. Specifically, increased light intensity of the stroboscope has been associated with photic induced abnormalities (Pantelakis et al 1962). Reduced background illumination may also enhance photosensitivity, although recently other investigators have suggested that background illumination has little significance. Flicker frequency is a major factor, as EEG abnormalities are best produced at a flash rate of 15–18 flashes per second, although several patients may respond to flicker frequencies outside this range. In the large study by Jeavons and Harding (1975), 11% of the photosensitive patients were sensitive at a flash rate of 5 flashes per second and 15% responded to a rate of 60 flashes per second. The response is loosely correlated with age, as children may respond to a wide range of flash frequencies and adults have a more specific response centering around 15 flashes per second (Newmark and Penry 1979).

The effect of eye closure on photosensitivity is unclear, although several photosensitive patients may have EEG abnormalities induced after eye closure alone (Jeavons and Harding 1975). The optimal eyelid position during photic stimulation has been widely discussed, but the open eyelid position is probably the most effective one (Panayiotopoulos 1974). The position of the eyes during stimulation is also varied, as nonmacular flicker stimulation sharply reduced the effectiveness of the stimulation (Jeavons and Harding 1975).

Other stimulation factors are also important. The impact of color of light has been widely investigated, but no color is consistently effective—although an individual patient may respond better to one or more specific hues. The combination of pattern stimulation with flicker is also controversial. Although Jeavons and Harding (1975) believe that the maximal responses are obtained with a combination of pattern and flicker stimulation, others have disputed this observation (Engel 1974, Wilkins et al 1980).

The EEG abnormality—the photoparoxysmal response—takes the form of several patterns (Table 13-3). The most significant characteristic of the photoconvulsive response for epilepsy is its duration. Spikes that persist after the conclusion of a flicker stimulus are strongly associated with seizures, whereas time-locked spikes are rarely associated with seizure activity (Reilly and Peters 1973). A generalized spike discharge that outlasts the flicker stimulus is almost diagnostic of a seizure disorder (Figure 13-1). Photic induced generalized spikes not outlasting the stimulus may be associated with clinical epilepsy, but 1% to 2% of the nonepileptic population may have this type of discharge as well. The nonepileptic individuals with this type of photic induced generalized discharge often have a strong family history of epilepsy.

Table 13-3
EEG Patterns Described as a Photoparoxysmal Response

EEG Pattern	Reference
Generalized spike-and-wave complex	Jeavons et al (1966)
Generalized multiple spike-and-wave complex	Pallis and Louis (1961); Ames (1971)
Generalized slow spike-and-wave complex	Chao (1962); Jeavons and Harding (1975)
Irregular spike-and-wave complex	Bickford et al (1953)

The use of the visual evoked response (VER) may help the analysis of photosensitivity, but the early data have not been conclusive. The VER is often abnormal in photosensitive patients but may also be abnormal in nonphotosensitive epileptic patients. The effect of antiepileptic medications on the VER is an important variable. An increased amplitude of the VER in several photosensitive patients may be related to flicker-induced occipital spikes (Hishikawa et al 1967), which has been observed in photosensitive patients (Jeavons and Harding 1975).

Several clinical factors have been associated with photosensitivity. First, female patients are more affected than males, and women outnumber men by a ratio of 3 to 4. This disparity is greatest among nonepileptic patients and patients with only photic induced seizures (Newmark and Penry 1979). In addition, age is also impor-

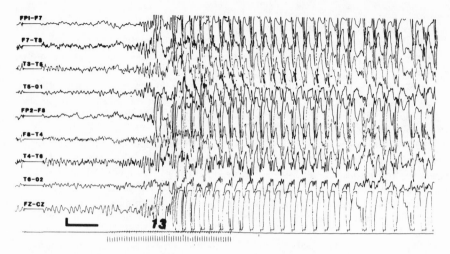

Figure 13-1 Photoparoxysmal response to a flash rate of 13 flashes per second in a 13-year-old girl.

tant. Photic induced abnormalities are almost always present in individuals below the age of 40, with the highest prevalence of abnormality in young women between the ages of 6 and 30. Children under the age of 6 are rarely photosensitive. In studies restricted to nonepileptic volunteers, photosensitivity is highest in the age group between 6 and 15, primarily among girls. The peak of prevalence of photosensitivity in these ages has not yet been explained and may be related to undisclosed maturational and endocrine factors.

Another important aspect of photosensitivity is the significance of inheritance. The frequency of photosensitivity in relatives of photosensitive patients is extremely high; as many as 40% to 50% of close relatives (siblings, parents, or offspring) may be photosensitive if the proper ages are tested (Newmark and Penry 1979). There have been several pedigrees with photosensitivity extending through three generations (Davidson and Watson 1956, Daly et al 1959). The 13 reported monozygotic twin pairs with photic induced seizures have an almost 100% concordance of EEG and seizure type. Photosensitivity is frequently present in patients with absence seizures, which may also be inherited (Newmark and Penry 1980). The possibilities of two separate genes or a single disorder with multiple manifestations must thus be raised. However, Doose et al (1973) have suggested that the inheritance of the paroxysmal response in patients with absence is separate from that of the generalized spike-and-slow-wave complex.

Other clinical factors are important in photosensitivity. Patients generally have normal intelligence and are free of significant neurologic dysfunction, although mental retardation may be present in 15% (Newmark and Penry 1979). Several neurologic syndromes have been associated with photosensitivity, including some storage diseases (Green 1971) and progressive myoclonic epilepsy. The resting EEG is normal in approximately one-half of photosensitive patients. A common abnormality is the generalized spike-and-wave complex after eye closure (Jeavons and Harding 1975), which is most often present in patients with clinical seizures. Photosensitive patients with additional spontaneous seizure disorders most often have a generalized seizure disorder, although in children this correlation between seizure type and photosensitivity is not as close as in adults (Hedenström and Schorsch 1966).

Several symptoms have been noted among nonepileptic photosensitive individuals. Severe headache has been reported (Scollo-Lavizzari 1971), but it is not known if headache is more frequent in photosensitive individuals than in the general population. The significance of alcoholism and alcohol withdrawal is also unclear. The photomyogenic response may appear after alcohol withdrawal (Gastaut et al 1958). Victor and Brausch (1967) have reported increased photic abnormalities in alcoholics after withdrawal of ethanol, but do not specifically describe photic induced seizures. Several psychiatric disorders have been found in photosensitive, adult patients, but no specific correlation has been made.

Several mechanisms have been suggested. As clinical syndromes associated with photosensitivity have usually included generalized or nonfocal cerebral dysfunction, a diffuse abnormality may be responsible. Patients with generalized seizures are prone to photosensitivity; and the progressive myoclonic epilepsies and the cerebral retinal degenerations, which have widespread cerebral abnormalities, are closely associated with photosensitivity.

Several investigators have attempted to determine the anatomical site of photosensitivity. Green (1968, 1969) has found an abnormal electroretinogram in several photosensitive patients, but this retinal finding may also be a reflection of cortical dysfunction. The visual cortex is often thought to be excessively excitable; clinical occipital signs such as visual field cuts are quite rare in photosensitive patients. Wilkins et al (1980) have examined the effect of different patterns on photosensitivity. Stripes are more epileptogenic than checkerboards, and the epileptogenesis increases if checks are progressively elongated in one direction to approximate stripes. Orientation of stripes may also be important (Wilkins et al 1980). Binocular stimulation, which may increase the number of activated cortical cells, is often more effective than monocular stimulation.

Pharmacologic manipulation of numerous CNS transmitters may affect photosensitivity significantly. Papio papio is a highly photosensitive baboon that also suffers from spontaneous seizures. Drugs that inhibit glutamate decarboxylase, the enzyme primarily responsible for degradation of γ-aminobutyric acid (GABA), markedly enhance the photosensitivity of Papio papio. This effect is not specific, however, as catecholamine antagonists may also exacerbate photosensitivity (Newmark and Penry 1979). Nevertheless, the efficacy of valproic acid (an effective drug for treatment of photosensitivity) may be secondary to its action and GABA activity.

A dopaminergic mechanism has been suggested by Quesney et al (1981). In five photosensitive epileptic patients, apomorphine (a dopamine receptor agonist) transiently blocked photosensitivity. Because the effect of apomorphine was not changed by naloxane (a narcotic antagonist), apomorphine's primary action was thought to be through the dopaminergic receptor. Apomorphine specifically blocked photosensitivity but did not affect spontaneous spike-and-wave discharges.

Several medications have been used to treat photosensitivity, but carefully controlled studies have not yet been performed. The efficacy of an antiepileptic drug is usually related to the induced seizure type rather than to photosensitivity per se. For example, photic induced generalized tonic-clonic seizures are most responsive to phenobarbital and phenytoin (Charlton and Hoefer 1964). These agents are ineffective against photic induced absence seizures (Robertson 1954). The best medications for photic induced absence attacks are clonazepam (Rail 1973), trimethadione (Bickford et al 1953), valproic acid (Jeavons et al 1977), and ethosuximide (Jeavons and Harding 1975), drugs that are usually effective against spontaneously occurring absence attacks. For photic induced myoclonic seizures, valproic acid is the preferred agent (Jeavons et al 1977). If more than one type of seizure is photic induced, seizure control is often not obtained, but valproic acid is perhaps the most effective agent.

In addition, conditioning therapy has been used successfully, primarily by Forster and colleagues (Forster and Campos 1964, Forster 1977). After repetitive monocular stimulation or stimulation with a brightly lit background that does not produce a photoparoxysmal response, a patient may be able to withstand previously epileptogenic photic stimulation without the induction of a seizure discharge. Several repetitive sessions are required to maintain the improvement. Because of the extensive training and expense required for treatment, the technique may not be useful for most patients. Tinted glasses that reduce the light intensity of the environment have been used successfully. These glasses may effectively prevent a photoparoxysmal response, but they may not be practical because of cosmetic, visual, and financial reasons. Monocular shielding is a technique advocated primarily by Jeavons and colleagues (Jeavons and Harding 1970). This treatment is not well suited for environmentally produced seizures, which may occur without a warning, but it may be an effective therapy in individuals who are primarily affected by the television.

OTHER VISUALLY INDUCED SEIZURES

Television-Induced Seizures

Several factors are important in the production of television-induced seizures. First, photosensitivity is usually present in patients with television-induced epilepsy. Among 299 patients with seizures induced by television, 40 had seizures produced by other environmental photic stimuli and all had photoparoxysmal response (Jeavons and Harding 1975). Two-thirds of the photosensitive patients reported by Jeavons and Harding (1975) had seizures induced by the television. A generalized tonic-clonic seizure is induced by a television in approximately 75% of susceptible patients, but myoclonic and absence seizures may also occur (Jeavons and Harding 1975). The patients who are affected by the television have clinical characteristics similar to those of other photic induced seizure patients. They are frequently young women, and only two patients over the age of 40 have been reported (Newmark and Penry 1979). Several have a family history of epilepsy or television-induced seizures. The method of television viewing is important in the production of the attack, as most patients have seizures when they are close to the set or when the individual is adjusting an out-of-focus set. The combination of a close viewing position and faulty television may be responsible for the majority of television-induced attacks.

Electroencephalographic testing has revealed EEG patterns that are similar to those of patients with photic induced seizures. Patients are often pattern sensitive (Stafansson et al 1977). Gastaut et al (1962) reported patients whose seizures historically occurred in front of a television set, but who could not reproduce a seizure in a laboratory setting. These investigators postulated that television-induced seizures may be caused by a combination of factors, including fatigue, ethanol, and menstrual hormonal factors that, when added to the photic stimulation of the television image, cause a seizure. In addition, the possibility of coincidence must be considered. Because many people spend several hours daily viewing the television, it is likely that a number of seizures may occur in front of the set regardless of the cause.

Self-Induced Seizures

The self-induced seizure is a different problem. Jeavons and Harding (1975) have described 30 photosensitive patients compulsively driven to the television. Five individuals admitted that they consciously used the television to induce a seizure. The other 25 did not desire seizures, but were, nevertheless, drawn toward the screen. In most patients with self-induced television epilepsy, the patient experiences a pleasurable sensation from the television screen, which then draws the photosensitive patient to sit near the screen, a position associated with seizures in susceptible individuals. Most patients with self-induced television epilepsy do not initiate the seizure by turning on the set but are unable to resist the set once it is on.

A second major method of self-precipitating seizures is hand-waving before a light source (Andermann et al 1962). In several intensive monitoring studies of hand-waving seizures, patients wave their hands across their eyes when emotionally distressed, inducing either an absence or generalized tonic-clonic seizure (Ames 1971). Robertson (1954) has reported several patients who are attracted to the sun, gaze at it, and then begin moving their arms before their eyes to produce a seizure. An important aspect of alleged self-induced hand-waving seizures is the possibility that several of these attacks may not be intentional. As reported by Ames (1974), a child thought to have self-induced seizures actually had attacks consisting of hand movements and deviations of the eye and head as part of the ictal event. In many instances, hand-waving is not a sufficiently efficient flicker source to produce a photic induced seizure. Ames (1971), using intensive monitoring procedures, has found that most patients have repetitive movements of the arms, which vary from two to five per second, lasting 1 to 4 seconds, a frequency that does not precipitate seizures in most sensitive patients.

A third major method of seizure induction is repeated blinking at a light source. Green (1966) has described electroencephalographically four patients whose seizures were initiated with blinking. Again, it is unclear if several of the patients may have suffered from blinking itself as a part of a seizure. Ames (1971) has observed a patient who was thought to be self-inducing her attacks by eyelid flutter but who actually had eyelid flutter and eye movement as part of the seizure.

The clinical characteristics of patients with alleged self-induced seizures are similar to other patients with photic induced attacks. There is a marked female preponderance, and most patients are children or young adults. Occasionally a family history of photosensitivity exists, but a family history of epilepsy is more common (Newmark and Penry 1979). Many patients have spontaneously occurring seizures in addition to the self-induced ones. The most common spontaneous seizure types are generalized tonic-clonic and absence seizures. Several patients with self-induced seizures have subnormal intelligence, and many have suffered from various psychiatric disorders. The type of attack elicited by self-induction is usually an absence or myoclonic seizure; generalized tonic-clonic seizures are rare, perhaps because the severity of the seizure reduces this type of self-induction.

Pattern-Evoked Seizures

Pattern presentation can be an effective precipitant of epileptiform discharges in

208

patients who may not otherwise be photosensitive. Patterns that have evoked seizures have included trousers, striped undershirts, a striped uniform of a milkman, screens, window curtains, rugs, a picket fence, telephone lines, the grating of escalator steps, upholstery, radiators, and a checkered tablecloth. All patients who have been tested with pattern-induced seizures have been responsive to pattern on the EEG, and several have had a photoparoxysmal response (Newmark and Penry 1979). The usual seizure evoked by pattern is generalized tonic-clonic, although myoclonic and elementary partial seizures have been reported. These patients are children or young adults, as are the patients with other visually evoked seizures; they may have family histories of epilepsy and usually do not have focal abnormalities. Because of the overlap of patients with photic induced seizures, pattern-induced seizures do not necessarily form a separate disorder.

Eye Closure

Seizures may be induced by eye closure. Electroencephalographic abnormalities are frequently found after eye closure in photosensitive patients, and clinical attacks including absence and generalized tonic-clonic seizures have been reported by a number of investigators (Gastaut and Tassinari 1966, Green 1968, Atzev 1962). The EEG abnormalities are usually associated with the act of closing the eye rather than with changes in the intensity of light caused by eye closure, as they may occur in total darkness. Passive eye closure by the examiner frequently does not induce EEG abnormalities. Patients with eye closure-induced seizures are typically young and female. Significant neurologic disorders may be present, including mental retardation and spontaneously occurring seizures (Newmark and Penry 1979). A family history of eye closure-induced epilepsy has been reported. However, eye closure-induced seizures usually do not form a specific syndrome, as patients with eye closure-epilepsy often have neurologic impairment and spontaneously occurring seizures as well.

Eye Movement

Seizures are extremely rarely precipitated by eye movement. Shanzer et al (1965) described a woman who had seizures upon extreme lateral gaze, an event that was first observed during an examination by her physicians of her cranial nerve function. The seizure lasted 1 minute and consisted of a conjugate shift of her eyes to the right upper gaze position, followed by abrupt loss of consciousness and clonic movements of her right limbs. Pathological examination revealed no explanation for this phenomenon. Vignaendra and Lim (1978) have described a patient who developed focal EEG discharges and complex partial seizures upon eye convergence. The discharges could be induced in darkness and after application of 5% cyclopentolate hydrochloride to the eyes.

Eye movement-induced attacks may also be symptoms of pseudoseizures. The author has evaluated a patient with alleged eye movement-induced seizures whose attacks, consisting of clonic jerking of the face and eyelids, were precipitated by lateral gaze to either side and were refractory to several antiepileptic medications. Several 6-hour intensive monitoring sessions and many routine electroencephalograms did not reveal any EEG abnormality. After an extensive hospitalization, the patient confessed that she voluntarily produced the attacks.

Partial seizures have been reportedly induced by gazing through a small opening

(Kawai and Fujii 1979). After the patient looked through a small opening with her left eye, clonic movements of her left arm and left eyelid would develop; these movements were followed by a sensation of absence of her left arm. Simultaneous electroencephalograms revealed enhanced spike activity in the right parietal area upon initiation of gaze, followed after 4 seconds of gaze by rhythmical spikes in the right parietal region, which were associated with left eye twitching and the feeling of absence of her arm.

Reading-Induced Seizures

A more common disorder has been seizures induced by reading. Patients with reading-induced seizures are usually free of neurologic impairment and are approximately equally divided between men and women; most are under 30 years of age (Newmark and Penry 1979). A typical attack is jaw myoclonus, which may be followed by a generalized tonic-clonic seizure if reading persists. Rarely, primary generalized tonic-clonic, absence, or elementary partial seizures may be precipitated. Attacks are often induced when a combination of factors are present. As examples, some patients may have seizures only after prolonged reading or fatigue, whereas others may have seizures only if the reading material is emotionally charged. Occasionally, the seizures may be associated with heavy use of tobacco or ethanol, or reading-induced seizures may occur only when the individual mouths his words. A family history of reading epilepsy is present in at least one-fourth of patients with this disorder (Newmark and Penry 1979).

Electroencephalographic studies do not always demonstrate a specific abnormality. Although most patients have normal nonreading EEGs, several patients have generalized spike or spike-and-wave activity and approximately 20% have a photoparoxysmal response. With prolonged reading, most patients will develop spike discharges, with the abnormality primarily restricted to the posterior head quadrants, either unilaterally or bilaterally.

Treatment of reading epilepsy is occasionally difficult. Although phenytoin is often ineffective, phenobarbital, ethosuximide, valproic acid, and clonazepam, as well as conditioning therapy, have been intermittently helpful (Geschwind and Sherwin 1967, Forster et al 1969, Hall and Marshall 1980, Murphy and Yamada 1981). Success with these therapies must be balanced against the fact that the disorder may be transient (Baxter and Bailey 1961).

In addition to the primary reading epilepsy, several patients have been described as suffering from secondary reading epilepsy (Bickford et al 1957), which includes patients with multiple seizure types who also have an abnormal resting EEG. In reports by Bickford et al (1957), one patient had seizures induced by patterns and another by intense concentration or calculation. Patients with secondary reading epilepsy may also have partial seizures and focal electroencephalographic abnormalities (Newmark and Penry 1979).

LANGUAGE-INDUCED SEIZURES

Associated with both visual evoked and auditory evoked seizures are the language-induced seizures. This disorder was first described by Geschwind and Sherwin (1967) and later by Stoupel (1968) and Bennett et al (1971) and includes patients whose seizures may be induced by reading, writing, or speaking. Typically, jaw myoclonus associated with focal epileptiform activity is induced by writing, by speaking, or by reading. In the patient described by Bennett et al (1971), the induction of seizures was unrelated to the patient's familiarity or comprehension of the text, text content, or the direction of visual scanning. Reading aloud had no effect and even nonsense syllables could activate both focal electroencephalographic abnormalities and clinical seizure activity.

A patient has been described with seizures induced by hearing speech. In this patient, described by Tsuzuki and Kasuga (1978), focal frontal spikes were elicited by verbal stimuli most specifically when the patient was addressed directly with emotionally charged speech. This patient also had spontaneous seizures, and it is unclear whether speech was a specific factor in precipitating her attacks. Although speech precipitated EEG abnormalities, she also demonstrated a significant diffuse encephalopathy and various noises and surprises precipitated her attacks.

An interesting type of language evoked seizures are seizures caused by writing (Sharbrough et al 1977, Ohtaka and Miyasaka 1977, Takahashi 1979). These seizures are variable, but most typically the patient has myoclonus, particularly of the hand that is writing, or absence attacks, with or without myoclonus. The electroencephalograms have been variable, with the evoked abnormalities consisting of either diffuse, generalized, 5-Hz, spike-and-wave bursts (Sharbrough et al 1977) or focal discharges (Takahashi 1979). Occasionally, the seizures can be provoked only if the writing is associated with anxiety or tension. Another report has described a patient who suffered from elementary partial seizures after an anastomosis of the superficial temporal to the left middle cerebral artery (Lee et al 1980). In this patient with a lesion in the left inferior motor area, the seizures consist of jerking of the jaw, cheek, periorbital muscles, and neck of the right side and are induced by reading aloud and by writing. They were not induced by simple movements of the throat or facial muscles or by nonlanguage intellectual performance such as calculation. Like the other patients, this individual had spontaneous seizures as well.

To summarize, the language-induced seizures have been primarily reported in adults or adolescents. At times they are associated with reading epilepsy and can be included in the secondary reading epilepsy syndrome. However, because of 1) the lack of a specific seizure type precipitated by the stress, 2) the multiple techniques required to precipitate an attack, and 3) the frequent presence of spontaneous seizures, the patients do not form a single syndrome. Treatment of a language-induced seizure is still uncertain because of the very few patients who have been reported. In most patients some success has been obtained with antiepileptic medication.

AUDITORY EVOKED SEIZURES

Sound-Induced Seizures

Auditory evoked seizures have been described for several years (Gowers 1901) and have been excellently reviewed by Forster (1977). The seizures caused by auditory stimuli may be broadly classified into two types: those that are stimulated by the sound itself and those that are provoked by startling sounds. Nonstartle auditory evoked epilepsy has been described by several investigators. Gastaut and Piravano (1949) reported four patients with absence seizures precipitated by intermittent high-intensity sound of 1 to 3000 Hz. The intermittent quality of the stimulation was essential for its epileptogenicity, as constant sounds of the same intensity had no effect. In a report by Forster (1977), a 17-year-old woman with complex partial seizures had attacks caused by the ringing of a telephone. Upon testing in the laboratory, EEG findings could not be demonstrated. In another patient, secondarily generalized tonic-clonic and complex partial seizures occurred after injury in an automobile accident; the seizures were precipitated by the voice of a local radio announcer. Upon laboratory testing, left temporal spikes or a clinical seizure appeared some, but not all, of the times the tape of the voice was presented to the patient. Other voices, including the scientist who worked with the patient in the Epilepsy Center, did not provoke an attack. It was concluded that the voice that precipitated the seizures had a specific prosody responsible for the attack.

Musicogenic Epilepsy

Related to auditory evoked seizures are the musicogenic epilepsies, which were first discussed by Critchley (1937). The seizure produced by music is most often a complex partial seizure or a secondarily generalized tonic-clonic seizure (Fujinawa et al 1977, Forster 1977, Newman and Saunders 1980). Prior to the music, the electroencephalogram may be normal, may have diffuse abnormalities, or may have temporal lobe abnormalities. Among patients with a temporal epileptiform focus, the left and right temporal areas are equally affected. During a seizure, the electroencephalographic findings are similar to those noted in complex partial seizures (Fujinawa et al 1977).

Several types of music have been responsible for producing seizures, from classical music to jazz, and a wide range of musical instruments have been involved. In a few patients, music is the only precipitant for the development of a seizure, but in most it is one of several precipitants. In some instances, the attacks are only loosely correlated with the music as in a seizure occurring 20 minutes after hearing the music (Lennox and Lennox 1960). In others the diagnosis of musicogenic epilepsy may be doubtful because of the possibility of pseudoseizures. In my experience, a patient with alleged music-induced attacks induced by concert music was tested clinically and electroencephalographically after listening to music from a concert piano. Although she developed a trance for several minutes, the electroencephalogram did not change from the normal premusic record.

The mechanism for musicogenic epilepsy is still unknown. A psychogenic cause, as mentioned in the preceding example, may be present in a few patients. Other factors that may be important include temporal or parietal lobe dysfunction, increased respiration during the music, or changes in cerebral circulation (Fujinawa et al 1977). The musical stimulus may be related to the other auditory stimuli, as in one patient (Poskanzer et al 1962) whose seizures, which were induced by church bells, were also induced by any sound within a specific frequency. Music that is emotionally significant to a patient may occasionally be more epileptogenic than music that is not (Poskanzer et al 1962, Toivakka and Lehtinen, 1965).

Therapy for musicogenic epilepsy is often only partially successful, but antiepileptic medication may be effective in some patients. Forster has tried conditioning therapy with a threshold alteration method. In this technique, a tape of the seizure-inducing music is presented to the patient until a seizure is evoked and then is continued through the postictal period until the patient returns to his normal clinical state (Forster 1977).

STARTLE-INDUCED SEIZURES

Some seizures are evoked by a combination of sensory stimulation and startle. Seizures produced by startle and an auditory stimulus have included myoclonic, clonic, elementary partial, secondarily generalized tonic-clonic, and complex partial seizures. The type of sound associated with the startle is usually not important for the induction of a seizure, but occasionally only a specific sound, including gunshots, dropped utensils, various alarm bells, and buzzers may be responsible. Startle-induced epileptiform discharges have included both focal spike-and-slow-wave discharges as well as irregular diffuse slow-spike-and-slow-wave complexes (Forster 1977). In a report of a startle-induced seizure (Bancaud et al 1968), depth electroencephalographic recording revealed epileptiform discharges originating from the supplementary motor area. Forster (1977) believes that startle-induced attacks are associated with temporal lobe dysfunction, causing excessive sensitivity to the afferent stimulation from the auditory messages. Startle seizures have been associated with focal neurologic disorders, as described by Wabayashi et al (1962), who observed focal jerks of the head followed by a generalized tonic-clonic attack in a woman with a homonymous hemianopsia and hemiplegia, and by Nakamura et al (1975), who described patients with Sturge-Weber syndrome and startle seizures. Although most reports describe abnormal and usually focal cerebral dysfunction, not all patients have focal abnormalities. Forster (1977) described at least two patients who suffered from a severe diffuse static encephalopathy.

Occasionally startle seizures may be precipitated by tactile or visual stimuli. Those attacks are often associated with severe encephalopathies, including subacute sclerosing panencephalitis. The prognosis of patients with startle attacks is poor primarily because of the associated severe encephalopathy, but it is unclear if startle seizures, specifically, have a poor prognosis.

A syndrome, of nonepileptiform startle-induced attacks has been reviewed by Andermann et al (1980). In the author's opinion, nonepileptiform startle disease is an autosomal dominant disorder, with hypertonia in infancy and later an unsteady gait. The episodes, which may be precipitated by sudden noises, movement, or sudden sensory stimuli, are characterized by falling to the ground without unconsciousness but with shaking of all limbs. In the very few patients who have been identified with this disorder, clonezapam has been effective. Characteristic electroencephalographic findings with this rare disorder have not been identified.

MOVEMENT-INDUCED SEIZURES

Seizures and other types of attacks involving motor abnormalities have been induced by limb movement. The types of attacks induced by movement do not necessarily form a single disorder, and several may not be seizures. An early, well-defined syndrome has been described by Lishman et al (1962), who described attacks precipitated by a quick movement of the legs, often in combination with an element of tension or anxiety. Occasionally, physical exercise may precipitate an attack (Burger et al 1972). The seizures may be variable but most typically consist of dystonia localized to one limb or confined to one side of the body. They may rarely consist of athetoid or ballistic movements. As summarized by Hishikawa et al (1973), approximately three-quarters of attacks are unilateral, although either side may be involved during a single attack. The episodes may be frequent and occur as often as 50 times per day, but an individual attack rarely lasts longer than 30 seconds. The electroencephalogram during an attack is usually normal, although epileptiform discharges have been reported.

The patient with movement-induced dystonia often has a normal neurologic examination and only rarely a history of epilepsy. He is often young; the age group between 10 and 20 is primarily affected. A family history may be present in as many as 60% of the individuals. The prognosis is often good, and many patients respond to low doses of carbamazepine, phenytoin, or phenobarbital.

The cause of movement dystonia is unknown. In a patient reported by Falconer et al (1963) with an epileptiform focus over the left hemisphere anterior to the rolandic fissure, removal of a scar controlled the attacks. Other investigators have suggested that the disorder is secondary to basal ganglia lesions (Hishikawa et al 1973). It is possible that some of the attacks may be supplementary motor seizures, whereas others have a different pathophysiology.

The syndrome of paroxysmal choreoathetosis is closely related to the movement dystonias and was first described by Mount and Reback (1940). This disorder differs from the movement dystonias in its early age of onset, ie, early childhood. The attacks are not precipitated by violent movement and may last longer than movement-induced dystonias, often up to several hours. The disorder may be resistant to therapy and is often inherited in an autosomal dominant pattern.

Elementary partial seizures may also be secondary to limb movement. In a report by Aquino and Gabor (1980), two patients with nonketotic hyperglycemia had focal tonic-clonic seizures that were induced by actual or attempted movement. These seizures resisted conventional antiepileptic therapy until appropriate therapy for the elevated blood glucose level was instituted. These seizures are distinct from the preceding ones as they occurred in older diabetic individuals who had partial motor seizures.

SENSORY EVOKED SEIZURES

Seizures evoked by somatosensory stimuli have been infrequently observed and do not form a single syndrome. Perhaps the best known of the sensory evoked attacks has been a familial syndrome entitled the *Jumping Frenchmen of Maine*, which was first described by William Beard in 1878 (Beard 1880). In the initial description of 50 individuals, including 14 men from four families of the Moosehead Lake region in Maine, several individuals jumped or jerked with either the hands or legs when a loud sound or unsuspected stimulus was given. In addition to the violent movement, the individuals usually emitted a sound. The attacks appeared frequently within a single day but would last only for a few seconds. The jumpers were observed primarily among men and boys; women were rarely involved, and children under the age of 4 were never involved. The prognosis was poor; as the original author stated, "Once a jumper, always a jumper." The attack was not associated with loss of consciousness and did not occur spontaneously.

The epileptic nature of these attacks is unclear, as the original report appeared before the development of electroencephalography; and subsequent reports have described normal EEGs. With prolonged observation, individuals have been noted to suffer from a single stereotypic flexion of the arms and trunk suggestive of myoclonic movements but without loss of consciousness.

Other sensory evoked attacks have been described. In a report by Goldie and Green (1959), an 18-year-old man with a left parietal angioma had a tingling in the right arm after the right side of his face was touched. Spike discharges in the left parietal area increased when the patient rubbed his face or even when he was asked to think about rubbing his face. In another report by Forster and Cleeland (1969), stimulation of the right thigh and abdomen produced attacks of stiffening of all limbs with simultaneous loss of consciousness. Electroencephalographic findings were nonspecific. In a case reported by Rothova and Roth (1963), tactile stimulation of the buttock and right thigh of the child produced epileptiform discharges in the right supplementary motor area. This child was successfully treated with antiepileptic medication. Perhaps the largest number of somatosensory evoked seizures has been a series of Indian patients, described by Mani et al (1974). In these patients, primarily children and adolescents, hot water poured on the head precipitated complex partial or generalized tonic-clonic seizures. Epileptiform electroencephalographic discharges were noted interictally in approximately one-third of the patients, but adequate ictal records were not performed. Over 50% of the patients had attacks that were reproducible in the epilepsy laboratories. Individuals whose seizures were precipitated only by a hot bath did not develop spontaneous seizures. Among patients with both spontaneous and hot bath seizures, the prognosis was not so clear.

Miscellaneous Sensory Evoked Seizures

Finally, a number of somewhat unusual stimuli have precipitated seizures. In a report by Behrman and Wyke (1958), a 58-year-old man had secondarily generalized tonic-clonic seizures after an aura of vertigo, ataxia, and tinnitus, precipitated by cold-water caloric testing in the right ear. Clonic jerking of the right arm and leg was accompanied by ictal changes in the electroencephalogram. The authors hypothesized that paroxysmal firing of hyperexcitable neurons in the brain stem reticular system was induced by the vestibular activity caused by the caloric testing.

Another unusual type of reflex seizure has been seizures associated with eating. Three cases have been described in a review of the literature (Robertson and Fariello 1979). In two of the three cases, seizures could be induced with the presentation of food only and were not secondary to motor or masticatory movements, salivation, or sensory stimulation of the oral cavity. In the most recent report, a 14-year-old boy with a right frontal subcortical astrocytoma, whose seizures consisted of left facial clonic movements occasionally spreading to the left hand and arm had attacks that were often but not always precipitated by eating. An electroencephalogram performed during a meal revealed rhythmical theta discharges followed by spike activity over the right frontal area. In this patient, surgical removal of the tumor and phenytoin, phenobarbital, and dexamethasone therapy successfully controlled the attacks. The authors have hypothesized that the etiology may be secondary to activation of hypothalamic nuclei that are involved in digestion. This hypothesis was not confirmed with depth electrode encephalography, and other attacks may be secondary to temporal lobe dysfunction, as has been suggested by Ahuja et al (1980) after clinical testing of three patients.

It has been postulated that seizures may be evoked in adults by sexual excitement. Kelly (1979) has described a 38-year-old man with complex partial seizures and a safety pin fetish who had complex partial seizures and epileptiform left temporal discharges precipitated by viewing a safety pin. Temporal lobectomy successfully treated both the fetish and the seizures. The possibility of pseudoseizures should also be considered. The author has examined a woman with a history of alleged orgasm-precipitated attacks who clearly had pseudoseizures and nonorganic neurologic symptoms.

Finally, some seizures may be evoked by decisions, as described by Cirignotta et al (1980). In two reports, generalized tonic-clonic and absence attacks were precipitated by episodes of anxiety provoked by decision making. Although the authors believed that the attacks were symptoms of an internal reflex epilepsy, the stimuli were sufficiently diverse (card games, chess, reading, and other anxiety-provoking activities) that the specific conclusions about this type of disorder are unobtainable. As patients frequently report increased seizure activity under periods of anxiety, the relationship between anxiety and epilepsy may be quite broad.

CONCLUSION

The sensory evoked seizures are a diverse but interesting group of attacks that are highly variable in both the types of evoked seizures and the required sensory stimuli. The best defined and most common disorder, the visually evoked seizures, are fortunately the most treatable. Several of the rarer types require extensive evaluation before they can be documented. Even the most studied of the sensory evoked seizures, the photic induced attacks, have not had a well-defined pathophysiology, although data have suggested that a combination of factors is involved.

BIBLIOGRAPHY

Adrian ED, Matthews BHC: The Berger rhythm: Potential changes from the occipital lobes in man. *Brain* 1934;57:355-385.

Ahuja GK, Mahandas S, Narayanaswamy AS: Eating epilepsy. *Epilepsia* 1980;21:85-89.

Ames FR: "Self-induction" in photosensitive epilepsy. *Brain* 1971;94:781-798.

Ames FR: Cinefilm and EEG recording during "hand-waving" attacks of an epileptic, photosensitive child. *Electroencephalogr Clin Neurophysiol* 1974;37:301-304.

Andermann K, Berman S, Cooke PM, et al (eds): Self-induced epilepsy. A collection of self-induced epilepsy cases compared with some other photoconvulsive cases. *Arch Neurol* 1962;6:49-65.

Andermann F, Keene DL, Andermann E, et al: Startle disease or hyperekplexia: Further delineation of the syndrome. *Brain* 1980;103:985-987.

Aquino A, Gabor AJ: Movement-induced seizures in nonketotic hyperglycemia. *Neurology* 1980;30:600-604.

Atzev E: The effect of closing the eyes upon epileptic activity of the brain. *Electroencephalogr Clin Neurophysiol* 1962;14:561.

Bancaud J, Talairach J, Bonis A: Physiopathogenesis of startle epilepsy (an epilepsy of the supplementary motor area). *Electrocephalogr Clin Neurophysiol* 1968;24:490.

Baxter DW, Bailey AA: Primary reading epilepsy: *Neurology (Minneap)* 1961;11:445-449.

Beard GM: Experiments with the "Jumpers" or "Jumping Frenchmen" of Maine. *J Nerv Ment Dis* 1880;7:487-490.

Behrman S, Wyke BD: Vestibulogenic seizures. A consideration of vertiginous seizures, with particular reference to convulsions produced by stimulation of labyrinthine receptors. *Brain* 1958;81:529-541.

Bennett DR, Mavor H, Jarcho LW: Language-induced epilepsy: Report of a case. *Electroencephalogr Clin Neurophysiol* 1971;30:159.

Bertha H, Lechner H: Das Krankheitsbild der Photogenen Epilepsie. *Wien Klin Wochenschr* 1956;68:954-962.

Bickford RG, Daly D, Keith HM: Convulsive effects of light stimulation in children. *Am J Dis Child* 1953;86:170-183.

Bickford RG, Klass DW: Sensory precipitation and reflex mechanisms, in Jasper HH, Ward AA Jr, Pope A (eds): *Basic Mechanisms of the Epilepsies*. Boston, Little Brown & Co, 1969, pp 543–564.

Bickford RG, Whelan JL, Klass DW, et al: Reading epilepsy: Clinical and electroencephalographic studies of a new syndrome. *Trans Am Neurol Assoc* 1957;81:100–102.

Brausch CC, Ferguson JH: Color as a factor in light-sensitive epilepsy. *Neurology (Minneap)* 1965;15:154–164.

Burger LJ, Lopex RI, Elliott FA: Tonic seizures induced by movement. *Neurology (Minneap)* 1972;22:656–659.

Chao D: Photogenic and self-induced epilepsy. *J Pediatr* 1962;61:733–738.

Charlton MH, Hoefer PFA: Television and epilepsy. *Arch Neurol* 1964;11:239–247.

Cirignotta F, Cicogna P, Lugaresi E: Epileptic seizures during card games and draughts. *Epilepsia* 1980;21:137–140.

Cobb S: Photic driving as a cause of clinical seizures in epileptic patients. *Arch Neurol Psychiatr* 1947;58:70–71.

Critchley M: Musicogenic epilepsy. *Brain* 1937;60:13–27.

Daly DD, Bickford RG: Electroencephalographic studies of identical twins with photoepilepsy. *Electroencephalogr Clin Neurophysiol* 1951;3:245–249.

Daly DD, Siekert RG, Burke EC: A variety of familial light sensitive epilepsy. *Electroencephalogr Clin Neurophysiol* 1959;11:141–145.

Davidson S, Watson CW: Hereditary light sensitive epilepsy. *Neurology (Minneap)* 1956;6:235–261.

Doose H, Gerken H: Possibilities and limitations of epilepsy prevention in siblings of epileptic children, in Parsonage MJ (ed): *Prevention of Epilepsy and Its Consequences*. London, International Bureau for Epilepsy, 1973, pp 32–35.

Doose H, Gerken H, Horstmann T, et al: Genetic factors in spike-wave absences. *Epilepsia* 1973;14:57–75.

Engel J: Selective photoconvulsive responses to intermittent diffuse and patterned photic stimulation. *Electroencephalogr Clin Neurophysiol* 1974;37:283–292.

Ernst J: Un cas d'épilepsie photosensible avec phénomène d'aimentation visuelle. *J Sci Med Lille* 1969;87:559–564.

Falconer MA, Driver MV, Serafetinides EA: Seizures induced by movement: Report of a case relieved by operation. *J Neurol Neurosurg Psychiatry* 1963;26:300–307.

Forster FM: *Reflex Epilepsy, Behavioral Therapy and Conditional Reflexes*. Springfield, IL, Charles C Thomas Publisher, 1977, p 318.

Forster FM, Campos GB: Conditioning factors in stroboscopic-induced seizures. *Epilepsia* 1964;5:156–165.

Forster FM, Cleeland CS: Somatosensory evoked epilepsy. *Trans Am Neurol Assoc* 1969;94:268–269.

Forster FM, Paulsen WA, Baughman FA: Clinical therapeutic conditioning in reading epilepsy. *Neurology (Minneap)* 1969;19:717–723.

Foster H: Letter to the editor. Photic fit near a helicopter. *Lancet* 1975;2:186.

Fujinawa A, Kawai I, Ohashi H, et al: A case of musicogenic epilepsy. *Folia Psychiatr Neurol Jpn* 1977;3:463–472.

Gastaut H, Pirovano E: Epilepsy induced with intermittent auditory stimulation. *Arch Psicol Neurol Psichiat* 1949;10:297–316.

Gastaut H, Regis H, Bostem F: Attacks provoked by television, and their mechanism. *Epilepsia* 1962;3:438–445.

Gastaut H, Tassinari CA: Triggering mechanisms in epilepsy. The electroclinical point of view. *Epilepsia* 1966;7:85–138.

Gastaut H, Trevisan C, Naquet R: Diagnostic value of electroencephalographic abnormalities provoked by intermittent photic stimulation. *Electroencephalogr Clin Neurophysiol* 1958;10:194–195.

Geschwind N, Sherwin I: Language-induced epilepsy. *Arch Neurol* 1967;16:25-31.

Goldie L, Green JM: A study of the psychological factors in a case of sensory reflex epilepsy. (Psychological factors in reflex epilepsy.) *Brain* 1959;82:505-524.

Goodkind R: Myoclonic and epileptic attacks precipitated by bright light. *Arch Neurol Psychiatr* 1936;35:868-874.

Gowers WR: *Epilepsy and Other Chronic Convulsive Diseases.* New York, William Wood and Co, 1885, p 255.

Green JB: Self-induced seizures. Clinical and electroencephalographic studies. *Arch Neurol* 1966;15:579-586.

Green JB: Seizures on closing the eyes. Electroencephalographic studies. *Neurology (Minneap)* 1968;18:391-396.

Green JB: Neurophysiological studies in Batten's disease. *Dev Med Child Neurol* 1971;13:477-489.

Green JB: Photosensitive epilepsy. The electroretinogram and visually evoked response. *Arch Neurol* 1969;20:191-198.

Hall JH, Marshall PC: Clonazepam therapy in reading epilepsy. *Neurology (Minneap)* 1980;30:550-551.

Hedenström I, Schorsch G: Photosensibilität im EEG bei Epileptikern und bei Oligophrenen mit seltenen Anfällen. *Arch Psychiatr Nervenkr* 1966;208:147-161.

Herrlin K-M: EEG with photic stimulation: A study of children with manifest or suspected epilepsy. *Electroencephalogr Clin Neurophysiol* 1954;6:573-589.

Herrlin K-M: Epilepsy, light-sensitivity and left-handedness in a family with monozygotic triplets. *Pediatrics* 1960;25:385-399.

Hishikawa Y, Furuya E, Yamamoto J, et al: Dystonic seizures induced by movement. *Arch Psychiatr Nervenkr* 1973;217:113-138.

Hishikawa Y, Yamamoto J, Furuya E, et al: Photosensitive epilepsy: Relationships between the visual evoked responses and the epileptiform discharges induced by intermittent photic stimulation. *Electroencephalogr Clin Neurophysiol* 1967;23:320-334.

Hutt SJ, Lee D, Ounsted C: Digit memory and evoked discharges in four light-sensitive epileptic children. *Dev Med Child Neurol* 1963;5:559-571.

Jeavons PM: Nosological problems of myoclonic epilepsies in childhood and adolescence. *Dev Med Child Neurol* 1977;19:3-8.

Jeavons PM, Clark JE, Maheshiwari MC: Treatment of generalized epilepsies of childhood and adolescence with sodium valproate ("Epilim"). *Dev Med Child Neurol* 1977;19:9-25.

Jeavons PM, Harding GFA: Television epilepsy, letter to the editor. *Lancet* 1970;2:926.

Jeavons PM, Harding GFA: *Photosensitive Epilepsy. A Review of the Literature and a Study of 460 Patients.* London, William Heinemann Medical Books, 1975, p 121.

Jeavons PM, Harding G, Bower BD: Intermittent photic stimulation in photosensitive epilepsy. *Electroencephalogr Clin Neurophysiol* 1966;21:308.

Kawai I, Fujii S: Ictal body scheme disturbance induced by looking through a small opening. *Epilepsia* 1979;20:535-540.

Keith HM, Aldrich RA, Daly DD, et al: A study of light-induced epilepsy in children. *Am J Dis Child* 1953;83:408-409.

Kelly D: Case history: Operations and the sexual drive. *Br J Sex Med* 1979;66:66.

Lee SI, Sutherling WW, Persing JA, et al: Language-induced seizure. A case of cortical origin. *Arch Neurol* 1980;37:433-436.

Lennox WG, Lennox MA: *Epilepsy and Related Disorders.* Boston, Little Brown & Co, 1960, p 265.

Lishman WA, Symonds CP, Whitty CWM, et al: Seizures induced by movement. *Brain* 1962;85:93-108.

Livingston S: *Comprehensive Management of Epilepsy in Infancy, Childhood and Adolescence.* Springfield, IL, Charles C Thomas Publishing, 1972, p 657.

Mani KS, Mani AJ, Ramesh CK, et al: Hot water epilepsy: Clinical and electroencephalographic features. Study of 60 cases. *Neurology (Bombay)* 1974;20:237-240.

Mount LA, Reback S: Familial paroxysmal choreoarthetosis: Preliminary report on a hitherto undescribed clinical syndrome. *Arch Neurol Psychiatry* 1940;44:841-847.

Murphy MJ, Yamada T: Clonazepam therapy in reading epilepsy. *Neurology* 1981;31:233.

Nakamura M, Kanai H, Miyamoto Y: A case of Sturge-Weber syndrome with startle epilepsy. *No To Shinkei* 1975;27:325-331.

Newman P, Saunders M: A unique case of musicogenic epilepsy. *Arch Neurol* 1980;37:244-245.

Newmark ME, Penry JK: *The Genetics of Epilepsy: A Review.* New York, Raven Press, 1980, p 122.

Newmark ME, Penry JK: *Photosensitivity and Epilepsy: A Review.* New York, Raven Press, 1979, p 230.

Ohtaka T, Miyasaka M: On a case of language induced epilepsy precipitated mainly by writing. *Psychiatr Neurol Jpn* 1977;79:587-601.

Pallis C, Louis S: Television-induced seizures. *Lancet* 1961;1:188-190.

Panayiotopoulos CP: Effectiveness of photic stimulation on various eye-states in photosensitive epilepsy. *J Neurol Sci* 1974;23:165-173.

Pantelakis SN, Bower BD, Jones HD: Convulsions and television viewing. *Br Med J* 1962;225:633-638.

Penry JK, Porter RJ, Dreifuss FE: Simultaneous recording of absence seizures with video and electroencephalography. *Brain* 1975;98:427-440.

Poskanzer C, Brown E, Miller H: Musicogenic epilepsy caused only by a "discrete" frequency band of church bells. *Brain* 1962;85:77.

Quesney LF, Andermann F, Gloor P: Dopaminergic mechanism in generalized photosensitive epilepsy. *Neurology* 1981;31:1542-1544.

Rail LR: The treatment of self-induced photic epilepsy. *Proc Aust Assoc Neurol* 1973;9:121-123.

Rao KS, Prichard JS: Photogenic epilepsy. *J Pediatr* 1955;47:619-623.

Reilly EL, Peters JF: Relationship of some varieties of electroencephalographic photosensitivity to clinical convulsive disorders. *Neurology (Minneap)* 1973;23:1050-1057.

Robertson EG: Photogenic epilepsy: Self-precipitated attacks. *Brain* 1954;77:232-251.

Robertson WC, Fariello RG: Eating epilepsy associated with a deep forebrain glioma. *Ann Neurol* 1979;6:271-273.

Rothova N, Roth B: A case of focal reflex epilepsy induced by tactile stimuli. *Cesk Neurol* 1963;26:33-35.

Scollo-Lavizzari G: Prognostic significance of "epileptiform" discharges in the EEG of non-epileptic subjects during photic stimulation. *Electroencephalogr Clin Neurophysiol* 1971;31:174.

Servit Z, Machek J, Stercova A, et al: Reflex influences in the pathogenesis of epilepsy in the light of clinical studies. *Epilepsia* 1962;3:315-322.

Shanzer S, April R, Atkin A: Seizures induced by eye deviation. *Arch Neurol* 1965;13:621-626.

Sharbrough FW, Westmoreland BF, Campa HK: Writing epilepsy. *Electroencephalogr Clin Neurophysiol* 1977;43:1875.

Stoupel N: On the reflex epilepsies: Epilepsy caused by reading. *Electroencephalogr Clin Neurophysiol* 1968;25:416-417.

Takahashi T: A case of graphogenic epilepsy induced by writing associated with psychic tension. *No To Shinkei* 1979;31:159-165.

Temkin O: *The Falling Sickness: A History of Epilepsy from the Greeks to the Beginnings of Modern Neurology,* ed 2. Baltimore, Johns Hopkins Press, 1971, pp 1-49.

Toivakka E, Lehtinen OJ: Musicogenic epilepsy. A case report. *Acta Neurol Scand* 1965;(suppl)13:529-533.

Tsuzuki H, Kasuga I: Paroxysmal discharges triggered by hearing spoken language. *Epilepsia* 1978;19:147-154.

Victor M, Brausch C: The role of abstinence in the genesis of alcoholic epilepsy. *Epilepsia* 1967;8:1–20.

Vignaendra V, Lim CL: Epileptic discharges triggered by eye convergence. *Neurology (Minneap)* 1978;28:589–591.

Wabayashi J, Kurita H, Yoshida J: A case of startle epilepsy. *Psychiatr Neurol (Japan)* 1962; 64:1101.

Wadlington WB, Riley HD Jr: Light-induced seizures. *J Pediatr* 1965;66:300–312.

Whitty CWM: Photic and self-induced epilepsy. *Lancet* 1960;1:1207–1208.

Wilkins AJ, Binnie CD, Darby CE: Visually induced seizures. *Prog Neurobiol* 1980;15:85–117.

CHAPTER 14

Status Epilepticus

Fritz E. Dreifuss

DEFINITIONS OF THE CONDITION

Status epilepticus may be defined as a seizure that persists for a sufficient length of time or is repeated frequently enough that recovery between attacks does not occur. Status epilepticus may be divided into two seizure types: partial (eg, Jacksonian) or generalized (eg, absence status or tonic-clonic status). When very localized motor status occurs, it is referred to as epilepsia partialis continua.

The *Dictionary of Epilepsy* (Gastaut 1973) defines status epilepticus as a "condition characterized by an epileptic seizure that is sufficiently prolonged or repeated at sufficiently brief intervals so as to produce an unvarying and enduring epileptic condition." A series of attacks in which consciousness is gained between the episodes is called serial seizures. The occurrence of serial seizures may evolve into status epilepticus. Therefore, from the practical point of view, serial seizures should be treated with the same concern as status epilepticus.

One usually regards status epilepticus as occurring when seizures continue for 30 minutes (Rothner and Erenberg 1980), though some would speak of it when two or more seizures occur without the regaining of consciousness and others would not regard "the fixed and enduring condition" to obtain for one hour (Gastaut et al 1967).

CLASSIFICATION OF SEIZURE TYPE

Status epilepticus may be divided into the following seizure types:
I. Generalized status epilepticus, including
  A. Convulsive seizures
    1. tonic-clonic status epilepticus
    2. tonic status epilepticus
    3. clonic status epilepticus
    4. myoclonic status epilepticus

  B. Nonconvulsive generalized status epilepticus, including absence status or so-called spike-wave stupor

II. Partial status epilepticus
  A. Simple partial status, including somatomotor status epilepticus, which includes both 1, 2 and 3.
    1. epilepsia partialis continua
    2. a condition characterized by paroxysmal, lateralized, epileptic discharges (PLEDs)

3. dysphasic status epilepticus also may occur (Sato and Dreifuss 1973).

B. Complex partial status epilepticus or "psychomotor status" is characterized by a nonconvulsive confusional state with automatisms

HISTORICAL BACKGROUND

According to Hunter (1959/60), status epilepticus was not much discussed until the 19th century. He quotes occasional reports including that of Willis (1667), who recognized the potential danger of repeated seizures, and that of Morgagni (1761), who reported death following a series of convulsions. Pritchard (1822) recognized quite clearly the danger of recurrent seizures without recovery of consciousness. It was Calmeil (1824) who coined the phrase *état de mal* and stated at that time that état de mal may be distinguished from a succession of seizures by the failure of the patient to recover consciousness between attacks.

Hunter discussed the relationship between the introduction of anticonvulsant medication and the increased incidence of status epilepticus. Hughlings Jackson (1880) warned that the withdrawal of bromide medication caused convulsive seizures and recommended that the "doses of drugs given should be diminished in number and quantity very gradually." Whereas previous accounts of status epilepticus were quite sporadic (Temkin 1971), by the 1870s it was recognized as a common mode of death in epileptics in institutions. Drug withdrawal as a cause of status epilepticus was also referred to by Gowers (1901) and by Turner (1907). Other common precipitating factors that were recognized included gross brain disease and acute inflammatory disorders.

The prevalence of generalized tonic-clonic status epilepticus varies in different series between 3% (Janz 1961, 1969) and 15% (Heintel 1972). Lennox (1960) reported that approximately one-half of his patients with status epilepticus only had one episode, approximately one-third had two to four episodes, and approximately 17% had more than four episodes of status epilepticus during their epileptic lifetime.

Generalized tonic-clonic status epilepticus may be the first manifestation of epilepsy, or it may be a complication of an ongoing epileptic illness. In most series, the prevalence of status epilepticus in symptomatic epilepsy is considerably higher than in so-called cryptogenic epilepsy, though in the series of Aicardi and Chevrie (1970), they are evenly divided. In the studies of Janz (1969) and of Hunter (1959/60), approximately two-thirds were in the symptomatic group, and in Whitty and Taylor's series (1949), nearly 90% were thus distributed.

CAUSE

The cause differed greatly in various studies, depending on the age group under review. Thus, in adult series, tumor, trauma, vascular disease, and infection were the most prevalent causes. In children, on the other hand, status epilepticus was frequently seen in patients with chronic static encephalopathy or a chronic progressive encephalopathy. In these cases sudden withdrawal of anticonvulsant medications was the most common precipitating factor. The remainder of the symptomatic group had acute brain injury associated with meningitis, encephalitis, or dehydration (Aicardi and Chevrie 1970). The occurrence of fever in both the symptomatic and the idiopathic groups is a common antecedent to the development of status epilepticus. The withdrawal of drugs other than anticonvulsant medications, such as barbiturates, tranquilizers, analgesics, and alcohol, and sleep deprivation may be responsible for precipitating status epilepticus among those so predisposed. It would therefore seem that status epilepticus occurs quite frequently among those who have structural brain disease. Acute brain disease may present with status epilepticus. In long-standing conditions, status epilepticus punctuates an ongoing epileptic disturbance. Janz (1964) has found that the majority of lesions to which status epilepticus may be attributed are in the frontal lobes.

OUTCOME

The outcome of status epilepticus is extremely guarded. The mortality rate has varied widely in different series. In the series of Aicardi and Chevrie (1970), the mortality rate was 11%. In addition, one-third of the patients were left with definite neurologic residuals, and one-half were mentally retarded. The idiopathic group fared no better than those in whom identifiable causes were found. The prognosis was worse for those whose convulsions lasted more than 1 hour or who had seizures that occurred in association with fever and that lasted more than 30 minutes. In the series of Janz (1969), the mortality rate was 6.6%. The lethality of the outcome and the incidence of residual neurologic dysfunction was related to the duration of status epilepticus and the number and severity of the attacks (Heintel 1972, Rowan and Scott 1970). Oxbury and Whitty (1971), in whose series mortality rate was 8.3%, reported that all the patients who died during the acute phase, regardless of cause, had severe pathological abnormalities of a potentially fatal nature. Few patients die during status epilepticus. Those that do die of circulatory collapse and respiratory arrest. Most patients die in the postconvulsive coma of status epilepticus complications or later of the conditions that caused the status epilepticus.

Most patients die of cardiac or circulatory disturbances and cerebral edema, electrolyte disturbances, aspiration pneumonia, or complications caused by medication administered for the treatment of status epilepticus. The neurologic consequences of the metabolic disorders, which include lactic acidosis, CO_2 narcosis, hyperkalemia, hypertension, hypoglycemia, and shock, account for the preponderance of mortality and morbidity, including residual neurologic sequelae (Wasterlain 1974, 1981). Meldrum and co-workers (Meldrum 1973ab, Meldrum et al 1983) demonstrated ischemic neuronal changes involving neocortex, hippocampus, and cerebellum. They related these changes to times during the seizure that correspond to periods of hyperpyrexia, hypoxia, hypotension, and acidosis. Metabolic studies have shown that a marked increase in regional glucose metabolic rate occurs throughout the brain during status epilepticus, with only the substantia nigra being excepted from this metabolic demand. The infant brain is considerably more vulnerable than any other brain.

It is possible that a major cause of ischemic cell damage is related to increased intracellular calcium concentration caused by a calcium influx that exceeds the capacity of the cell to deal with it in an appropriate manner.

Although much of the discussion of status epilepticus will hinge on generalized tonic-clonic status, other forms of status epilepticus require elaboration.

STATUS EPILEPTICUS IN THE NEONATE

According to Kellaway (1983), neonatal convulsions may consist of clonic seizures (frequently focal or hemiclonic, or bilateral but asynchronous), myoclonic seizures (as a consequence of cerebral hypoxia), and tonic postural seizures (frequently associated with neonatal hypoxia; occur in infants with depressed forebrain function that may in part be the result of brain stem disinhibition). He also describes electrical status with no clinical accompaniment but with, nevertheless, a poor prognosis for cerebral development.

TONIC ATTACKS IN CHILDHOOD

Generalized tonic seizures are seen in the childhood age groups, both as the manifestations of infantile spasms and as manifestations of Lennox-Gastaut syndrome. In Lennox-Gastaut syndrome, drop attacks are most frequently the hallmark of the syndrome. However, tonic seizures sometimes continue for prolonged periods and may be prominent and associated with prolonged stupor. Similarly, clonic seizures and so-called myoclonic astatic seizures may occur in the form of status with prolonged stupor. In other cases, stupor in the face of a paucity of movement may be seen associated with a decrease in postural tone.

ABSENCE STATUS

The term *petit mal status* was first used by Lennox and Lennox (1960) in describing the seizure of a child in whom 3-Hz, regular, spike-and-wave discharges accompanied a mild clinical confusion. This was subsequently elaborated. In addition, similar patients were found to present in middle age with isolated absence status, but unlike the children, patients in this older group often lacked a history of previous absence.

In true absence status there is a confused or dreamy state. Electrographically the absence attack may be prolonged or the absences may occur so frequently that there are no definite interruptions to the attack. Such an attack may last for hours or even days. During this time the patient moves around as if in a daze, may answer questions momentarily, and may engage in quasi-purposeful activity, though in a confused manner. The EEG shows spike-and-wave or polyspike-and-wave discharges of a virtually continuous nature.

PARTIAL STATUS EPILEPTICUS

Simple Partial Status Epilepticus: Epilepsia Partialis Continua

In this condition, there is focal convulsive activity of a prolonged nature and preserved consciousness. This condition was described by Kojewnikow in 1895. In some cases, the condition becomes generalized; but in between tonic-clonic seizures, the epilepsia partialis continua persists.

In adults, the condition is frequently caused by either a tumor or vascular insufficiency of a focal area of cortex. In children, this condition may be the result of a so-called chronic encephalitis (Rasmussen and McCann 1968) or of Lafora body encephalitis. The latter, though a generalized progressive disease, may present for prolonged periods of time as epilepsia partialis continua, though with an obviously progressive course. Occasionally cysticercosis may present in this manner. The typical course of epilepsia partialis continua in a child suffering from "chronic encephalitis" is as follows: the epilepsia partialis continues for weeks, months, or even years, during which time the affected extremity becomes progressively paretic. Ultimately, when the child is hemiplegic, the seizure frequently stops. In cases of

Lafora body encephalitis, the seizures ultimately become multifocal.

Complex Partial Status Epilepticus

Complex partial seizures may occur with such frequency that the attacks merge into so-called psychomotor status. The attacks may be characterized by what Scott and Masland (1953) described as aura continua, a prolonged dreamy state, or rapidly repetitive complex partial seizures. Aura continua consists of epigastric, olfactory, or other aura (described under complex partial seizures or under simple partial seizures), with psychic manifestations, depending on whether or not unconsciousness is disturbed. A prolonged dreamy state is associated with a clouding of consciousness, a postictal amnesia, and behavior that may be, for the moment, apparently purposeful but poorly sequenced. When a patient is engaged in conversation, he appears to respond in slow motion and on occasion inappropriately. The electroencephalogram usually shows focal abnormalities with slowing or spike discharges arising from a temporal lobe and occurring on a continuous basis.

TREATMENT OF STATUS EPILEPTICUS

Generalized Tonic-Clonic Status

Because of the hazards of status epilepticus, immediate intervention is necessary. Untreated status epilepticus rarely stops spontaneously. Thus, the condition constitutes a medical emergency and convulsions must be stopped quickly to prevent permanent brain damage or death (Wasterlain 1981).

Prompt general care measures to maintain circulatory status should be instituted. Respiration and circulation must be attended to; hypoglycemia and hypoxia must be corrected. Respiratory obstruction has to be avoided. An oral airway may suffice, but intubation may be necessary. Blood pressure should be maintained. Most deaths result from cardiac failure and the hypoxia, hypotension, and acidosis that accompany a hypermetabolic state, ie, due to continued seizures increase the myocardial load. An intravenous line should now be established and blood drawn for determination of blood levels of glucose, urea nitrogen, electrolytes, CBC, calcium, and magnesium, and for a toxic screen and anticonvulsant drug levels. An intravenous injection of 25–50% glucose solution (1 g/kg) is given, and 100 mg of thiamine is administered intramuscularly. An intravenous infusion of isotonic saline should be started. When the results of the studies return, any severe metabolic acidosis should be corrected by the administration of bicarbonate. At this stage, a specific therapy should be employed to stop the seizures. Treatment for status epilepticus is best carried out in an intensive care unit, and medications are administered intravenously.

Diazepam and Phenytoin

The drug of choice for early termination of seizures is diazepam (Baily and Fenichel 1968, Browne and Penry 1973, Gastaut et al 1965, Lombroso 1966, Meldrum and Brierley 1973a), which is administered in a dose of 0.25–0.4mg/kg up to 10 mg total, at a rate not exceeding 1 mg/min. Because of rapid distribution of diazepam, the blood level obtained decreases rapidly. Administration of intravenous diazepam may be repeated up to three times, at intervals of 15–20 minutes. The drug is insoluble and should not be mixed with other fluids. It should be injected into the intravenous tubing being used to administer normal saline. During administration of diazepam, blood pressure, respiration, and cardiac functions should be monitored. Apnea and hypotension are side effects and are more likely to occur if the patient has previously received a barbiturate. For this reason, it is very important for the referring physician to make sure that a list of previously administered medications accompanys the patient to the emergency room.

Because of the evanescent effect of diazepam, a long-acting drug should be administered immediately after the injection of diazepam. This second drug is usually phenytoin, which is administered in a dose of 10–15 mg/kg up to 1 g total (Albani 1982, Leppik 1979, Wilder et al 1977). In older children and adults, phenytoin is administered at the rate of up to 50 mg/min. Small children are infused at the slower rate of 0.5–1 mg/kg per minute (Dreifuss 1982). Again, the drug is administered into the saline intravenous tubing because phenytoin tends to precipitate in a dextrose solution and because it cannot be diluted into the reservoir bottle. Intravenous phenytoin reaches peak blood levels within 15 minutes, and adequate therapeutic levels are maintained for 24 hours (Wilder et al 1977).

The side effects of intravenous phenytoin include cardiac slowing or arrhythmia, which may necessitate a reduction of infusion rate. This complication may be worsened by systemic acidosis and hypercalcemia. On the other hand, phenytoin produces very little depression of the level of consciousness and of respiration.

The use of diazepam and phenytoin is important because diazepam is eminently suited to rapid termination of seizures but not to long-term therapy. The second drug must be administered early enough to avoid what would otherwise be a therapeutic gap. On the next day, medication can be given by the oral route.

If seizures continue, phenytoin dosage may be increased up to 20 mg/kg. If seizures still recur, phenobarbital may be given intravenously up to a dose fo 20 mg/kg at a rate no faster than 100 mg/min. During administration of phenobarbital, respiration and blood pressure monitoring are necessary. Near the upper dosage levels, mechanical ventilation may be necessary. The side effects of phenobarbital are drowsiness; and the drug has to be given in doses that cause depression of the level of consciousness and occasionally hypotension. The maximum brain concentration of this drug is not reached until after approximately 1 hour. The long half-life of the drug may lead to toxic accumulation when large doses are used repeatedly. Phenobarbital has no particular advantages over phenytoin and diazepam and has the disadvantages inherent in depression of consciousness and respiratory function. These side effects increase the hazard to the patient and may well delay the diagnosis of the underlying cause of the status epilepticus.

Paraldehyde

Use of paraldehyde is an honored tradition in the treatment of status epilepticus, though it is now rarely used as a primary medication for this condition. Paraldehyde has been given intramuscularly, intravenously, or by rectal administration. The disadvantages of intramuscular administration are delayed action (30 to 60 minutes) and possible muscle necrosis at the injection site. The initial dose is 5–10 mL.

The drug is prepared for intravenous administration by mixing 5 mL in 95 mL of 5% dextrose in ½ normal saline. This solution is administered by slow intravenous drip in a dose of 0.2 mg/kg. Side effects caused by too rapid administration include hiccup, tachycardia, and pulmonary edema. A dose of 0.3 mL/kg diluted in peanut oil (1:10) has been found to be rapidly effective when administered rectally, though it tends to be irritating to the rectal mucosa.

The chief advantage of paraldehyde is the margin of safety existing between the anticonvulsant dose and the lethal dose. Its disadvantages were noted earlier and also include the need to use a fresh solution for each dose as this drug is decomposed to acetic acid by light.

Lidocaine

Lidocaine (dispensed as 0.5%, 1%, and 2% solutions in 5% glucose or normal saline for intravenous administration) has been used in the treatment of status epilepticus. At present, this is not a drug of first choice, although it is frequently successful. In treatment of cardiac arrhythmias, this drug is frequently administered in the first few hours following a myocardial infarction. One of the principal advantages of lidocaine is rapidity of action—usually within 0.5 minute. If the patient with status epilepticus does not respond rapidly, administration of this drug should be discontinued. The dosage for intravenous administration is 2-3 mg/kg (1% solution). For administration by infusion, 4-6 mg/kg per hour is recommended (Gamstorp 1983).

The advantages of lidocaine are the rapidity of its action and the absence of sedation. Its disadvantage is that it does not lend itself to prolonged therapy.

Valproate

Rectal administration of valproate (30-60 mL/kg) has been successfully used in the management of status epilepticus (Vajda et al 1978).

General Treatment Measures

Following control of seizure activity, the patient must be started on adequate "running" doses of the appropriate anticonvulsant drug. If phenobarbital is used, the patient's unconscious state may be considerably prolonged, and repeated plasma drug level determinations will be necessary.

Despite the use of an appropriate drug regimen, seizures may continue. General anesthesia should then be considered. A short-acting anesthetic agent, such as a barbiturate, should be administered for at least 2 hours. Anesthesia and muscle relaxation should be considered not only when anticonvulsant drugs are ineffective, but also when respiratory insufficiency and cardiac and circulatory collapse are imminent. An advantage of barbiturate anesthesia is a lowering of the increased intracranial pressure, which is frequently a complication of prolonged seizures. Halothane is contraindicated because of this complication.

In addition to the emergency measures and the effort to control seizures, general treatment measures include treatment of cerebral edema. Complications arising from cerebral edema include interference with cerebral perfusion and accumulation of lactate (Wasterlain 1974, 1981). In the absence of contraindications, cerebral edema may be treated with mannitol (2 g/kg administered over a period of 4 hours), furosemide (up to 200 mg in a 24-hour period), or dexamethazone (4 mg every 6 hours).

Immediately after institution of treatment, the cause of the status epilepticus should be sought. The patient's history, the results of a careful physical examination, and, if indicated, a spinal tap and CT scan should be obtained. As mentioned earlier, if the patient is a known epileptic, the most likely cause of status epilepticus is drug noncompliance or an intercurrent febrile illness. However, there are some patients who will present de novo with status epilepticus that has no obvious cause. A child presenting with status epilepticus for the first time should be suspected of having a serious intracranial lesion.

Treatment of Tonic, Clonic, and Myoclonic Status

Tonic, clonic, and myoclonic status epilepticus respond to some extent to treatment with diazepam and clonazepam (Gastaut et al 1965). Some physicians recommend phenobarbital or phenytoin. However, valproic acid is now considered to be the drug of choice in these seizure forms.

Treatment of Absence Status

The drug of choice in the treatment of absence status is diazepam. It is administered intravenously in the same manner as in the treatment of generalized tonic-clonic status. Administration of diazepam results in cessation of absence status in over 90% of cases. However, this control may be transient (Browne and Penry 1973). For long-term therapy, the drug of choice is valproic acid administered in a dose of 30-60 mg/kg. Older patients who suffer from absence status without a previous history of absence seizures likewise respond dramatically to the intravenous administration of diazepam. However, the drugs of choice for long-term prevention of recurrence are phenytoin or phenobarbital. This drug response may reflect the fact that many of these so-called abnormalities are focal interictally. This finding raises the question whether secondary bilateral synchrony is the cause of the spike-wave stupor.

Treatment of Epilepsia Partialis Continua

The long-term treatment of epilepsia partialis continua with most anticonvulsants is relatively unsatisfactory. However, the attacks may sometimes be assuaged by the administration of diazepam intravenously. Phenytoin, carbamazepine, and clonazepam have all been employed with varying degrees of success. The treatment of partial seizure status is of less urgency than that of generalized seizure status because this disorder is considerably less threatening to the body's homeostatic mechanisms. Therefore, the physician is able to weigh the benefits and the risks of aggressive anticonvulsant drug management.

Treatment of Status Epilepticus in the Neonate

Maintenance of an adequate airway and an adequate glucose concentration are of greatest importance in emergency management of neonatal seizures. Although the clinical manifestations of neonatal status epilepticus are frequently subtle, variable, and nondramatic, the metabolic requirements of the infant are greatly increased over the resting level. Therefore, the seizures, though appearing mild, are of great metabolic consequence and require authoritative intervention. Glucose (3-5 mg/kg, 25-30% solution) should be administered as soon as the IV line has been established. A further 0.5-1 g/hr should be maintained. However, steps should be taken to avoid hyperhydration of hypohydration. Calcium and magnesium are not usually administered unless serum levels of these electrolytes are low.

Phenobarbital is administered in a dose of 15-20 mg/kg IV to achieve a blood level of approximately 20-25 mg/L. The maintenance dosage is 3-5 mg/kg/day. Phenobarbital has a longer half-life in neonates than in older children.

If phenytoin is used, the initial dose is 15–20 mg/kg. This dose should not be given at a rate faster than 3 mg/kg/min. Maintenance doses should be given intravenously because of unpredictable adsorption of this drug in the small infant.

Some authors (Gamstorp 1982) recommend a diazepam drip of 0.3–0.4 mg/kg/hour intravenously for up to 1 week, or lidocaine, 4 mg/kg/hour up to a total of 10 mg/kg, if necessary.

Accurate diagnosis is necessary because some apparent neonatal seizures may be manifestations of forebrain depression (Kellaway 1983) with brain stem release phenomena rather than being true seizures. Duration of therapy is also dictated by diagnostic considerations, upon which judgment of the probable natural history will be based. It is becoming apparent that long-term anticonvulsant therapy is needed in only a small proportion of infants with neonatal convulsions and that trial medication withdrawal may be undertaken within a week, unless there is evidence of central nervous system dysfunction. A further consideration must be the as-yet undetermined potential effects of prolonged antiepileptic drug therapy on the developing nervous system. This is a further deterrent to prophylactic anticonvulsant therapy in the absence of proof of its efficacy.

BIBLIOGRAPHY

Aicardi J, Chevrie JD: Convulsive status epilepticus in infants and children. *Epilepsia* 1970; 11:187–197.

Albani M: Phenytoin in infancy and childhood, in Escueta AV, Wasterlain CG, Porter RJ (eds): *Status Epilepticus*. New York, Raven Press, 1983, pp 457–464.

Bailey DW, Fenichel GM: The treatment of prolonged seizure activity with intravenous diazepam. *Pediatr Pharmacol Ther* 1968;73:923–927.

Browne TR, Penry JK: Benzodiazepines in the treatment of epilepsy. *Epilepsia* 1973;14:277–310.

Dreifuss FE: Treatment of status epilepticus, in Swaiman K, Wright F (eds): *Neurology in Childhood*. St. Louis, Mosby & Co, 1982.

Gamstorp I: Treatment of neonatal status epilepticus, in Pippenger CE, Morselli P (eds): *Antiepileptic Drugs in Childhood*. New York, Raven Press, 1983 (in press).

Gastaut H, Roger J, Lob H: *Les États de Mal Épileptiques*. Paris, Masson, 1967.

Gastaut H, Naquet R, Poire R, et al: Treatment of status epilepticus with diazepam (Valium). *Epilepsia* 1965;6:167–182.

Gastaut H: *Dictionary of Epilepsy. Part 1. Definitions*. Geneva, World Health Organization, 1973.

Gowers WR: *Epilepsy and Other Chronic Convulsive Diseases*. London, J & A Churchill, 1901.

Heintel H: *Der Status Epilepticus. Seine Ätiologie, Klinik and Letalität*. Stuttgart, Fischer, 1972.

Hunter RA: Status epilepticus: History, incidence and problems. *Epilepsia* 1959/60;1:162–188.

Jackson JH: Digitalis with bromide of potassium in epilepsy. *Br Med J* 1880;32.

Janz D: Conditions and causes of status epilepticus. *Epilepsia* 1961;2:170–177.

Janz D: *Die Epilepsein*. Stuttgart, Georg Thieme Verlag, 1969.

Janz D: Status epilepticus and frontal lobe lesions. *J Neurol Sci* 1964;1:446–457.

Kellaway P, Hrachory RA: Status epilepticus in newborns: A perspective on neonatal seizures, in Escueta AV, Wasterlain CG, Porter RJ (eds): *Status Epilepticus*. New York, Raven Press, 1983, pp 93–99.

Lennox WG, Lennox MA: *Epilepsy and Related disorders*. Boston, Little Brown & Co, 1960.

Leppik IE, Sherwin AL: Intravenous phenytoin and phenobarbital: Anticonvulsant action, brain content and plasma binding in rat. *Epilepsia* 1979;20:201–207.

Lombroso CT: Treatment of status epilepticus with diazepam. *Neurology* 1966;16:629–634.

Meldrum BS, Brierley JB: Prolonged epileptic seizures in primates: Ischemic cell changes and its relation to ictal pathophysiological events. *Arch Neurol* 1973a;28:11–17.

Meldrum BS, Horton RW: Physiology of status epilepticus in primates. *Arch Neurol* 1973b; 28:1–9.

Meldrum BS: Metabolic factors during prolonged seizures and their relation to nerve cell death, in Escueta AV, Wasterlain CG, Porter RJ (eds): *Status Epilepticus.* New York, Raven Press, 1983, pp 261–275.

Oxbury JM, Whitty CWM: Causes and consequences of status epilepticus in adults: A study of 86 cases. *Brain* 1971;94:733–744.

Rasmussen T, McCann W: Clinical studies of patients with focal epilepsy due to "chronic encephalitis." *Trans Am Neurol Assoc* 1968;93:89.

Rothner AD, Erenberg G: Status epilepticus. *Pediatr Clin North Am* 1980;27:593–602.

Rowan AJ, Scott DP: Major status epilepticus. *Acta Neurol Scand* 1970;46:573–584.

Sato S, Dreifuss FE: Electroencephalographic findings in a patient with developmental expressive aphasia. *Neurology* 1973;23:181–185.

Scott JG, Masland RL: Occurrence of continuous symptoms in epilepsy patients. *Neurology* 1953;3:297–301.

Temkin O: *The Falling Sickness. A History of Epilepsy from the Greeks to the Beginnings of Modern Neurology,* ed 2. Baltimore, Johns Hopkins Press, 1971.

Turner WA: *Epilepsy.* London, Mcmillan, 1907.

Vajda FJE, Symington GR, Bladin PF: Rectal administration of sodium valproate in status epilepticus. *Neurology* 1978;28:897–899.

Wasterlain CG: Mortality and morbidity from serial seizures. *Epilepsia* 1974;15:155–176.

Wasterlain CG: Status epilepticus, in *Seminars in Neurology.* New York, Thieme & Stratton, 1981, vol 1, pp 87–94.

Whitty CWM, Taylor M: Treatment of status epilepticus. *Lancet* 1949;2:591–594.

Wilder BJ, Ramsey RE, Willmore LJ, et al: Efficacy of I.V. phenytoin in the treatment of status epilepticus: Kinetics of central nervous system penetration. *Ann Neurol* 1977;1:511–518.

CHAPTER 15

Pharmacologic Management of Epilepsy in Childhood

J. Chris Sackellares

Epilepsy is a common disorder among children, affecting approximately 4 or 5 out of every 1000 people below the age of 20 (Hauser and Kurland 1972, Cavazzuti 1980). The incidence and prevalence rates for epilepsy among children provide some measure of the magnitude of epilepsy as a health care problem, but the serious impact of the disorder upon the individual child and his or her family is more difficult to quantitate.

Over the past three decades, significant advances have improved the medical management of epilepsy. Numerous new antiepileptic drugs have become available since phenytoin was first introduced in 1938. Some of these drugs were found to be too toxic or to be ineffective and are no longer used except in rare circumstances. Others have proved to be both safe and effective. We also know more about the efficacy, toxicity, and pharmacology of the drugs used today. Through use of a common language to classify seizures and through improvement in the methodology for clinical trials, a vast literature has developed from which the physician can draw reasonably valid conclusions as to the likelihood of a given drug being effective in controlling a given type of seizure.

Our understanding of the basic mechanism of the epilepsies and of the mechanisms of action of antiepileptic drugs is limited. Therefore, our knowledge of drug efficacy is based upon empirical observations of the effect of a given drug in controlling seizures of a given type.

Through numerous acute and chronic clinical trials of antiepileptic drugs, profiles of potential toxic effects have been developed for most antiepileptic drugs in use today. The rather poor relationship between the dose and the biological effects of most antiepileptic drugs, and by contrast, the close relationship between blood levels and biological effects have been well established. As a result, antiepileptic drug assays are widely available through clinical laboratories.

The pharmacologic properties of most antiepileptic drugs have now been described in great detail. This information is being applied in the clinical setting on a day-to-day basis. The physician can draw upon this knowledge of therapeutic plasma level ranges, elimination half-lives, and potential drug–drug interactions to tailor his treatment to the individual patient. The most universally accepted classification of epileptic seizures is the International Classification of Epileptic Seizures (1981). According to the International Classification, seizures are divided into partial seizures, generalized seizures, and unclassified seizures. Partial seizures begin locally within one cerebral hemisphere. They are further divided into partial seizures with simple symptomatology, partial seizures with complex symptomatology, and partial seizures with secondary generalization. Generalized seizures begin simultaneously in both hemispheres. As a result, consciousness is usually altered at onset. Generalized seizures are further divided into absence seizures, tonic seizures, clonic seizures, tonic-clonic seizures, atonic seizures, and massive bilateral myoclonus. Unclassified seizures are those that are unclassifiable because of insufficient information.

Classification of epileptic seizures is useful for several reasons. Any given antiepileptic drug may be very effective in controlling one type of seizure, yet completely ineffective in controlling another type of seizure. The seizure type also has prognostic implications. Primary generalized tonic-clonic seizures and primary generalized absence seizures are more likely to respond to medical treatment than partial seizures. In a study of 40 patients with refractory seizures referred to the University of Virginia Medical Center, 6.5% had generalized tonic-clonic seizures; these seizures were either under control or occurred infrequently. By contrast, 4.25% had partial complex seizures occurring weekly, and 7.5% had daily partial complex seizures (Sutula et al 1981). A number of authors have reported that generalized tonic-clonic (grand mal) seizures are relatively more responsive to treatment (Craig and MacKinnon 1965, Fukuyama et al 1963). Partial complex seizures are somewhat less likely to respond to treatment (Fukuyama et al 1963, Livingston and Peterson 1956, Lundervold and Jabour 1962). However, if partial seizures fail to respond to medical treatment, surgical treatment may be an alternative. This is not the case for primary generalized seizures. The seizure type may also give some information as to cause. For example, a patient with partial seizures is more likely to have an identifiable structural lesion as the underlying cause of his seizures than a patient with primary generalized seizures.

ESTABLISHING THE DIAGNOSIS

The initial step in the management of epilepsy is to establish the diagnosis. This involves verification that the child is experiencing recurrent seizures, definition of the type of seizures the child is having, and determination of the severity of the disorder. In some cases, the diagnosis is straightforward. But the clinical manifestations of epileptic seizures are myriad. They include a variety of motor, sensory, cognitive, affective, and autonomic phenomena, many of which can be seen in other medical and psychiatric disorders. Different types of epileptic seizures may share similar clinical or electroencephalographic features, thus making classification difficult. For some types of seizures, it is even difficult to determine the frequency of occurrence because of the subtlety of the clinical manifestations, short duration, or extremely high frequency.

In spite of the development of sophisticated diagnostic procedures, the most powerful diagnostic tool is the medical history. The historical inquiry is directed toward defining the clinical manifestations of the seizures—the frequency, duration, and temporal patterns of the seizures—and identifying any environmental precipitants. The problem of classifying a given patient's seizures is compounded by the fact that he or she may be experiencing more than one kind of seizure. Furthermore, the same type of seizure may vary in clinical symptomatology. For example, a child with absence seizures may, on some occasions, have seizures manifested by alteration in consciousness only (absence simple). At other times, the child may have seizures manifested by mild clonic movements or automatisms in addition to altered consciousness (Porter et al 1975). The parents may give a confusing and seemingly contradictory account of the child's seizures. Each may emphasize certain aspects of the seizures and fail to report other details. The patient may have been unconscious during all or part of the seizure or may be amnestic for the event. In most instances, asking the parents to describe specific examples of several recent seizures, from beginning to end, is a fruitful approach to the history. The patient can add any subjective sensations he may have experienced, and the entire event can be clearly reconstructed.

A seizure may be arbitrarily divided into four phases: 1) prodrome, 2) signs and symptoms just prior to altered consciousness, 3) altered consciousness, 4) signs and symptoms occurring during alteration of consciousness, and 5) postictal signs and symptoms. All of these phases may not occur during any given seizure. For example, in simple seizures, consciousness is not lost. In a primary generalized seizure, there are no signs or symptoms prior to the loss of consciousness. Once detailed descriptions of several seizures have been obtained, the physician can develop working hypotheses as to the type or types of seizures that have occurred.

The next step is to estimate the frequency and duration of each type of seizure. For some seizures, such as tonic-clonic seizures, the parents can provide an accurate seizure count. For more subtle seizures, such as absence seizures, the seizure count may be drastically underestimated. It is also important to determine whether seizures occur randomly or periodically and whether they tend to occur singly or in clusters. If the seizures tend to occur in periodic clusters, this must be considered when evaluating the effects of a new drug regimen. It is important to document the seizure frequency and duration on the initial visit. This information provides an estimate as to the severity of the disorder and provides a baseline for comparison by which the results of treatment can be measured.

A number of factors may influence the patient or the parents' subjective assessments of seizure frequency or severity. One parent may give far different estimates than the other. The child may give still another estimate. It may not be possible to obtain sufficiently accurate and detailed seizure description or estimates of seizure frequency during the initial interview. It is therefore wise to ask the patient and his family to keep an accurate seizure log during the interval between visits. The log should include a description of each seizure, the date and time of occurrence, and any apparent precipitating events. A little time spent in instructing the family about what to look for often results in vastly improved historical data on subsequent visits.

THE EXAMINATION

Although the child with epilepsy may appear to be completely normal between seizures, a detailed general physical and neurologic examination remains an important diagnostic tool. The examination may provide clues as to the presence of underlying systemic or neurologic disorders and serves as a baseline by which to judge any adverse effects of medications.

Sensorium, orientation, coordination, the presence of nystagmus, and gait alteration should be carefully assessed during initial and follow-up examinations. If absence seizures are suspected, 3 minutes of hyperventilation may precipitate a seizure, providing a definitive diagnosis.

THE ELECTROENCEPHALOGRAM

The electroencephalogram (EEG) is used to confirm the diagnosis of epilepsy and to aid in the classification of the seizures. The standard EEG recording is performed while the patient is awake and alert. In most instances activation procedures are performed in addition to recording during the resting state. Standard activation procedures include hyperventilation for 3 minutes, intermittent photic stimulation, and sleep. Hyperventilation and photic stimulation are not only used to induce paroxysmal discharges in the EEG but are also useful in precipitating absence seizures. Photic stimulation may, if prolonged, precipitate generalized tonic-clonic seizures. This can usually be avoided by discontinuing the stimulus as soon as paroxysmal discharges occur in the tracing.

Paroxysmal discharges may be arbitrarily divided into ictal discharges and interictal discharges. Ictal discharges are those that are associated with clinical seizure phenomena, and interictal discharges are brief paroxysms unassociated with clinically detectable seizure activity. In general, interictal discharges are of shorter duration than ictal discharges. For instance, the generalized spike-wave discharges characteristic of absence seizures are associated with measurable prolongation of reaction time when they are 3 or more seconds in duration. However, in some cases, paroxysmal discharges lasting less than 1 second may be associated with clinical manifestations. Such is the case for generalized myoclonic seizures.

The frequency of abnormal routine EEG recordings among patients with seizures depends upon the type of seizures as well as the recording conditions. It has been estimated that without activation procedures, the EEG shows specific abnormalities in only 40% of patients with epilepsy (Gastaut and Tassinari 1975). Thus, a normal EEG does not exclude the diagnosis of epilepsy. The sensitivity of the routine EEG can be increased by activation procedures.

In patients with partial seizures, the characteristic finding on the interictal EEG is the presence of a localized spike, spike-wave, or sharp wave discharges recorded over one hemisphere. However, these discharges may occur bilaterally over both hemispheres, either synchronously or independently. The characteristic interictal EEG pattern in patients with generalized seizures is the generalized, bilaterally synchronous and symmetrical spike, spike-wave, or polyspike-wave discharges.

Ideally, one prefers to record ictal EEG paroxysms. The recording of paroxysmal discharges at the time of a clinical seizure is virtually diagnostic of epilepsy and in most cases provides sufficient information to classify the seizure. Of course, there is always the possibility that a given patient may be experiencing more than one type of seizure.

Newer intensive monitoring procedures have been developed to increase the likelihood of recording a paroxysmal discharge, to provide detailed objective information about the clinical and EEG manifestation of the seizures, and to provide data about seizure frequency and duration. These procedures are described in detail elsewhere in this book (see Chapter 17). They include prolonged EEG monitoring (PEM), using either radiotelemetry or cable telemetry, and EEG monitoring with simultaneous closed circuit television recording of the patient (EEG-CCTV). These procedures are useful tools in the management of seizures in children. They provide the opportunity to record ictal seizure events. Ictal paroxysms are seldom recorded during routine EEG recordings, which are usually from 20 to 30 minutes long (Bowden et al 1975, Woods et al 1975).

Electroencephalographic recordings with simultaneous closed circuit television recordings are particularly useful in differentiating among seizures with similar clinical characteristics. For instance, complex partial seizures may be difficult to distinguish from generalized absence seizures on clinical grounds alone. This is particularly true if detailed observation of the clinical symptoms are unavailable. Both types of seizures may be manifested by altered consciousness, mild clonic components, automatisms, and autonomic phenomena. The EEG-CCTV recordings on videotape enable the physician to review the clinical and EEG manifestations of the seizures simultaneously. They may also aid in differentiating pseudoseizures from epileptic seizures. Pseudoseizures are less common in children than adults, but well-documented cases of pseudoseizures in children have been reported (Holmes et al 1980). The EEG-CCTV recordings are also useful for providing documentation and quantification of infantile spasms.

Prolonged EEG monitoring performed for 6 to 12 hours provides an objective assessment of the frequency of generalized absence seizures. Parental reports of absence seizure frequency are often inaccurate (Browne et al 1974a). The brevity, high frequency, and subtle clinical signs of absence seizures make it difficult to accurately assess absence seizure frequency by clinical observation alone.

DRUG THERAPY

Treatment of epilepsy is a complex endeavor, the goal of which is to reduce the negative impact of the disorder on the quality of the patient's life, while minimizing the adverse effects of treatment. Each component of the treatment program should be evaluated in light of how well it contributes to attainment of that goal. Although seizures are the most obvious aspect of the disorder to reduce the quality of life for the epileptic, there are many other psychological, educational, and social complications in epilepsy that are less obvious but are just as important to the patient and his or her family. Failure to address these psychological and social problems may result in treatment failure, despite significant reduction in seizures. In this section we will consider the pharmacologic treatment directed toward seizure control. Seizure control is a key component of the treatment program directed toward reducing the disability caused by epilepsy.

Drug Efficacy

There are numerous drugs available for the treatment of epileptic seizures. There is really no "drug of choice" for the treatment of epilepsy. For any given patient, a number of factors should be considered when choosing the best drug to use. A major factor in the choice of an antiepileptic drug is the type of seizure one is treating. Some drugs, such as ethosuximide, are highly effective in controlling only one type of seizure (generalized absence), whereas others, such as valproic acid, are useful in a broad spectrum of seizure types. Thus, for a patient with only absence seizures, ethosuximide may be most appropriate, whereas for a patient with both absence and tonic-clonic seizures, valproic acid may be preferable. The use of these drugs is directed toward maximum control of seizures with minimum adverse effects.

Numerous studies of the efficacy of antiepileptic drugs have been published. Unfortunately, many older studies were uncontrolled and failed to correlate blood levels with clinical effects (Coatsworth 1971). Thus, observations made and conclusions drawn from these studies were limited. As a result, professional opinions as to the relative efficacy and safety of antiepilepsy drugs were based largely on personal experience and popular trends. In recent years, a number of studies have been published that utilize double blind-controlled protocols with careful monitoring of antiepileptic drug levels. Indications for each antiepileptic drug based on seizure are being established (Jeavons 1977, Porter and Penry 1978, Sherwin 1977), although for the less common types of seizures (such as tonic seizures and atonic seizures) the data are not sufficient to draw strong conclusions as to the relative efficacy of the various antiepileptic drugs.

It is convenient to group antiepileptic drugs into three groups: 1) drugs effective in generalized tonic-clonic seizures and all forms of partial seizures, 2) drugs effective in absence seizures, and 3) drugs with a broad spectrum of efficacy (Table 15-1). The use of the drugs in treating specific types of seizures will be discussed later.

Table 15-1
Spectrum of Efficacy for Commonly Used Antiepileptic Drugs

Generalized Tonic-Clonic and All Forms of Partial Seizures	Generalized Absence	Broad Spectrum of Efficacy
Carbamazepine	Ethosuximide	Valproic acid
Phenytoin	Trimethadione	Clonazepam
Phenobarbital		
Primidone		

Potential Toxicity

Potential adverse effects should also be considered when choosing an antiepileptic drug. In fact, with the large number of highly effective drugs available now, the relative toxicity of these drugs may be the most important of the factors to consider when choosing a drug. Antiepileptic drugs may affect any system of the body adversely, but they most commonly affect the central nervous system, gastrointestinal tract, liver, and hematopoietic systems. Acute or subacute toxic effects, such as nausea, drowsiness, or ataxia, are usually related to dosage or blood level. In most instances, these effects are usually related to dosage or blood level. In most instances, these effects can be alleviated by dosage adjustments. More chronic toxicity such as gingival hyperplasia, polyneuropathy, hirsutism, and folate deficiency occur over months to years and are also related to duration of therapy. Idiosyncratic reactions such as skin rashes and bone marrow depression may occur with any dosage. Their occurrence necessitates discontinuation of the drug.

The Side Effects of Anticonvulsant Drugs in the Pediatric Age Range

Some side effects of anticonvulsion medications are particularly likely to affect the young and may be sufficiently insidious to escape attention. These include 1) effects on learning and congitive function, 2) effects on behavior ranging from inattentiveness to the appearance of thought disorders and psychotic behavior, 3) exacerbation of seizures, and 4) the appearance of movement disorders.

EFFECTS ON LEARNING AND COGNITIVE FUNCTION. Lennox (1960) felt that approximately 5–15% of his patients suffered impairment of cognitive abilities as a result of anticonvulsant drugs. Trimble and Reynolds (1976) have reviewed this aspect of anticonvulsant therapy. They have implicated phenobarbital as a cause of difficulty with intellectual performance, even at blood levels in the therapeutic range. Phenytoin has been more often implicated as a factor in impaired cognitive function (Stores 1975), even at blood levels in the therapeutic range. In addition, a syndrome of progressive intellectual deterioration has been reported in patients taking phenytoin; this deterioration is not always reversible. The child's school performance progressively deteriorates independently of seizure frequency. On occasion, ethosuximide has been implicated in impairment of cognitive function, but controlled studies have not confirmed this. Though sodium valproate has not been used for a length of time sufficient to allow conclusions concerning long-term effects on behavior and educational progress, early studies indicate that this drug is remarkably free from side effects on cognitive ability, as is carbamazepine.

BEHAVIORAL CHANGES. Behavioral side effects of phenobarbital, particularly hyperactivity, have been well documented. Such behavior is frequently disruptive to the extent of being unacceptable. Behavioral changes have also been reported with clonazepam; these changes consist of hyperactivity, restlessness, short attention span, irritability, and aggression. Behavioral effects with ethosuximide have included psychotic episodes, and these are usually associated with high serum levels of the drug. Primidone produces behavioral side effects in a large proportion of patients, and these are different from the nondirected hyperactivity of phenobarbital in that the behavior is often described as "mean," indicating a more organized misbehavior.

EXACERBATION OF SEIZURES. This may occur with phenytoin, which may exacerbate myoclonic seizures and may also exacerbate generalized tonic-clonic seizures when the blood level reaches the toxic range.

ABNORMAL MOVEMENTS. The development of abnormal movements has been described with phenytoin; these movements consist of choreoathetosis and occasionally asterixis. Dystonia may complicate carbamazepine use, and patients on valproate tend to develop a tremor. Acute basal ganglia reactions with ethosuximide and with valproate have been reported.

Pharmacologic Properties

The pharmacologic properties of a drug may also be a factor in drug selection. The ideal drug should have a high therapeutic index (ratio of the therapeutic dose to toxic dose), pharmacokinetic characteristics that enable a single daily dosage regimen, a predictable and linear relationship between dose and blood level, and no interaction with other drugs. None of the currently available antiepileptic drugs meet all of these criteria. Thus, drug selection is usually based primarily upon the relative effectiveness of the drug in controlling the specific type of seizure as compared to the potential for adverse effects. However, knowledge of the basic pharmacokinetic properties of the chosen drug is mandatory if the drug is to be used effectively.

In recent years, detailed pharmacokinetic profiles have been developed for most of the currently available antiepileptic drugs. The role of the clinician is to apply this extensive knowledge to the practical problems of prescribing optimal dosage regimen for his patient. Many pharmacokinetic parameters are used to describe the time courses of drug and metabolite concentrations in biological fluids and tissues. Those parameters that are most useful to the clinician are summarized in Table 15-2. The half-life (or the corresponding first-order rate constant) is the most useful parameter for determining the dosage regimen (Wagner 1979). One can derive a rough estimate of the optimum loading dose, dosage interval, and maintenance dose from the half-life (Kruger-Thiemer 1965). The rule of thumb is to make the dosage interval equal to the half-life of elimination, the loading dose equal to twice the maintenance dose, and the maintenance dose equal to the minimum amount in the body necessary for effective therapy (Kruger-Thiemer 1965). This rule assumes a one-compartment model and a rate constent for absorption that is much larger than the elimination rate constant (Wagner 1979). Of course, other considerations such as the possibility of gastric irritation or the range between toxic and therapeutic blood levels must be considered. For instance, a drug such as ethosuximide, which tends to cause gastric irritation, may require shorter dosage intervals to enable use of smaller individual doses. Carbamazepine may require shorter dosage intervals than predicted by the preceding rule of thumb in order to maintain minimum plasma levels sufficient to control seizures while avoiding peak plasma levels high enough to cause transient side effects. In the case of carbamazepine, small fluctuations of concentration can result in significant changes in its biological effects.

Table 15-2
Pharmacokinetic Parameters

Parameter	Units	Definition
Apparent volume of distribution (V_d)	liters/kg	A calculated measure of the extent of a drug's distribution in the body
C_{max}	µg/mL	Peak plasma level
T_{max}	hours	Time required to achieve a peak plasma level
Elimination rate (k)	fraction/hour	Defines the rate of fall in plasma concentration
Plasma half-life ($t_{1/2}$)	hours	Time required for the plasma concentration to fall to one-half of the original concentration
Plasma concentration (level)	µg/mL	Concentration of the total amount of drug (bround to plasma protein plus unbound fraction)
Free fraction	µg/mL	Percentage of the drug that is dissolved in plasma water, not bound to plasma protein
Steady state		Stage at which the amount of drug absorbed is equal to the amount of drug eliminated over each dosage interval
V_{max}	mg/hr	Michaelis-Menten constant that represents the maximum velocity of the reaction
K_m	µg/mL	Michaelis-Menten constant that represents the concentration when the velocity of the reaction is half-maximal

For some drugs, chronic oral antiepileptic drug therapy may be initiated by administering an oral loading dose, thus achieving therapeutic plasma levels quickly. This approach is usually feasible for phenytoin or phenobarbital. Alternatively, the maintenance dosages may be instituted without administering a loading dose. In the latter case, a steady state will be achieved after a period of time equal to approximately five half-lives. For some drugs, an oral loading dose is not feasible. For example, an oral dose of ethosuximide is not recommended because of the likelihood of gastric irritation. Benzodiazepines such as clonazepam must be started in doses lower than the ultimate maintenance dose to allow tolerance of the sedative effects to occur. Carbamazepine is metabolized more slowly when first introduced than later, after it induces enzymes for its own metabolism. As a result, the initial dose should be small in comparison to the ultimate maintenance dose.

The elimination half-lives for antiepileptic drugs commonly used in childhood epilepsy are listed in Table 15-3. These values should be used as a rough guide because there may be considerable variation of elimination rates among individual patients. This interindividual variability is particularly important in the pediatric age group, because the half-life of many drugs (eg, phenytoin and phenobarbital) varies as a function of age.

Table 15-3
Pharmacologic Parameters of Antiepileptic Drugs*

Drug	Usual Dose (mg/kg/day)	Therapeutic Range (μg/mL)	Half-Life (Hours)	Protein Bound (%)
Carbamazepine	10–15	5–12	9–19	70
Phenytoin	5–10†	10–20	1.2–100	90
Phenobarbital	4–6	15–40	37	40
Primidone	12–25	5–10	12	<50
Ethosuximide	15–35	40–100	30	0
Valproic acid	15–60	50–100	6–18	90
Clonazepam	0.05–0.2	20–80 (ng/mL)	20–40	<50
Diazepam	—‡	Not determined	9–54	95

*These pharmacologic parameters are estimates and vary remarkably among individual patients and among patients of various ages. They should be used only as general guidelines for therapy. The half-life for carbamazepine changes with time because of autoinduction. The half-life of phenytoin is dose dependent. The half-lives of all drugs are affected by drug–drug interactions. Drug–drug interactions can also affect plasma protein binding.
†For the treatment of status epilepticus, phenytoin is administered intravenously in a dose of 15 to 18 mg/kg. The maximum infusion rate in adults is 50 mg/min.
‡Diazepam is rarely used as an oral maintenance drug. The intravenous dose of diazepam required for treating status epilepticus ranges from 0.07 mg/kg to 1.25 mg/kg in children and 2.5 to 10 mg (total dose) in adults. The actual dose used should be based on the clinical response.

Many of the published half-lives or elimination rates for antiepileptic drugs are based upon pharmacokinetic studies in adults. The manner in which children utilize drugs is remarkably different from that of adults. Children below the age of 11 years metabolize phenytoin, phenobarbital, primidone, carbamazepine, and ethosuximide more rapidly (Pippenger 1978). There is a tendency for children treated for epilepsy to become more lethargic or mentally dull or to have an exacerbation of seizures as they approach puberty. This problem may arise as drug utilization patterns change with age (Pippenger 1978). These changes in drug utilization translate into differences of half-life. Thus, as the child approaches puberty, the same dosage in milligrams per kilogram may result in significantly higher steady-state plasma levels. The problem can be avoided by alerting the patient and family to the potential problems and by carefully monitoring drug levels.

The pharmacokinetic behavior of phenytoin presents additional problems to the clinician because of the nonlinear relationship between dosage and plasma level, because of its capacity-limited elimination. The elimination of phenytoin follows Michaelis-Menten kinetics; the half-life is dosage dependent (Arnold and Gerber 1970, Atkinson and Shaw 1973, Garrettson and Jusko 1975, Gerber and Wagner 1972, Richens and Dunlop 1975).

The relationship between plasma levels and dose for phenytoin is described by the following equation:

$$Ro = V_{max} \, P/(K_m + P)$$

where Ro is the dose, P is the plasma concentration, and V_{max} and K_m are the Michaelis-Menten constants.

Because the metabolism of phenytoin follows Michaelis-Menten kinetics, the relationship between dose and plasma level is not linear. The implications of this nonlinear relationship are illustrated in Figure 15-1. At lower doses, small increments in the maintenance dose result in small increases in steady-state plasma levels of phenytoin. At higher doses, the same small increments in dose will lead to marked increases in plasma phenytoin levels and unexpected toxicity.

Because both K_m and V_{max} for phenytoin vary among individual patients, the dose required to achieve any given plasma concentration will vary. Chiba et al (1980) calculated the Michaelis-Menten constants for phenytoin in 104 children ranging from 6 months to 16 years of age. Values for K_m were highly variable (3.7 $\pm$ 4.3 g/mL) but did not correlate with age. Values of V_{max} ranged from 6 to 25 mg/kg/day and varied inversely with age.

The usual maintenance dose of phenytoin is between 5 and 10 mg/kg/day. However, because of the wide individual variability of phenytoin metabolism, the plasma levels resulting from a given dose are unpredictable. Figure 15-2 illustrates the range of plasma levels that can result in different patients from dosages within the usual dosage range. In Figure 15-2C, K_m is very high. If V_{max} is low, a dose of 5 mg/kg/day would result in plasma levels within the therapeutic range, whereas a dose of 9 mg/kg/day would result in toxic levels. If K_m is low (Figure 15-2A), higher doses are required to achieve therapeutic plasma levels. One can predict the optimal dose of phenytoin for an individual by measuring the steady-state plasma level for two different dosages, then calculating the values for K_m and V_{max}. The desired plasma level can then be entered into the preceding formula, and the optimal dosage calculated. This method is time consuming when done by hand, but the task can be simplified by using a graphic method described by Ludden et al (1977) or by using a programmable calculator (King and Kaul 1980). This approach has been demonstrated to be useful for preventing phenytoin toxicity in children (Chiba et al 1980).

Figure 15-1 The expected steady-state plasma level for phenytoin (μg/mL) is plotted against the daily maintenance dose (mg/kg/day) for a patient with "average" Michaelis-Menten kinetics (K_m = 4 μg/mL; V_{max} = 10 mg/kg/day). The nonlinear relationship between dose and plasma level is illustrated.

Figure 15-2 Steady-state plasma phenytoin concentration is plotted against V_{max} for three different dosages of phenytoin. **A** K_m is low (0.5 μg/mL). **B** K_m is mid-range (3 μg/mL). **C** K_m is high (7 μg/mL).

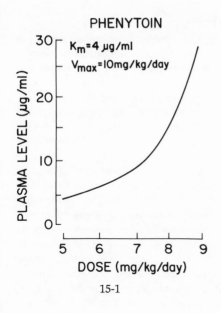

15-1

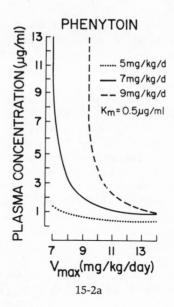

15-2a

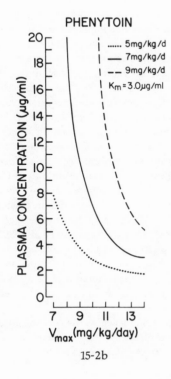

15-2b

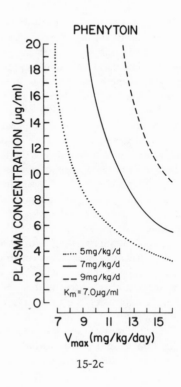

15-2c

USE OF ANTIEPILEPTIC DRUG BLOOD LEVELS

The effects of antiepileptic drugs upon the central nervous system are dependent upon the amount of drug present in the brain. Because it is impossible to measure brain concentrations, plasma concentration (blood levels) are used as an estimate of the amount of drug present in the brain. The therapeutic range is the range of plasma concentrations for which optimal seizure control is most likely to occur without undue side effects. Plasma levels above this range are likely to cause side effects, whereas plasma levels below this range are likely to be inadequate for optimal seizure control. The therapeutic ranges have been established for most antiepileptic drugs. These ranges are not often based upon rigorous statistical analysis, but, in practice, they serve as a useful guide to therapy (Eadie and Tyrer 1980). The usual therapeutic ranges for commonly used antiepileptic drugs are shown in Table 15-3.

It should be borne in mind that the optimal plasma level for any given patient may fall at any point within the therapeutic range and, in some instances, may fall outside the usual therapeutic range. For example, the established therapeutic range for ethosuximide is 40 to 100 $\mu g/mL$. In some instances, absence seizures may not be controlled with plasma levels just above 40 $\mu g/mL$ but may come under complete control with levels in the upper therapeutic range (Sato et al 1981). In some patients, intolerable side effects may occur even though plasma levels are within the usual therapeutic range. Clinical signs of toxicity, in spite of "therapeutic" plasma levels, are particularly common in patients receiving several antiepileptic drugs concomitantly (Sutula et al 1980). Although one cannot invariably predict the optimum drug level for an individual patient, clinical effects correlate better with plasma levels than with dosage.

Once a steady-state drug concentration is reached, the fluctuation range of plasma concentrations during the dosage interval remains essentially constant. The minimum concentration occurs just prior to a dose. The maximum concentration occurs at a time that is dependent upon the absorption rate and elimination rate of the drug and is, therefore, harder to predict. Therefore, in general, one should usually sample blood for drug levels at the end of a dosage interval, just prior to the next dose. For drugs with relatively long half-lives, relative to the dosage interval, such as phenobarbital, the steady-state plasma level fluctuates within a narrow range. By contrast, drugs such as valproic acid and carbamazepine may fluctuate markedly during the dosage interval. For the latter drugs, careful attention to sampling time with respect to the dosage interval is particularly important. Transient toxic effects (particularly diplopia, drowsiness, and headache) commonly occur when the plasma carbamazepine level reaches a peak, following an oral dose (Hoppener et al 1980). Furthermore, there may be wide swings between minimum and maximum plasma levels of carbamazepine. These fluctuations are particularly large when carbamazepine is given along with other antiepileptic drugs (Hoppener et al 1980). When transient toxic effects occur following a dose, it may be useful to obtain additional samples at the time when side effects first occur to document the plasma level at which side effects occur in that patient. The drug regimen should then be altered, either by decreasing the total daily dose or by decreasing the dosage interval (eg, changing from a twice daily to a thrice daily schedule).

Clinical laboratories usually report antiepileptic blood levels as the concentration of the total drug (ie, both the plasma protein-bound fraction and the free fraction). In most situations, the concentration of total drug in the plasma adequately reflects brain concentration and correlates well with biological effects.

Phenobarbital is an example of an antiepileptic drug that is not highly bound to plasma protein. In humans, approximately 40% of total serum phenobarbital is bound to serum albumin (Goldberg 1980). In contrast, approximately 97% of phenytoin is bound to plasma proteins (Barth et al 1976). Valproic acid is also highly protein bound (Taburet and van der Kleijn 1977, Cramer and Mattson 1979, Klotz and Antonin 1977, Gugler and Mueller 1978). For drugs that are highly bound to plasma proteins, conditions causing a decrease in protein binding can result in significant changes in the free fraction in the plasma. Because the free fraction is that portion that is available for entry into the brain and metabolism, an increase in the free fraction can cause changes in the biological effects and pharmacokinetics. Booker and Darcy (1975) showed better correlation between free phenytoin concentrations and clinical toxicity than between total serum level and toxicity. Thus, in some circumstances, direct measurement of the free fraction in the plasma may be advisable. Patients with hypoalbuminemia may show toxic effects when total phenytoin levels are in the therapeutic range as a result of a relative excess of unbound drug (Boston Collaborative Drug Surveillance Program 1973). Uremia may cause reduction in the binding of phenytoin to serum proteins (Odar-Cederlof and Borga 1974). This reduction in binding results in an increase in the free fraction and enhanced activity of phenytoin. The overall effect is that total phenytoin concentrations may be low while the biologically active free fraction remains within the therapeutic concentration. Drug–drug interactions may also alter protein binding. For example, phenytoin and valproic acid compete for plasma protein binding sites, increasing the free fraction of both drugs (Cramer and Mattson 1979). Therefore, in conditions such as uremia or hypoalbuminemia, or when there is a potential for drug–drug interactions affecting protein-binding, the free fraction of phenytoin or valproic acid may provide a better guide for therapy than total drug levels.

Follow-up of Treatment

The child with epilepsy should be examined at intervals to assess the effects of treatment. The interval between visits will vary considerably, depending upon the severity of the seizures, the response to treatment, the potential for adverse drug effects, and whether the drug regimen is being changed or has been stabilized. The interval examination is used to assess seizure control, to identify adverse effects of treatment, to assess the current therapeutic regimen, and to plan future diagnostic and therapeutic intervention.

The assessment of seizure control depends upon an accurate history. As indicated earlier, the patient, the family, and the physician are biased observers. Subjective estimates of the degree of seizure control should be, whenever possible, supplemented by diaries or logs upon which each seizure is recorded. In some instances (eg, absence seizures), prolonged EEG monitoring may be required to obtain an accurate estimate of the effects of treatment upon seizure frequency and duration. Subjective opinions regarding seizure control should not be ignored, however. If more objective seizure counts do not correlate with the patient's subjective opinion, there is probably a reason. For example, the patient may be taking his medications sporadically. Psychological or social factors may also color the patient's report of seizure control. Or, the patient and family members may need more education in recognizing seizures.

Evidence of antiepileptic drug toxicity should be sought at each visit. Although the utility of antiepileptic drug level assays has been emphasized, the patient's report of subtle side effects should be taken seriously, even in the face of "therapeutic" drug levels. The patient himself, either through careful history taking or through the physical examination, remains the best source of information as to the effect of drug therapy. Laboratory data are meaningful only in the context of the clinical findings.

Polypharmacy

The practice of concurrent use of multiple antiepileptic drugs is firmly ingrained in the practice of neurology. In a European survey, Guelen et al (1975) found that among 11,700 patients from 15 centers epileptic patients were receiving an average of 3.2 drugs per patient. Polypharmacy is particularly common in the treatment of patients with refractory seizures. Among 40 patients admitted to an epilepsy unit for refractory seizures, 85% were receiving at least two drugs, 55% were receiving three or more drugs, and 15% were receiving four or more drugs at the time of admission (Sutula et al 1981). Reynolds and Shorvon (1981) have suggested that a number of factors contribute to the practice of polypharmacy, including the chronicity and prognosis of epilepsy, the wide availability and choice of drugs, lack of agreement as to the most suitable choice of drugs for different seizures, traditional approaches to drug treatment, and limits of efficacy of available antiepileptic drugs. Although evidence supporting the necessity of polypharmacy is lacking, there is data indicating that polypharmacy is unnecessary in a large number of cases. In a retrospective analysis of 50 adult epileptic outpatients who were taking two anticonvulsant drugs, Shorvon and Reynolds (1977) found evidence that seizure control had improved in 36%. The same authors (Shorvon and Reynolds 1979) reported the results of a prospective study in which polypharmacy was reduced to monotherapy in 20 of 40 adult patients. During the subsequent year, seizure control was improved in 55%, unchanged in 28%, and worse in 17%. There was also clinical evidence for improvement of mental function in this group of patients. In the study by Sutula et al (1981), the average number of antiepileptic drugs per patient was reduced from 2.55 to 1.95 over a period of approximately 8 weeks. Furthermore, the reduction in the number of antiepileptic drugs was associated with reduced seizure frequency in most patients.

There is also evidence that polypharmacy may have adverse intellectual effects. Shorvon and Reynolds (1979) reported clinical evidence for improved alertness, reduction of depression anxiety, fatigue, and improved behavior and intellectual function in many of the patients following the reduction of polypharmacy. The changes were based on clinical observations. More recently, Giordani et al (1983) reported improvement in objective tests of cognitive and intellectual performance following intensive diagnostic and therapeutic intervention in patients with refractory seizures. Although the improvement in cognitive and intellectual measures did not correlate with reduction in seizure frequency, there was significant correlation with reduction in the number of antiepileptic drugs.

Another problem with polypharmacy is drug–drug interactions (see Table 15-4). Virtually all the antiepileptic drugs can interact with other antiepileptic drugs to alter pharmacokinetics. Phenobarbital is a strong inducer of microsomal enzymes. Phenytoin and phenobarbital compete for the same enzymes that are involved in their biotransformation; valproic acid interacts with phenytoin, phenobarbital, carbamazepine, and ethosuximide. Phenytoin enhances the biotransformation of primidone to phenobarbital. Many drugs, including phenytoin and phenobarbital, appear to reduce steady-state plasma levels of valproic acid (Sackellares et al 1981). Thus, drug–drug interactions confound the predictions of plasma levels and biological effects, severely complicating the pharmacologic management of epilepsy. Drug–drug interactions may also cause serious side effects that do not relate to the plasma concentrations of the drugs involved. For example, in some patients, administration of valproic acid to patients receiving other antiepileptic drugs can induce a profound stuporous state not directly attributable to drug levels (Sackellares et al 1979).

Table 15-4
Interactions among Antiepileptic Drugs

Affected Drug	Change in Level	Interacting Drug	Putative Mechanism
Carbamazepine	Lowered	Phenobarbital Phenytoin Primidone	Increased metabolism
Clonazepam	Lowered	Phenobarbital	Increased metabolism
	Raised	Phenytoin	Decreased metabolism
Valproate	Lowered	Carbamazepine	
Phenobarbital	Raised	Valproate	Decreased metabolism
Phenytoin	Lowered	Cambamazepine Clonazepam Phenobarbital	Increased metabolism
	Raised	Valproate	Free fraction due to protein binding
		Ethosuximide	Decreased metabolism
		Phenobarbital	Substrate competition
Primidone	Raised	Valproate	Decreased metabolism
	Lowered	Phenytoin	Increased metabolism

INDIVIDUAL DRUG THERAPY

Although there are approximately 15 anticonvulsant drugs on the market at the present time, many have been virtually discarded as relatively ineffective or relatively toxic. The following drugs are the principal ones in use at the present time.

Phenobarbital

Phenobarbital was introduced in 1912 and has been one of the most widely used anticonvulsants. It is successful against the tonic components of major seizures and has a powerful effect in protecting against maximal electroshock convulsions. Phenobarbital is well absorbed and has a high lipid solubility, assuring it an affinity for the central nervous system. It acts as a depressant in multisynaptic pathways, probably by augmenting presynaptic inhibition and depressing posttetanic potentiation.

After oral administration, peak blood levels and peak brain levels are reached in 10–12 hours. Excretion is predominantly via the kidney, though some glucuronic acid conjugation takes place in the liver.

Drug metabolism enzymes are induced in the liver, and this may have a bearing on habituation to the drug. Acute withdrawal may precipitate seizures. Phenobarbital has the ability to induce microsomal liver enzymes responsible for the metabolism of bilirubin and steroids, as well as other drugs including phenytoin and warfarin sodium. The simultaneous administration of sodium valproate leads to an increased level of phenobarbital. The half-life of the drug is 50–150 hours, and the administration of successive doses before elimination of the previous dose leads to accumulation until a plateau is reached at a stage when intake and elimination are equal (known as the steady state). For phenobarbital, steady state is achieved in approximately 3 weeks. There is some individual variation in the relationship of dose to blood level so that the blood level cannot be reliably predicted from the administered dose. The therapeutic blood level range lies between 10 and 30 μg/mL.

Phenobarbital has been recommended for control of generalized tonic-clonic seizures and for partial seizures of either the simple or the complex type and is used also in the prophylaxis of febrile convulsions where such prophylactic therapy is indicated.

Because of its long half-life, the drug may be administered in one daily dose, but divided doses are usually administered.

The idiosyncratic side effects include skin rashes and drug fever. Side effects from overdose include drowsiness and irritability and in children exacerbation of hyperactivity.

In emergency situations such as status epilepticus, the drug is injected intravenously (see Chapter 14).

Phenytoin

Phenytoin was introduced in 1938. It appears to have an action on the cell membrane, where it enhances the extrusion of sodium ions from the cell by stimulating sodium-potassium ATPase and by its action on the sodium pump mechanism. It may also suppress the elevation of cyclic nucleotide levels that are induced by depolarization by inhibiting the influx of sodium and calcium, which may be associated with transmitter release.

Phenytoin is well absorbed from the gastrointestinal tract and is predominantly metabolized in the liver by parahydroxylation. The metabolic product is excreted in the urine. Phenytoin is 90% protein bound and has a half-life averaging 24 hours after oral administration. Enzyme induction due to the simultaneous administration of other drugs tends to reduce blood levels. The steady-state blood level is achieved after approximately 4–6 days, and this can be shortened with an initial loading dose of three times the daily maintenance dose at the beginning of treatment. The therapeutic blood level range of phenytoin is 10–20 μg/mL. The drug has been considered to be the drug of choice in generalized tonic-clonic seizures and in partial seizures, both elementary and complex, although it is preferred in the treatment of elementary partial seizures. It may be administered in a single dose. In children, the dosage recommendation is 5–8 mg/kg/day, and there is a relatively wide margin of safety between the therapeutic and the lethal dose levels. In status epilepticus, it is given intravenously as described in Chapter 14. Side effects include hypersensitivity reactions consisting of skin rash, fever, lymphadenopathy, and sometimes splenomegaly and jaundice. Dose-related side effects include cerebellar and brain stem dysfunction with vertigo, ataxia, diplopia, slurred speech, and depression of consciousness. Abnormal movements sometimes occur, and chronic overdose may result in depletion of Purkinje cells.

Prolonged administration may lead to gum hypertrophy, interference with immunoglobulin production, coarsening of the facial features, folate deficiency with or without macrocytic anemia, lymph node enlargement, interference with vitamin D metabolism, interference with contraceptive hormones, and interference with the immune system with the development of systemic lupus erythematosus.

Primidone

Primidone was introduced in 1952 and is closely related structurally to phenobarbital. It is readily absorbed from the gastrointestinal tract within approximately 3 hours. Phenobarbital is one of its metabolic products, and another pharmacologically active product is phenylethylmalonamide. The drug is not protein-bound and has a half-life of approximately 12 hours. Primidone is therefore administered in several doses. It is useful in generalized tonic-clonic seizures and partial seizures, although there is probably no specific benefit of primidone over other drugs in the treatment of complex partial seizures. The drug dose seems to be quite effective in massive adolescent myoclonus associated with generalized tonic-clonic seizures. Therapeutic blood levels are 5–10 μg/mL. The drug should be administered initially in a very small dose, with gradual increase in the dosage to approximately 20 mg/kg/day in children. The most frequently encountered side effects (such as ataxia, vertigo, and nausea) are dose related.

Carbamazepine

Carbamazepine, introduced in 1962, is an iminostilbine derivative. It is absorbed slowly and reaches peak plasma levels in approximately 3 hours. It is approximately 70% protein-bound and has a 12-hour half-life requiring, therefore, divided dose administration. The only by-product, carbamazepin-10,11-epoxide, is pharmacologically active. The drug inhibits maximal electroshock seizures in animals and has potent inhibitory effects on polysynaptic pathways.

The drug is administered in doses of up to 25 mg/kg and has a therapeutic blood level range between 6 and 12 μg/mL. It is effective against generalized tonic-clonic seizures and against partial seizures, particularly complex partial seizures. Various drug interactions occur with carbamazepine, including lower blood levels in the face of phenytoin, phenobarbital, and valproic acid; in combination therapy, frequent blood level estimations are necessary. The drug tends to induce its own breakdown, so that with long-term administration, increases in dosage may be necessary.

Side effects include dizziness, drowsiness, ataxia, and nausea, which appear to occur 1–3 hours after the administration dose and may be modified by modifying the dosage regimen. Long-term side effects include hepatic impairment and bone marrow depletion, which are quite unusual but which mandate occasional blood studies for their early detection.

Carbamazepine is closely related structurally to the tricyclic antidepressants, and there may be psychotropic or antidepressant effects associated with its administration.

Clonazepam

This drug, a benzodiazepine, is rapidly absorbed after oral administration; it reaches peak plasma concentrations in 1 hour. It is excreted primarily as oxazepam

248

after breakdown in the liver. It has a half-life of approximately 18 hours, and it is usually administered in divided doses. Tolerance develops quite rapidly, and breakthrough seizures may occur.

The drug has been used particularly in the treatment of absence seizures and of myoclonic seizures refractory to ethosuximide or valproate. Although it is a very potent anticonvulsant, it has two serious side effects: 1) it causes significant behavioral changes, and 2) withdrawal of the drug has to be accomplished extremely slowly because of the tendency for rebound generalized tonic-clonic seizures to occur.

The dosage ranges from 1 to 20 mg per day and it is usual to begin with 0.05 mg/kg and gradually increase this to 0.2 mg/kg/day.

Diazepam

Diazepam is predominantly used intravenously as an anticonvulsant, though it may be used in large doses orally for myoclonic seizures. It is particularly effective intravenously in the treatment of alcohol withdrawal seizures as well as status epilepticus (see Chapter 14). On intravenous administration, the dose is 0.25–0.4 mg/kg up to 1 mg/kg, delivered at a rate of 1 mg/min; at this dosage it has a rapid but brief effect.

Ethosuximide

Ethosuximide is a succinimide drug. It was introduced in 1958. Gastrointestinal absorption is rapid, peak blood levels are reached 4 hours after ingestion, and there is little protein binding. The half-life varies between 30 and 60 hours, depending on age, with a mean half-life of 48 hours. Ethosuximide blood levels are closely related to dosage. The therapeutic blood level range is 40–100 μg/mL. Ethosuximide protects against metrazole-induced seizures and clinically is effective against absence seizures. Children can tolerate 25–30 mg/kg/day, and the usual dose range is 500–1500 mg, depending on size. Seventy-five percent of patients with uncomplicated absence seizures respond favorably to ethosuximide, but those whose absence seizures are on the basis of structural neurologic disease do less well.

Side effects include overdose effects characterized by anorexia, nausea, vomiting, drowsiness, headaches, and hiccups. Chronic administration may result in leukopenia and pancytopenia, and periodic blood counts should be performed. Idiosyncratic side effects include erythema multiforme and the Stevens-Johnson syndrome. Occasionally, systemic lupus erythematosus results.

Valproic Acid and Sodium Valproate

Valproic acid and sodium valproate are anticonvulsants with a structural formula (a short-chain carboxylic acid) that is considerably different from that of the other anticonvulsants. Valproic acid was originally used as an organic solvent. Its mechanism of action appears to depend largely on its interference with the degradation of γ-aminobutyric acid, an action that leads to increased brain concentrations of this inhibitory neurotransmitter. Valproic acid is most effective in generalized seizures, ie, absence seizures, myoclonic seizures, and generalized tonic-clonic seizures. Some effect has been noted in partial seizures, particularly complex partial seizures. In absence seizures, the drug is at least as effective as ethosuximide, and in myoclonic seizures it is considerably more effective. Moreover, both absence and myoclonic seizures that do not respond to either ethosuximide or valproic acid may respond to a combination of the two agents. Therapeutic blood level range is 50–100 μg/mL, and this is usually achieved with a dosage of between 20 and 60 mg/kg/day.

Side effects include drowsiness, gastrointestinal discomfort, and change in appetite with either increase or decrease in weight. There may be some hair loss, which is usually transient. The most disturbing side effect is an unheralded liver failure, which, though rare, is frequently fatal and of which there have so far been approximately 60 instances. Pancreatitis has also been reported. On the other hand, the drug is sufficiently effective to continue to be one of the most useful new agents in the treatment of epilepsy. It is recommended that patients taking this drug have liver function studies at regular intervals. Interference with platelet aggregation, though not usually of clinical significance, should be considered, particularly where elective surgery is contemplated.

Drug interactions include increasing blood levels of phenobarbital and occasional decreasing blood levels of phenytoin with an increase in the free-level phenytoin because of the competition for protein binding. Like phenytoin, valproate is approximately 90% protein bound.

Trimethadione

This drug is an oxazoladine dione that has proved useful in the treatment of absence seizures. However, its potential toxicity (particularly with regard to bone marrow depletion and nephrosis) is such as to make this a much less popular agent than the other drugs used in the treatment of absence.

Trimethadione is readily absorbed from the gastrointestinal tract and is metabolized by the elimination of one methyl group. The dose is approximately 20 mg/kg in children.

The side effects include sedation, gastrointestinal symptoms, and hemeralopia, which is characterized by a peculiar glare that is seen around objects. Skin rash, exfoliative dermatitis, and bone marrow depression as well as the nephrotic syndrome and the development of SLE and occasionally of myasthenia gravis militate against its continued use now that more effective and safer drugs are available.

Acetazolamide

Acetazolamide is a sulfonamide drug that inhibits the enzyme carbonic anhydrase. It has some anticonvulsant properties, usually as an adjunctive drug in patients with generalized seizures and particularly in those whose seizures are related to the menses. It is also useful in Lennox-Gastaut syndrome on occasion, in a dose of 250 mg daily.

Clorazepate

Clorazepate is a benzodiazepine and is related to diazepam. It is a potentially useful adjunctive drug in the treatment of complex partial seizures in combination with carbamazepine.

Bromides

Though now rarely used, bromides were the only anticonvulsants available between 1857 and 1912, and they continue to be quite effective. With the introduction of blood level estimations, the unpleasant toxic side effects of bromides can largely be avoided. Bromides are rapidly and completely absorbed in the small intestine and have a plasma half-life of approximately 12 days, although this can be altered by changing the chloride concentration. A mixture of triple bromides is still occasionally used for otherwise intractable convulsive seizures in a therapeutic dose of from 1 to 2 grams 3 times a day, yielding blood levels of 80–120 mg/dL. Side effects include drowsiness, psychotic behavior, and skin rashes.

TREATMENT OF SEIZURES COMMONLY OCCURRING IN CHILDREN

Generalized Absence Seizures

Generalized absence seizures are characterized by periods of altered consciousness that begin abruptly and end abruptly and that typically last for 10 seconds in duration and rarely last for over 30 seconds. Other symptoms, including mild clonic movements, automatisms, autonomic phenomena, and increased or decreased postural tone, may accompany altered consciousness.

The seizures usually begin after 2 years of age, and more often begin between the ages of 5 to 7 years of age. Absence seizures usually occur more than once a day. The high frequency of these seizures has made it possible to study the clinical phenomenology of the seizure in detail, using concomitant EEG and videotaped television recording of the patients (Porter, Penry and Dreifuss 1975). Detailed analysis of split-screen EEG-TV recording techniques have demonstrated that consciousness may be altered to varying degrees. In some cases, the patient may be totally unresponsive to verbal and visual stimuli and be amnestic for words spoken during the event or instructions given during the seizures. In other instances, the patient may be unable to respond to instructions; but immediately after the seizure he may be able to recall words, phrases, and instructions given during the event. In many instances, the patient may be able to continue performing a simple task such as pressing a telegraph key at the sound of an electronic whistle. However, the response time for stimuli occurring during the spike-wave discharge is prolonged as compared to the response time interictally (Browne et al 1974a). In some instances, continuous visuomotor tasks may be impaired but to a lesser degree than when the patient momentarily closes his eyes (Goode et al 1970). Using EEG-CCTV techniques, we have documented several examples of patients responding verbally to simple questions, such as, "What is your name?" or "Where do you live?" In these instances, the patient's responses tend to be brief, simple, and slower than normal. We have frequently observed that patients may continue a task such as reading or counting aloud, eating or card-playing, but in a slow and uncoordinated manner. Because the patient may partially retain his ability to respond to external stimuli, it is difficult to accurately ascertain the frequency and duration of absence seizures. In some instances, the diagnosis cannot be established with certainty without concomitant EEG and clinical observations during seizures. As a result, accurate estimation of seizure frequency from reports of family members and teachers is not possible. One may need to rely upon more objective measures such as long-term radiotelemetered EEGs or ambulatory cassette EEG recordings to supplement historical reports of seizure frequency. Reaction time studies have demonstrated that measurable impairment of response to auditory stimuli occurs with even brief generalized spike-wave discharges (Browne et al 1974b).

Once the seizure frequency has been documented, appropriate antiepileptic drug therapy can be initiated. Ethosuximide has been regarded as the drug of choice for the treatment of absence seizures (Carter and Gold 1968). Valproic acid is also effective in controlling absence seizures (Simon and Penry 1975, Pinder et al 1977, Villareal et al 1978). Double blind-controlled studies, comparing ethosuximide to valproic acid, indicate that the two drugs are equally effective in controlling absence seizures (Suzuki et al 1972, Sato et al 1982). Valproic acid may be a better choice for patients who are experiencing other types of seizures in addition to absence seizures, because it is effective in controlling several other types of seizures as well. However, recent reports of rare instances of severe and sometimes fatal hepatotoxicity and pancreatitis and of serious blood dyscrasias in some patients receiving valproic acid emphasize the need for judicious use of this drug (Camfield et al 1979, Jacobi et al 1980, Coulter and Allen 1980, Coulter et al 1980, Smith and Boots 1980). In a double-blind study comparing valproic acid to ethosuximide, 44.4% of previously untreated patients with absence seizures were rendered seizure free with ethosuximide; and in 87.5%, seizures were completely controlled with valproic acid. The efficacy of the two drugs was not significantly different (Sato et al 1982). In a long-term follow-up study of the same group of patients, complete seizure control was achieved in 98% of cases with either valproic acid or valproic acid and ethosuximide.

The usual dose of ethosuximide required for control of absence seizures ranges from 15 to 25 mg/kg/day, and the therapeutic range is between 40 and 100 μg/mL (Browne et al 1975). There is marked individual variation in the relationship between dose and plasma level (Penry et al 1972). In some patients, seizures not controlled with blood levels in the lower therapeutic range may be controlled with higher levels without causing significant side effects. Because of the propensity of the drug to cause nausea and vomiting, the drug should be given in two or three divided doses each day. The starting doses should be low. Dosage increments can be made, usually weekly, as required. The usual dose of valproic acid is 15–60 μg/kg/day. It is usually given in three divided doses daily, but some authors have suggested a twice a day regimen. The proposed therapeutic range is 50–1000 μg/mL.

Valproic acid may produce drowsiness, nausea, and vomiting, particularly during the first week of therapy. The symptoms can be avoided by starting with low doses (10–15 μg/kg/day) and gradually increasing the dose every 3 to 4 days as required. If valproic acid is given to a patient receiving ethosuximide, side effects may occur as a result of a drug interaction that causes the plasma level of ethosuximide to rise (Cramer and Mattson 1979).

Other drugs that may be effective in treating absence seizures include trimethadione and clonazepam. Once seizures are thought to be controlled on the basis of historical reports, a follow-up long-term EEG recording may be useful in confirming seizure control.

Generalized Tonic-Clonic and Partial Seizures

Generalized tonic-clonic seizures involve both cerebral hemispheres simultaneously at the onset of the seizures. They are characterized clinically as symmetrical tonic extension of the neck, trunk, and extremities, followed by clonic symmetrical jerking of facial musculature, neck, trunk, and extremities. These movements usually last for 1 to 2 minutes and are followed by postictal flaccidity of muscles, with gradual return of consciousness over several minutes. There is often postictal drowsiness and confusion.

At times, the tonic phase is preceded by bilateral clonic jerking. Partial seizures (those beginning within one cerebral hemisphere) may generalize to become tonic-clonic seizures. In these cases, the EEG may show a focal onset of seizure discharge and then spread to involve both hemispheres. The initial clinical symptoms may be motor, sensory, cognitive, affective, or autonomic, depending upon the site of the original focus. Partial seizures with secondary generalization usually respond to the same drugs as primarily generalized seizures but are usually more difficult to control.

Partial simple and partial complex seizures also occur in children. Like partial seizures with secondary generalizations, these seizures begin locally within one cerebral hemisphere. They are often more difficult to control than primarily generalized seizures.

Generalized tonic-clonic seizures and partial seizures (including partial complex seizures, partial elementary seizures, and partial seizures with secondary generalization) respond to a number of drugs, including carbamazepine, phenytoin, phenobarbital, and primidone. Clonazepam may be effective in this group of seizures (Browne 1976), and valproic acid has been shown to be effective when used adjunctively (Simon and Penry 1975, Pinder et al 1977). There are few controlled studies comparing the efficacy of these drugs for any given seizure type, and the relative efficacy of these drugs has not been determined conclusively. The "drug of choice" remains a personal preference. In view of the lack of data on relative efficacy, it seems reasonable to base the choice of drug on other factors. Some physicians prefer phenobarbital because of the low incidence of severe adverse reactions. Others prefer to avoid phenobarbital because of its propensity for causing mental dullness and for exacerbating hyperactivity in some children. The elimination half-life of phenobarbital is shorter in children (37 hours) than in adults (73 hours) (Garrettson and Dayton 1970). Thus, children may require higher doses, relative to body weight, to achieve the same steady-state plasma phenobarbital levels. In neonates, the elimination half-life of phenobarbital is initially very long (115 hours), but it rapidly decreases after 4 weeks of therapy (67 hours) (Pitlick et al 1978). Eadie and co-workers (1977) found that the relationship between dose and steady-state plasma levels of phenobarbital were statistically different for different age groups. Their age groups were 1) less than 4 years (excluding neonates); 2) 4–14 years, 3) 15–40 years, and 4) over 40 years of age. The usual therapeutic plasma level ranges from 15 to 40 µg/mL. However, because of the insidious onset of toxic side effects and variations in individual tolerance, the upper end of the therapeutic range has been reported to be different by different authors (Pippenger and Rosen 1975, Feldman et al 1975, Loiseau et al 1977).

Infantile Spasms (see Chapter 6)

Infantile spasms usually occur in the first year of life and rarely occur after the age of 2 years. They are manifested clinically by sudden, lightning-like flexor, and occasionally extensor, spasms of the neck, trunk, and extremities. Characteristically, the interictal EEG shows hypsarrhythmia, and the spasms are usually associated with a brief generalized electrodecremental pattern. Currently, the treatment of choice is ACTH. The recommended dose ranges from 40 to 80 units per day, given intramuscularly. However, a study by Hrachovy et al (1980) suggests that doses of 20 to 30 units per day may be sufficient to control infantile spasms in some patients. The duration of treatment varies from 5 weeks to several months. While spasms cease in up to 80% of patients, they may recur in approximately 39% (Pollark et al 1979). Intellectual deterioration is usually associated with infantile spasms. Even in a patient whose spasms respond to treatment with ACTH, most patients continue to show evidence of mild to severe mental retardation (Pollack et al 1979). Prednisone (2 mg/kg/day) has also been shown to be effective in the control of infantile spasms in 25% of patients (Hrachovy et al 1979). Valproic acid given in a dose of 20 mg/kg/day was reported to control spasms in 4 of 18 infants and to reduce the frequency by 50% in 8 others (Pavone et al 1981). Other drugs such as clonazepam, valproic acid, and nitrazepam have been reported to be effective, controlling spasms in a few cases. There is some evidence that early treatment with ACTH may be important in minimizing the degree of mental deterioration. In some instances, spasms have been controlled by treatment with pyridoxine. Benign myoclonus of early infancy (Lombroso and Fejerman 1977) should be distinguished from infantile spasms because of its lack of association with other seizure phenomena and good prognosis.

Febrile Convulsions (see Chapter 12)

Febrile convulsions represent another problem unique to childhood. Febrile convulsions are divided into simple febrile seizures and epilepsy triggered by fever. Simple febrile seizures are brief generalized convulsions (less than 15 minutes in duration), with no focal components, which occur during a febrile illness. The neurologic examination reveals an apparently normal child, and the EEG, performed at least 5 days after a seizure, is normal. There is often a family history of febrile convulsions (Millichap 1968). Simple febrile convulsions should be differentiated from epilepsy triggered by seizures. Prolonged seizures, seizure with focal signature, abnormalities seen during neurologic examination, an abnormal EEG, and a family history of epilepsy are evidence of the latter disorder. The incidence of recurrent febrile convulsions of both types can be reduced by chronic prophylactic treatment with phenobarbital. The use of chronic phenobarbital therapy for simple febrile convulsions is controversial. The potential adverse effects of phenobarbital therapy should be weighed against the risk of recurrent convulsions.

Phenytoin appears to be ineffective in preventing simple febrile convulsions. Valporic acid was found to be as effective as phenobarbital. The need for performing lumbar punctures in children presenting with febrile convulsions is debated. However, there have been well-documented cases of meningitis presenting as febrile convulsions, without signs of meningeal irritation (Ratcliffe and Wolf 1977).

THERAPEUTIC FAILURE

If seizures fail to respond to antiepileptic drug therapy, it is important to re-evaluate the case in detail, looking for factors that may have been overlooked or initial clinical impressions that were incorrect. For instance a drug that has been found to be ineffective in the past may not have been used in a dose sufficient to achieve adequate blood levels. In many cases drugs that were not tolerated in the past because of a toxic effect may have been initiated at too high a dose or may have caused toxic effects because of synergistic toxicity or overlooked drug interactions. The same drug may be well tolerated when used alone or in combination with different drugs. In some cases, a potentially effective drug may have been overlooked. In a few instances, the drugs chosen were based on erroneous classification of the seizures.

On occasion, patients will report symptoms as seizures when, in fact, they are not. Patients may learn to recognize their absence seizures as brief lapses in attention. Once the absences are controlled, they may continue to report normal attentional lapses or daydreaming as seizures. In the case of partial complex seizures, patients may focus on the affective component (eg, anxiety) of their aura and then report the same affective states as seizures, even when they occur under normal circumstances.

In a study of a group of 40 patients with refractory seizures, intensive monitoring of seizures, clinically and electrographically, as well as careful monitoring of antiepileptic drug levels led to the discovery of several factors that contributed to treatment failure. By addressing these problems, seizure control was improved, and the number of antiepileptic drugs were reduced in most of the patients (Sutula et al 1981). Subtherapeutic antiepileptic drug levels is one possible reason for treatment failure. Because of the wide availability of plasma antiepileptic drug level assays, this problem can be easily identified and corrected. Noncompliance by the patient or family members responsible for administering the medications is also a factor that may contribute to treatment failure. Noncompliance is not difficult to identify, but one must be cautious about attributing subtherapeutic drug levels to noncompliance. Other factors, such as poor absorption from the gastrointestinal tract, an unusually fast rate of drug metabolism, or drug interactions, frequently account for persistently low blood levels. In the aforementioned study, noncompliance was documented in only one case (Sutula et al 1981). However, this was a series in which patients with a history of noncompliance were not included.

There are numerous reasons for noncompliance, and the reasons vary from case to case. Therefore, there is no uniformly effective way of dealing with noncompliance. In some cases, the patient changes to his own regimen because the prescribed regimen had been ineffective in controlling seizures and may have caused side effects. In some instances, these side effects are subjective or transient and may not be associated with objective signs of toxicity. In these cases, the physician may need to adjust medications to eliminate the side effects. At times, the problem of noncompliance may be addressed by educating the patient as to the reasons for adhering to a strict daily drug regimen. In some cases the dosage schedule can be changed to times that are more convenient for the patients. Children are often reluctant to take their medicine at school. Rearranging the schedule to enable the patient to take medicine after arriving home from school can be an important step in enhancing compliance.

When seizures fail to respond to appropriate therapy, evaluation of the underlying cause is in order. A number of progressive neurologic disorders, including brain tumor and metabolic and degenerative disorder can present with seizures. Discussion of the vast array of disorders of the nervous system and the systemic disorders that can cause seizures is beyond the scope of this chapter.

Another problem that can account for refractory seizures and that is found in 47.5% of the cases studied by Sutula et al (1981) is erroneous seizure classification. Erroneous seizure classification may lead to an inappropriate choice of drugs. This is a particularly common problem in the case of absence seizures and partial complex seizures. The symptomatology of these two seizure types is so similar that they are often confused. Furthermore, they respond to different groups of drugs. Another problem in diagnosis is that of pseudoseizures. Seizure-like behavior, presumably occurring on a psychological basis, is sometimes seen in children as well as in adults (see Chapter 17). To confound the problem, most patients with pseudoseizures also have epileptic seizures (Holmes et al 1980). There are a number of clinical features that may be used to distinguish pseudoseizures from epileptic seizures. However, in many cases, intensive monitoring, using prolonged EEG monitoring or prolonged EEG with simultaneous closed circuit television monitoring, of the patient may be required before the diagnosis can be made with any degree of certainty.

DISCONTINUING ANTIEPILEPTIC DRUG THERAPY

Once seizures have been brought under control, the quesiton arises as to when antiepileptic drugs should be withdrawn. There are a number of reasons why discontinuation of antiepileptic drugs is desirable. The potential for either acute or chronic toxic effects has been discussed earlier. There is also evidence that antiepileptic drugs may impair cognitive functions, cause slow learning, and behavior problems in children (Camfield et al 1979). The psychosocial implications of successful withdrawal of antiepileptic drugs are also important. If antiepileptic drugs can be withdrawn without recurrence of seizures, the child will no longer have to live with the social stigma of epilepsy or be subject to the limitations society continues to place on the epileptic. Recent studies have provided very useful prognostic data that can aid the physician in determining whether a given child is at reasonably low risk of recurrent seizures if drugs are withdrawn. In a study of 68 children in whom antiepileptic drugs were withdrawn after a seizure-free period of 4 years, 74% remained seizure free (Emerson et al 1981). These patients were between the ages of 6 and 22 years when their medication was discontinued. These authors found no significant difference in the risk of release for different seizure types. However, the number of patients with any given seizure type was small. Several factors, including IQ below 70, early age at seizure onset, number of generalized tonic-clonic seizures prior to remission, high therapeutic levels of antiepileptic drugs, and definitively abnormal EEGs predicted higher risk of seizures after withdrawal of medications. However, multivariate analysis found the number of generalized tonic-clonic seizures before control and the EEG to be the factors important in predicting outcome. This study also found that most relapses recurred shortly after medications were withdrawn. The recurrence rate found in this study was similar to that found by several other investigators (Holowach et al 1972, Zenker et al 1957, Juul-Jensen 1964). Annegers et al (1979) found that 10 years after diagnosis, the probability of completing a 5-year seizure-free period without medication was 40% in the group whose seizures began between the ages of 10 and 19 years. This may be translated as a 40% chance of entering a 5-year seizure-free period without medication 5 years after the diagnosis is made. On the basis of the preceding studies, it would seem reasonable to consider discontinuing medications after a patient has been seizure-free on medication for 4 to 5 years, if the EEG does not show definitive abnormalities. The decision whether or not to discontinue medication for a given patient must, of course, be based upon social and psychological features as well. If medications are discontinued, it is advisable to begin tapering the dose of one drug while maintaining the blood levels of the other drug or drugs. If seizures do not recur, the remainder of the drugs can be withdrawn sequentially.

BIBLIOGRAPHY

Annegers JF, Hanser WA, Elveback LR: Permission of seizures and relapse in patients with epilepsy. *Epilepsia* 1979;20:729–737.

Arnold K, Gerber N: The rate of decline of diphenylhydantoin in human plasma. *Clin Pharmacol Ther* 1970;11:121–134.

Atkinson AJ, Shaw JM: Pharmacokinetic study of a patient with diphenylhydantoin toxicity. *Clin Pharmacol Ther* 1973;14:521–528.

Barth N, Alvan O, Borga O, et al: Two-fold interindividual variation in plasma protein binding of phenytoin in patients with epilepsy. *Clin Pharmcokinet* 1976;1:444–452.

Booker HE, Darcy B: Serum concentrations of free diphenylhydantoin and their relationship to clinical intoxication. *Epilepsia* 1975;14:177–184.

Boston Collaborative Drug Surveillance Program: Diphenylhydantoin side effects and serum albumin levels. *Clin Pharmacol Ther* 1973;14:529–532.

Bowden AN, Gilliatt RW, Wilson RG: The place of EEG telemetry and closed-circuit television in diagnosis and management of epileptic patients. *Proc R Soc Med* 1975;68:246–248.

Browne TR: Clonazepam: A review of a new anticonvulsant drug. *Arch Neurol* 1976;33: 326–332.

Browne TR, Dreifuss FE, Dyken PR, et al: Ethosuximide in the treatment of absence (petit mal) seizures. *Neurology* 1975;25:515–524.

Browne TR, Penry JK, Porter RJ, et al: Responsiveness before, during, and after spike-wave paroxysms. *Neurology (Minneap)* 1974a;24:659–664.

Browne TR, Penry JK, Porter RJ, et al: A comparison of clinical estimates of absence seizure frequency based on prolonged telemetered EEG's. *Neurology (Minneap)* 1974b;24: 381–382.

Camfield PR, Bagnell P, Camfield CS, et al: Pancreatitis due to valproic acid. *Lancet* 1979; 1:1198.

Camfield CS, Chaplin S, Doyle A, et al: Side effects of phenobarbital in toddlers: Behavioral and cognitive aspects. *J Pediatr* 1979;95:361–365.

Carter S, Gold A: Medical intellegence: Current concepts. Convulsions in children. *N Engl J Med* 1968;278:315–317.

Cavazzuti GB: Epidemiology of different types of epilepsy in school age children of Modena, Italy. *Epilepsia* 1980;21:57–62.

Chiba K, Ishizaki T, Miura H, et al: Michaelis-Menten pharmacokinetics of diphenylhydantoin and application in the pediatric age patient. *J Pediatr* 1980;96:479–484.

Coatsworth JJ: *Studies on the Clinical Efficacy of Marketed Antiepileptic Drugs.* NINCDS monograph no. 12. Washington, DC, US Government Printing Office.

Commission on Classification and Terminology, International League against Epilepsy: Proposed revision of clinical and electroencephalographic classification of epileptic seizures. *Epilepsia* 1981;22:480–501.

Coulter DL, Allen RJ: Pancreatitis associated with valproic acid therapy for epilepsy. *Ann Neurol* 1980;7:92.

Coulter DL, Wu H, Allen RJ: Valproic acid therapy in childhood epilepsy. *JAMA* 1980;244: 785–788.

Craig WS, MacKinnon JM: Convulsions in infancy and childhood—Part 2. *Br Med J* 1965; 5:433–499.

Cramer JA, Mattson RH: Valproic acid: In vitro plasma protein binding and interaction with phenytoin. *Ther Drug Monitor* 1979;1:105–116.

Eadie MJ, Landen CM, Hooper WD, et al: Factor influencing plasma phenobarbitone levels in epileptic patients. *Br J Clin Pharmacol* 1977;43:541–547.

Eadie MJ, Tyrer JH: *Anticonvulsant Therapy: Pharmacological Basis and Practice,* ed 2. New York, Churchill Livingstone, 1980, pp 9–18.

Emerson R, D'Souza BJ, Vining EP, et al: Stopping medications in children with epilepsy: Predictors of outcome. *N Engl J Med* 1981;304:1125–1129.

Feldman RG, Pippenger CE, Florence ML: The relation of anticonvulsant drug levels to complete seizure control. *Epilepsia* 1975;16:203–204.

Fukuyama Y, Arima M, Nagahata M, et al: Medical treatment of epilepsies in childhood: A long-term survey of 801 patients. *Epilepsia* 1963;4:207–224.

Garretson LK, Jusko J: Diphenylhydantoin elimination kinetics in overdosed children. *Clin Pharmacol Ther* 1975;17:481–491.

Garretson LK, Dayton PG: Disappearance of phenobarbital and diphenylhydantoin from serum of children. *Clin Pharmacol Ther* 1970;11:674–679.

Gastaut H, Tassinari CA (ed): Clinical EEG. Part A. Epilepsies, in Redmond A (editor-in-chief): *Handbook of Electroencephalography and Clinical Neurophysiology.* Amsterdam, Elsevier, vol 13, 1975.

Gerber N, Wagner JG: Explanation of dose-dependent decline in diphenylhydantoin plasma levels by fitting to the integral form of the Michaelis-Menten equation. *Res Commun Chem Pathol Pharmacol* 1972;3:455–466.

Giordani B, Sackellares JC, Miller SM, et al: Changes in neuropsychological test performance following improved seizure control and elimination of barbiturate anti-epileptic drugs. *Neurology* 1983, in press.

Goldberg MA: Phenobarbital: Binding, in Glaser GH, Penry JK, Woodbury DM (eds): *Antiepileptic Drugs: Mechanisms of Action.* New York, Raven Press, 1980, pp 501–504.

Goode DJ, Penry JK, Dreifuss FE: Effects of paroxysmal spike-wave on continuous visual-motor performance. *Epilepsia* 1970;11:241–245.

Guelen PJM, van der Kleijin E, Woudstra U: Statistical analysis of pharmacokinetic parameters in epileptic patients clinically treated with antiepileptic drugs, in Schneider H, Janz D, Gardner-Thorpe C, et al (eds): *Clinical Pharmacology of Antiepileptic Drugs.* Berlin, Springer Verlag, 1975, pp 1–10.

Gugler R, Mueller G: Plasma protein binding of valproic acid in healthy subjects and in patients with renal disease. *Br J Clin Pharmacol* 1978;5:441–446.

Hauser WA, Kurland LT: Incidence prevalence, time trends of convulsive disorders in Rochester, Minnesota: A community survey. *US DHEW NINCDS*, Monograph 14, Publication 73-390. Bathesda, MD, 1972, E66:41–43.

Holmes GL, Sackellares JC, McKienernan J, et al: Evaluation of childhood pseudoseizures using EEG telemetry and videotape monitoring. *J Pediatr* 1980;97:554–558.

Holowach J, Thurston DL, O'Leary J: Prognosis in childhood epilepsy: Follow-up study of 148 cases in which therapy had been suspended after prolonged anticonvulsant control. *N Engl J Med* 1972;286:169–174.

Hoppener RJ, Kuyer A, Meijer JWA, et al: Correlation between daily fluctuations of carbamazepine serum levels and intermittent side effects. *Epilepsia* 1980;21:341–350.

Hrachovy RA, Frost JD Jr, Dellaway P, et al: A controlled study of ACTH therapy in infantile spasms. *Epilepsia* 1980;21:631–636.

Hrachovy RA, Frost JD Jr, Kellaway P, et al: A control study of prednisone therapy in infantile spasms. *Epilepsia* 1979;20:403–407.

Jacobi G, Thorbeck R, Ritz A, et al: Fatal hepatotoxicity in child on phenobarbitone and sodium valproate, Letter to editor. *Lancet* 1980;29:712–713.

Jeavons PM: Choice of drug therapy in epilepsy. *Practitioner* 1977;219:543–556.

Juul-Hensen P: Frequency of recurrence after discontinuation of anticonvulsant therapy in patients with epileptic seizures. *Epilepsia* 1964;5:352–363.

King W, Kaul AF: Determining phenytoin dosage with the use of a programmable calculator. *Drug Intel Clin Pharm* 1980;14:686–693.

Klotz U, Antonin RH: Pharmacokinetics and bioavailability of sodium valproate. *Clin Pharmacol Ther* 1977;21:736–743.

Kruger-Thiemer E: Pharmacokinetics and dosage concentration relationships, proceedings of the 3rd international pharmacological meeting, July 24–30, 1966, in *Physico-Chemical Aspects of Drug Actions.* Vol. 7, New York, Pergamon Press, vol 7, 1965, pp 63–113.

Lennox WF, Davis JP: Clinical correlates of the fast and slow spike-wave electroencephalogram. *Pediatrics* 1950;5:626–644.

Lennox WG, Lennox MA: *Epilepsy and Related Disorders.* Boston, Little Brown & Co, 1960, pp 689–691.

Livingston S, Peterson D: Primidone (mysoline) in the treatment of epilepsy. *N Engl J Med* 1956;254:327.

Loiseau P, et al: Intérêt du dosage des anticonvulsants dans le traitment des epilepsies. *Nouv Press Med* 1977;6:813–817.

Lombroso CT, Fejerman N: Benign myoclonus of early infancy. *Ann Neurol* 1977;1:138–143.

Ludden TM, Allan JR, Valutsky WA, et al: Individualization of phenytoin dosage regimens. *Clin Pharmacol Ther* 1977;21:287–293.

Lundervold A, Jabour JT: A correlation of clinical, electroencephalographic, and roentgenographic findings in children with epilepsy. *J Pediatr* 1962;60:220–223.

Millichap JG: *Febril Convulsions.* New York, Macmillan, 1968.

Odar-Cederlof I, Borga O: Kinetics of diphenylhydantoin in uremic patients: Consequences of plasma protein binding. *Eur J Clin Pharmacol* 1974;7:31–37.

Pavone L, Incorpora G, LaRosa M, et al: Treatment of infantile spasms with sodium dipropylacetic acid. *Dev Med Child Neurol* 1981;23:454–461.

Penry JK, Porter RJ, Dreifuss FE: Ethosuximide: Relation of plasma levels to clinical control, in Woodbury DM, Penry JK, Schmidt RP (eds): *Antiepileptic Drugs.* New York, Raven Press, 1972, pp 431–441.

Penry JK, Porter RJ, Dreifuss FE: Simultaneous recording of absence seizures with video tape and electroencephalography. A study of 374 seizures in 48 patients. *Brain* 1975;98:427–440.

Pinder RM, Brogden RN, Speight TM, et al: Sodium valproate: A review of its pharmacological properties and therapeutic efficacy in epilepsy. *Drugs* 1977;13:81–123.

Pippenger CE: Pediatric clinical pharmacology of antiepileptic drugs: A special consideration, in Pippenger CE, Penry JK, Kutt H (eds): *Antiepileptic Drugs: Quantitative Analysis and Interpretation.* New York, Raven Press, 1978, pp 315–319.

Pippenger CE, Rosen TS: Phenobarbital plasma levels in neonates. *Clin Perinatol* 1978;2:111–115.

Pitlick W, Painter M, Pippenger CE: Phenobarbital pharmacokinetics in neonates. *Clin Pharmacol Ther* 1978;23:346–450.

Pollack MA, Zion TE, Kellaway P: Long-term prognosis of patients with infantile spasms following ACTH therapy. *Epilepsia* 1979;20:255–260.

Porter PJ, Penry JK: Efficacy and choice of antiepileptic drugs, in Meinardi H, Rowan AJ (eds): *Advances in Epileptology.* Amsterdam, Swets & Zeitlinger, 1977, pp 220–231.

Ratcliffe JC, Wolf SM: Febrile convulsions caused by meningitis in young children. *Ann Neurol* 1977;1:285–286.

Reynolds EH, Shorvon SD: Monotherapy or polypharmacy for epilepsy? *Epilepsia* 1981;22:2–10.

Richens A, Dunlop A: Serum phenytoin levels in management of epilepsy. *Lancet* 1975;2:247–248.

Sackellares JC, Lee SI, Dreifuss FE: Stupor following administration of valproic acid to patients receiving other antiepileptic drugs. *Epilepsia* 1979;20:697–703.

Sackellares JC, Sato S, Dreifuss FE, et al: Reduction of steady state valproate levels by other antiepileptic drugs. *Epilepsia* 1981;22:437–441.

Sato S, White B, Penry JK, et al: Valproic acid versus ethosuximide in the treatment of absence seizure. *Neurology* 1982;32:157–163.

Sherwin AL: Pharmacological principle in the management of patients with epilepsy, in Meinardi H, Rowan AJ (eds): *Advances in Epileptology.* Amsterdam, Swets & Zeitlinger, 1977, pp 211–219.

Shorvon SD, Reynolds EH: Reduction in polypharmacy for epilepsy. *Br Med J* 1979;2:1023–1025.

Shorvon SD, Reynolds EH: Unnecessary polypharmacy for epilepsy. *Br Med J* 1977;1:1635–1637.

Simon D, Penry JK: Sodium di-N-propylacetate (DPA) in the treatment of epilepsy: A review. *Epilepsia* 1975;16:549–573.

Smith FR, Boots M: Sodium valproate and bone marrow suppression. *Ann Neurol* 1980; 8:197–199.

Stores G: Behavioral effects of anti-epileptic drugs. *Devel Med Child Neurol* 1975;17:647–658.

Sutula TP, Sackellares JC, Miller JQ, et al: Intensive monitoring in refractory epilepsy. *Neurology* 1981;31:243–247.

Suzuki M, et al: A double-blind comparative trial of sodium dipropylacetate and ethosuximide in epilepsy, in children, with special emphasis on pure petit mal seizure. *Med Prog (Jpn)* 1972;82:470–488.

Taburet AM, van der Kleijn E: Plasma protein binding of 2-N-propylpentanoate. *Pharm Weekblad* 1977;112:356–361.

Trimble MR, Reynolds EH: Anticonvulsant drugs and mental symptoms. *Psychol Med* 1976;6:169–178.

van der Kleijn E, Guelen PJM, van Wijk C, et al: Clinical pharmacokinetics in monitoring chronic medication with antiepileptic drugs, in Schneider H, Janz D, Gardner-Thorpe C, et al (eds): *Clinical Pharmacology of Antiepileptic Drugs*. New York, Springer-Verlag, 1978, pp 11–33.

Villareal HJ, Wilder BJ, Willmore LT, et al: Effect of valproic acid on spike and wave discharges in patients with absence seizures. *Neurology* 1978;28:886–891.

Wagner JG: *Fundamentals of Clinical Pharmacokinetics*. Hamilton, IL, Drug Intelligence Publications, Inc, 1979.

Woods I, Ives JR, Gloor P: Prolonged EEG recordings in patients with generalized epilepsy. *Electroencephalogr Clin Neurophysiol* 1975;39:295.

Zenker C, Croh C, Roth G: Probleme und Erfahrungen beim Absenzen antikonvulsiver Therapie. *Neue Osterreich Z Kinderheilkund* 1957;2:152–163.

CHAPTER 16

Surgical Management of Epilepsy in Childhood

Fritz E. Dreifuss

SURGICAL TREATMENT OF EPILEPSY

The era of neurosurgical management of epilepsy was ushered in by Horsley in 1886 with the removal of an area of cicatrization. Long prior to this, there had been reports of trephination for epilepsy, and the elevation of depressed fractures was practiced in medieval times. The modern era was largely initiated by the Montreal School. When Penfield began cortical excision surgery, temporal lobe ablations formed a minor proportion of the total surgical procedures (Rasmussen 1975ab). By the mid-1940s, 25%; by the 1950s, 50%; and, more recently, more than two-thirds of all the operations performed represented temporal lobe ablations. Jensen (1975) and Crandall (1977) reviewed the status of temporal lobectomy, which constitutes at least 85% of all surgical procedures for the amelioration of epilepsy at this time.

Surgical treatment of epilepsy can be divided into 1) prophylactic surgery, 2) removal of epileptogenic lesions, 3) removal of epileptic foci, and 4) interference with spread.

Prophylactic Surgery

Prophylactic surgery includes the elevation of depressed skull fractures and the exploration and debridement of open head wounds.

Removal of Epileptogenic Lesions

The removal of epileptogenic lesions includes the removal of brain tumors, subdural hematomas, arteriovenous malformations and focal gliosis (Falconer and Cavanagh 1967, Mathieson 1975). The operation of hemispherectomy (Krynauw 1950) for treatment of intractable seizures associated with infantile hemiplegia and for Sturge-Weber disease (Alexander and Norman 1960) and epilepsia partialis continua caused by "chronic encephalitis" (Rasmussen and McCann 1968) represents the ultimate in ablative surgery for large destructive brain lesions. It has been found that intractable seizures and intractable behavior and learning problems in patients with infantile hemiplegia or Sturge-Weber disease may respond favorably to the removal of the damaged hemisphere, which may be acting as an inhibitor to the function of the undamaged hemisphere. Because of postoperative problems, including cerebral hemosiderosis, obstructive hydrocephalus, and accumulation of fluid in the cavity, this operation became less popular over the years. However, technical refinements and the introduction of shunts for the hemispherectomy cavity have improved the outlook for patients thus operated on (Rasmussen 1975). Topectomy (ie, the removal of limited portions of a hemisphere containing an epileptogenic lesion) may be successful in ameliorating intractable partial seizures, particularly in the younger age groups.

Removal of Epileptogenic Foci

The removal of epileptic foci is, at this time, the most frequent operation for amelioration of intractable epilepsy. As a practical matter, this is more or less synonymous with anterior temporal lobectomy (Jensen 1975, Crandall 1975, Rayport 1977, Falconer 1967, Van Buren et al 1975). Falconer introduced the concept of operating on patients in the younger age groups prior to the development of educational and sociological handicaps, which develop pari passu with the intractability of the process and which might be prevented by the early successful abolition of the underlying seizure disorder. Because of the natural tendency for seizures to improve with age, it is essential to develop rather rigid criteria for consideration of elective surgery in children. Moreover, as stated by Rayport (1977), the surgical facilities for the evaluation and treatment of persons potentially eligible for temporal lobe resection do not exist in sufficient numbers and careful selection procedures are essential also on that score.

Criteria for consideration for surgical management are presented in the following list.

1. Seizures must be intractable to medical therapy, which must have been pursued vigorously with an appropriate medication regimen, good compliance, and blood levels well up into the therapeutic range. The number of seizures must be such as to disrupt normal living; this usually implies multiple seizures per month.

2. The seizures must originate in a well-circumscribed region of brain that can be removed without risk of producing a major or disabling neurologic handicap. Seizures must be partial, either simple partial or complex partial. This implies that the seizures are usually located in the temporal lobe. Evidence for localization of the epileptic focus is obtained from the history, from the patient, and from observers. The seizure repertoire must point to constancy of the clinical picture relative to localizational criteria. Electroencephalographic studies must include both interictal and ictal recordings. Ictal recordings are considerably more reliable in terms of lateralization of the focus responsible for seizures than are interictal foci, which may be present on the same side as the ictal focus but may occasionally be seen contralaterally. The presence of bilateral interictal foci does not invalidate the patient from consideration, as one side may be considerably more active than the other. If noninvasive methods have left doubt as to the localization of the focus, depth electrode recordings may be resorted to (Engel et al 1981, Bancaud et al 1965, Walter 1975). These studies have shown that even ictal recordings from the scalp may produce false localizing evidence. Radiographic studies may be helpful. The plain skull film may show asymmetry of the middle fossae or intracranial calcifications. A CT scan is helpful in further elucidation of these anomalies. Position emission tomography is a useful adjunct in the evaluation of persons with partial seizures because the technique shows areas of cerebral hypometabolism, which indicate the interictal seizure state, or foci of hypermetabolism during the seizure, Engel (1983).

Neuropsychological tests will frequently aid in the lateralization of the cerebral dysfunction. Moreover, the neuropsychological evaluation will assess whether or not a brain lesion can be removed without undue risks of producing neurologic deficits such as aphasia or amnesia.

Sodium amytal injected into the carotid arteries for evaluation of speech dominance and memory is a vital part of the preoperative assessment (Blume et al 1973).

3. Mental retardation and psychosis are contraindications of surgery. The patient who has complex partial seizures and psychosis cannot expect improvement in the latter (Taylor 1972).

With careful patient selection, the operation of temporal lobectomy can be expected to yield seizure control in approximately 70% of patients with previously intractable seizures. The mortality and morbidity are now quite low.

Interference with Spread

Section of the corpus callosum (Wilson et al 1978) is gaining in popularity. This procedure is reported to be effective in reducing the incidence of generalized seizures in patients with partial seizures. The focus is predominantly in one hemisphere. The neuropsychological consequences of corpus callosum sections have been well described but they probably are not of overriding significance in relation to the gaining of seizure control. The open craniectomy corpus callosum section technique is attended by a significant risk, and the population suitable for this type of surgical intervention requires further definition.

ROLE OF SURGICAL THERAPY

In a review of epilepsies in the pediatric age group, the present role of surgical therapy has to be kept in perspective. Our Comprehensive Epilepsy Program is responsible for the treatment of approximately 3500 children each year. Of these, approximately 100 are evaluated in the long-term intensive monitoring milieu of the Diagnostic, Treatment, and Rehabilitation Unit. Of these, in turn, four or five patients are assessed as needing neurosurgical intervention (such as a temporal lobectomy) other than that needed for the treatment of underlying lesions that are detected during the evaluative process.

BIBLIOGRAPHY

Alexander GL, Norman RM: *The Sturge-Weber Syndrome.* Bristol, J Wright & Son, 1960.

Bancaud J, et al: *La Stereo-electroencephalographie dans l'Epilepsie.* Paris, Masson & Cie, 1965.

Blume WT, Grabow JD, Darby FL, et al: Intracarotid amobarbital test of language and memory before temporal lobectomy for seizure control. *Neurology* 1973;23:812–819.

Crandall PH: The role of neurosurgery in the treatment of medication-refractory epilepsy, in Commission for the Control of Epilepsy and Its Consequences: *Plan for Nationwide Action on Epilepsy.* Washington, DC, DHEW, 1977.

Crandall PH: Postoperative management and criteria for evaluation, in Purpura D, Penry JK, Walter RD (eds): *Advances in Neurology.* New York, Raven Press, vol 8, 1975, pp 265–279.

Engel J Jr, Rausch R, Lieb JL, et al: Correlation of criteria used for localizing the epileptic foci in patients considered for surgical therapy of epilepsy. *Ann Neurol* 1981;9:215–224.

Engel J Jr, Kuhl DE, Phelps ME: Regional brain metabolism during seizures in humans, in Esculta AV, Waterlain CG, Porter RJ (eds): *Status Epilepticus.* New York, Raven Press, 1983, pp 141–148.

Falconer MA: Surgical treatment of temporal lobe epilepsy. *NZ Med J* 1967;66:539–544.

Falconer MA, Cavanagh JB: Clinico-pathological considerations of temporal lobe epilepsy due to small focal lesions. A study of cases submitted to operation. *Brain* 1959;82:482–504.

Horsley V: Brain surgery. *Br Med J* 1886;2:670–675.

Jensen I: Temporal lobe surgery around the world. *Acta Neurol Scand* 1975;52:354–373.

Krynauw RA: Infantile hemiplegia treated by removing one cerebral hemisphere. *J Neurol Neurosurg Psychiatry* 1950;13:243–267.

Mathieson G: Pathological aspects of epilepsy with special reference to the surgical pathology of focal cerebral seizures, in Purpura DP, Penry JK, Walter RD (eds): *Advances in Neurology*. New York, Raven Press, vol 8, 1975, pp 107–138.

Rasmussen T: Surgical treatment of patients with complex partial seizures, in Penry JK, Daly DD (eds): *Advances in Neurology*. New York, Raven Press, vol 11, 1975, pp 414–449.

Rasmussen T: Cortical resection in the treatment of focal epilepsy, in Purpura DP, Penry JK, Walter RD (eds): *Advances in Neurology*. New York, Raven Press, vol 8, 1975a, pp 139–154.

Rasmussen T, McCann W: Clinical studies of patients with focal epilepsy due to "chronic encephalitis." *Trans Am Neurol Assoc* 1968;93:89–94.

Rayport M: The role of neurosurgery in medication-refractory epilepsy, in Commission for the Control of Epilepsy and Its Consequences: *Plan for Nationwide Action on Epilepsy*. Washington, DC, DHEW, 1977.

Taylor DC: Mental state and temporal lobe epilepsy: A correlative account of 100 patients treated surgically. *Epilepsia* 1972;13:727–765.

Van Buren JM, Ajmone Marson C, Mutsuga N, et al: Surgery of temporal lobe epilepsy, in Purpura DP, Penry JK, Walter RD (eds): *Advances in Neurology*. New York, Raven Press, vol 8, 1975, pp 155–196.

Walter RD: Principles of clinical investigation of surgical candidates, in Purpura DP, Penry JK, Walter RD (eds): *Advances in Neurology*. New York, Raven Press, vol 8, 1975.

Wilson DH, Reeves A, Gazzaniga M: Division of the corpus callosum for uncontrollable epilepsy. *Neurology* 1978;28:649–653.

CHAPTER 17

The Comprehensive Epilepsy Program in Diagnosis and Management

Fritz E. Dreifuss

THE ROLE OF THE COMPREHENSIVE EPILEPSY PROGRAM IN THE MANAGEMENT OF THE PATIENT WITH INTRACTABLE SEIZURES

The principal goals in the treatment of persons with epilepsy include:

1. The elimination of seizures.
2. Prevention, including prevention of epilepsy, prevention of seizures, and prevention of consequences of seizures.
3. The achievement of these goals at the least cost in terms of surgical damage, drug toxicity, and major expense.

The need to eliminate seizures is predicated on the assumption that these are deleterious to the organism, either directly by causing further neuronal impairment or through mechanisms such as kindling, which perpetuate themselves if untreated, or indirectly by causing physical, social, psychological, vocational, and recreational impairment and thereby irreversibly altering the quality of life and ability to cope of the individual.

The rubric of prevention encompasses prevention of epilepsy, prevention of seizures, and prevention of consequences of seizures (Commission for the Control of Epilepsy and Its Consequences 1977). These goals are to be achieved by elimination of epileptogenic events such as head injuries, nervous system infections by agents that cannot be prevented by immunization, early and vigorous management of treatable inflammatory illnesses such as meningitis, prevention of birth trauma by better antenatal care and obstetrics, and prevention of early teenage pregnancies.

Seizures may be prevented by the early and adequate application of appropriate anticonvulsant therapy (either pharmacologic or surgical) and by the avoidance and elimination of precipitating factors. These factors include sleep deprivation and other influences known to be instrumental in seizure provocation in individual cases, such as exposure to photic stimulation and to certain sounds and other reflex precipitating influences. Prevention of consequences of seizures includes prevention of neurologic consequences, ie, the neuronal changes induced by uncontrolled seizures. These neuronal changes include pathological changes, such as cell death, and physiological changes, such as the development of self-perpetuating and mirror foci. Psychosocial consequences, including social, educational, and vocational handicaps should not be allowed to develop and, if they have developed, they should not be allowed to continue.

Whichever means of therapy are applied, whether surgical or pharmacologic, a major goal has to be the achievement of the aforementioned objectives at the least possible cost to the patient. Costs can be measured in terms of brain damage resulting from an investigative and surgical approach to the underlying problem and from drug toxicity, which may vitiate a satisfactory result of seizure control. Brain damage occurs when the nature and the amount of medication that has to be administered to achieve seizure control is such as to render the patient *hor de combat* as a result of intolerable side effects. Also, expense of treatment may be a major consideration, and occasionally a compromise may have to be achieved between the medication regimen deemed ideal and that deemed economically feasible in a particular set of circumstances, a compromise that may make the difference between compliance and noncompliance, and thus, between tolerable seizure control that may be short of ideal and abandonment.

A Comprehensive Epilepsy Program is the ultimate resource for the integration of multidisciplinary efforts in the areas of health care delivery, education, and research (Dreifuss 1980). It extends to all levels of care and includes regional, diagnostic, and follow-up services and mobilization of community resources, such as the voluntary agencies, the educational, vocational and rehabilitative services, and the local medical referral resources. Some patients require acute intensive care or the service of an acute care inpatient unit. Central to a Comprehensive Epilepsy Program is a specialized diagnostic, treatment, and rehabilitation unit with facilities for intensive monitoring and intensive application of all diagnostic and treatment modalities required for those who, by virtue of their epilepsy or the secondary effects thereof, are unable to compete effectively in the field of education, independent living or rehabilitation. Such a unit is usually geared to a considerably longer period of hospitalization than is customary in the acute care unit of a hospital. The unit encompasses intensive monitoring capability and the activities of a clinical research center. It also encompasses educational facilities with outreach components, postgraduate courses on advances in epilepsy management, courses for allied health professionals, inservice programs for teachers and counselors, and sessions for patient and parents. The participation of social workers, educatonal consultants, and vocational rehabilitative counselors adds immeasurably to the quality of life of patients and may also directly influence the degree of seizure control (Figure 17-1).

Investigative Intensive Monitoring

One of the major roles of intensive monitoring is the accurate identification of individual seiure types. The new International Classification of Epileptic Seizures (Commission on Classification and Terminology 1981) aids in the identification of seizure types, in the communication between physicians about seizures, and in the management of seizures, which is enhanced by the application of specific anticonvulsant drugs to specific seizure types. Anticonvulsant drugs are becoming increasingly targeted on certain varieties of seizures with the result that therapy is becoming less empirical. Observation of seizures, however, frequently does not allow an accurate and definitive elucidation of the type of seizure under observation. Capture of the seizure on videotape with simultaneous EEG display allows the observer to focus on the seizure, to replay it, and to accurately classify it (Figure 17-2). This technique has added to management, particularly in patients whose seizures have never previously been accurately documented and whose seizures had been rela-

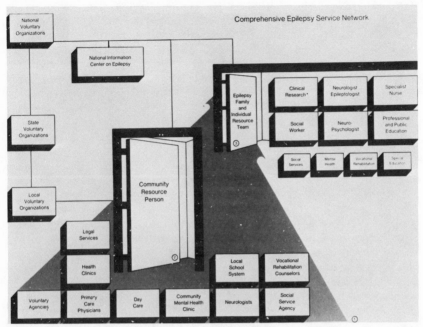

Figure 17-1 Organization of a Comprehensive Epilepsy Program. Adapted from Report of the Commission for the Control of Epilepsy and Its Consequences.

tively intractable. For example, distinction between absence seizures and complex partial seizures with loss of consciousness only and between absence seizures with automatisms and complex partial seizures with automatisms, ranks among the most difficult of neurologic differential diagnoses without the use of intensive monitoring. A misdiagnosis here may have major consequences (Dreifuss 1975). For example, a child with absence seizures with automatisms might be falsely diagnosed as suffering from complex partial seizures. Treatment with an inappropriate drug causes delay in the amelioration of the condition and the possibility of unnecessary side effects.

Differential Diagnosis

One of the reasons seizures present as an intractable problem is that the seizure may be only a part of the overall predicament. The patient may be suffering from pseudoseizures, ie, seizure caused by nonorganic neurologic dysfunction. Pseudoseizure may be the result of malingering, of hysteria, and of other physiological disturbances. They frequently occur in persons who have epilepsy and occasionally in persons who do not. They represent episodic clinical events resembling epileptic seizures that are not, however, associated with ictal or postical changes in the electroencephalogram when the clinical events and the electroencephalograms are simultaneously recorded. Not only will the presence of pseudoseizures lead to a markedly inflated seizure count, but it will also lead, unless recognized, to postponement of appropriate psychological intervention. Such patients are subjected to increasing doses of potentially toxic medications. Intensive monitoring with simultaneous display of the patient's seizure activity and EEG is an extremely important tool for

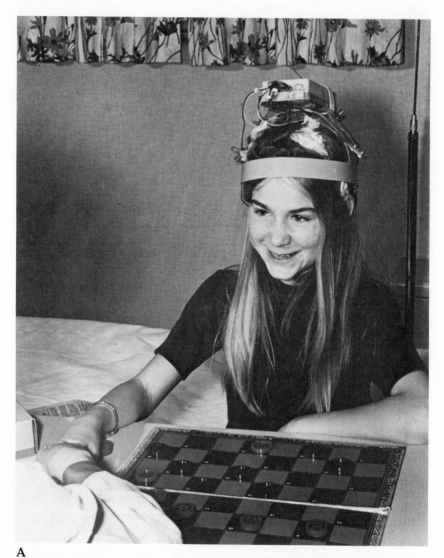

A
Figure 17-2 Intensive monitoring using **A** EEG telemetry and **B** split-screen video technique.

the accurate identification, not only of seizures, but also of pseudoseizures; it enables the appropriate therapy to be used in the individual case.

One of my patients was a young woman who had had recurrent hospitalizations for intractable status epilepticus. She had been intubated so many times in various emergency rooms that she had developed laryngeal stenosis and had been told that she could no longer be intubated. Over the course of many months, she had received large doses of intravenous diazepam and phenytoin to control her episodes of status epilepticus. She was ultimately referred to the Epilepsy Center from a city approximately 800 miles away, a trip that required an airplane journey with a change of aircraft. On the first plane, she had a seizure sufficiently severe to jeopardize the plane's

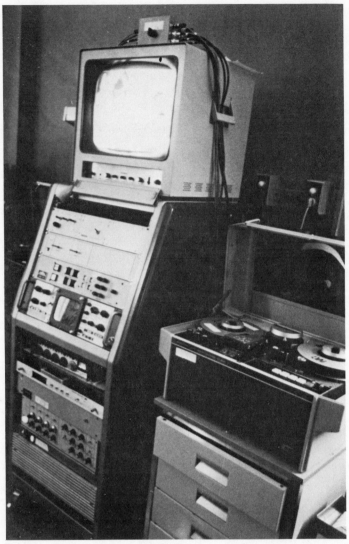

B

itinerary. On the second plane, she had a similar attack, but the stewardess, fortunately, was able to give an accurate account of what appeared to have been a
pseudoseizure. Subsequent intensive monitoring revealed several seizures, none of
which had an EEG accompaniment and none of which was convincing as an epileptic
seizure. The patient subsequently was taken off anticonvulsant medications, entered
psychotherapy, and has since then remained free of seizures. Parenthetically, this
case illustrates the usefulness of educating airplane attendants in the recognition and
management of seizure disorders occurring under their purview. This is one of the
educational functions of the Comprehensive Epilepsy Program.

It should be stressed that the majority of persons with pseudoseizures also have epilepsy. Unraveling of this complex skein leads to the best results because the individual seizure types are recognized and the therapy most appropriate to each is applied. Table 17-1 illustrates the differential diagnostic features of seizures and pseudoseizures. This distinction becomes important even in children as young as 3 and 4 years of age (Holmes et al 1980, Finlayson and Lucas 1979, Schneider and Rice 1979).

Table 17-1
Characteristics of Epileptic Seizures and Pseudoseizures

Characteristic	Epilepsy	Pseudoseizures
Ictal EEG abnormality	Usually paroxysmal, with postictal slow	None
Incontinence	Common	None
Postictal behavior	Always in tonic-clonic Common in complex partial seizures	None
Behavior in seizures	Stereotyped; no direct violence	Frequently combative Obscenities common
Exacerbation by stress	Occasional	Common
Relief by manipulation of medication	Frequent	Rare

Intensive monitoring occasionally identifies other episodic disturbances. Respiratory and cardiac monitoring in addition to the EEG will identify cases of breath-holding, cardiac or vasovagal syncope, and the various types of apnea. For children, important differential diagnostic features, which may be clarified with intensive monitoring, are outlined in Table 17-2.

Table 17-2
Differential Diagnosis of Seizures

Syncope	Sleep syndromes
Cardiac	Terrors
Vasovagal	Myoclonus
Reflex	Hallucinations
Hydrocephalic attacks	Paralysis
Vertigo	Walking
Periodic syndrome of children	Hemiplegic migraine
Hyperventilation	Hysteria
Breath-holding	

Syncope is usually not difficult to diagnose. It results from inadequate cerebral perfusion, which is usually caused by blood pressure falls and which usually occurs in the upright position. In the majority of children, syncope occurs as a result of an emotionally traumatic experience, prolonged standing at attention, or exposure to heat. Some convulsive movements are occasionally seen, particularly if there is a delay in attaining recumbency, ie, if someone tries to prop up the child after he or she had fainted.

More sinister are the cardiac syncopes, which may be caused by sudden obstruction of cardiac output (eg, by an atrial myxoma or a ball valve thrombus) or by sudden changes in cardiac rhythm such as may occur with cardiac asystole (Stokes-Adams syndrome). Changes in cardiac rhythm may occur as a result of the so-called "long QT syndrome," which may lead to ventricular fibrillation and sudden death (Romano et al 1963, Ward 1964). Patients with syncope almost invariably become extremely pale; their pulse slows and may be imperceptible.

Hydrocephalic attacks have been observed in two patients, one of whom had an Arnold Chiari malformation and the other an aqueductal stenosis with shunt obstruction. The attack in each case was quite sudden, with cessation of activity, staring, pupil dilatation, buckling of the knees, and unconsciousness with stertorous respiration. The first stage was followed by restlessness, and after 15 and 25 minutes, respectively, the patients regained consciousness via a period of confusion and severe headache. Hypotension, bradycardia, and cerebral slowing accompanied these attacks.

Vertigo may be confused with seizures in a child too young to describe the sensation; and, conversely, epilepsy may present as paroxysmal vertigo, including sensations of falling in space and floating, as well as rotary sensations in a horizontal or vertical plane. True epileptic vertigo is accompanied by focal electroencephalographic changes during the attack (Eviatar and Eviatar 1977).

The periodic syndrome in children encompasses several types of episodes, some of which are epileptic, and others of which have an undetermined cause. Almost certainly many of them represent childhood migraine, which is considerably more common than generally supposed. Intensive monitoring is extremely useful for identifying the nature of the attack. Symptoms under this heading include severe recurrent paroxysmal headaches with or without visual disturbancs. Occipital seizures in children frequently present with distortions or loss of vision. Such a symptom might be difficult to distinguish from migraine. However, the situation is clarified by electroencephalography, which almost invariably shows marked occipital lobe epileptic discharges in this syndrome. Small children frequently do not complain of visual phenomena as part of the migraine syndrome. In older children, typical migraine visual phenomena may be described. Recurrent attacks of abdominal pain, sudden unexplained changes in behavior or personality, numbness and tingling in the extremities on one side of the body, and even hemiplegia and aphasia may occur as migraine phenomena, and these may be quite difficult to distinguish from focal seizures with EEG corroboration. Recurrent attacks of abdominal pain and vomiting, which sometimes occur often enough to produce dehydration and which occasionally occur at regular intervals of 20 to 40 days, usually represent migraine. Occasionally, however, the attacks are associated with transient disturbances of consciousness and focal or generalized spike-wave abnormalities in the electroencephalogram (Douglas and White 1971). In these cases, which represent the rare syndrome of abdominal epilepsy, anticonvulsant drugs may be of benefit (O'Donohoe 1971). In the majority of patients with a migraine variant, long-term administration of propranolol is likely to be of greater benefit. The situation becomes particularly troublesome when two conditions coexist, as in one of my patients. This 6-year-old child had classic, nocturnal, rolandic, benign childhood seizures and abdominal migraine, with attacks every 3 weeks. Intensive monitoring is extremely valuable in sorting out such a situation.

Hyperventilation syncope is occasionally seen in children, particularly adolescents, and is usually quite easily reproduced by getting the patient to hyperventilate. Here, the cause is usually not difficult to discern with an adequate history.

Differential diagnosis of breath-holding spells may be difficult without intensive monitoring. Where the history of classic cyanotic breath-holding is clear, the diagnosis is quite easy. The child is either injured or thwarted or its feelings are in some way hurt; it will cry and cry until it stops breathing. It continues to forcibly contract its thorax despite a closed glottis. Cyanosis occurs, and the child may then relax, give a few jerks, and have a postictal lethargy for a few seconds, with a suffused face and complete exhaustion. The pallid form of breath-holding, however, is more difficult to identify (Lombroso and Lerman 1967). This syndrome probably represents several conditions, including reflex syncope. Here a child may sustain a mild injury (usually a blow on the head of no great moment); the child will usually give a cry or gasp and fall limp and pale, with some circumoral cyanosis and occasionally some jerking of the extremities. Some of these attacks are probably breath-holding spells; others are reflex syncope; and others are epileptic. Because breath-holding attacks usually occur very frequently, EEG confirmation with a prolonged, cassette-recorded EEG is quite feasible. Some apneic spells are the result of limbic system epileptic discharge, and this type of disturbance will response to anticonvulsant medications. Monitoring of these patients should include electrocardiographic recordings, as sudden cardiac arrhythmias may terminate fatally.

Sleep syndromes are difficult to elucidate without objective recording. Here again, prolonged electroencepahlography with simultaneous video observation may prevent diagnostic errors. Enuresis, sleep walking, night terrors, and somniloquy are all frequently seen in children, as are hypnogogic myoclonic jerks (Dement et al 1975). The latter frequently occur in light sleep, the others in deep sleep. Night terrors characteristically occur during stage IV sleep and can be quite easily identified in this way from seizures, particularly those of the "rolandic epilepsy" variety. In both of these conditions, the child may look terrified. However, only in night terrors (which usually occur in younger children) will the child wake up screaming and show the autonomic changes of fear. Episodic hypersomnia may be seen in narcolepsy and in sleep apnea syndromes. Narcolepsy is usually seen in older age groups but may occur in children. It may present with the classic triad of symptoms: uncontrollable daytime sleepiness, cataplexy, (or sudden loss of muscle tone associated with emotional precipitants) and hypnogogic or sleep paralysis, which is often associated with a frightening hallucinatory "visitation" experience, occasionally of an autoscopic kind.

Sleep apnea occurs in response to airway obstruction and occasionally is caused by central alveolar hypoventilation. In the nursery, the distinction between central sleep apnea and apnea due to neonatal seizures may be a difficult one without EEG monitoring. Normal apneas of sleep seen in REM sleep are less than 10 seconds in duration. Central sleep apneas are repetitive, exceed 10 seconds in duration, and occur in NREM sleep, with many episodes in a single night. There is sometimes a family history of sleep apnea (Schiffman et al 1980).

Elucidation of episodic behavioral disturbances is another reason for intensive monitoring. Occasionally spike-wave stupor will present as an episodic behavioral disturbance with confusion and occasionally psychotic behavior. When this occurs, electroencephalographic monitoring during an episode of disturbed behavior will reveal the disturbance to be the result of so-called spike-wave stupor. This condition is readily controlled by the intravenous administration of anticonvulsant drugs, such as diazepam.

In a Comprehensive Epilepsy Program setting, intensive monitoring is to objectively enumerate seizures when this is required for the evaluation of the effectiveness of anticonvulsant drugs, particularly in drug trials. Intensive monitoring was first introduced in the context of drug studies comparing new anticonvulsant drugs with existent agents for the treatment of absence seizures (Penry et al 1975). The seizure count provided by observers is notoriously unreliable in other than generalized tonic-clonic seizures. The simultaneous evaluation of seizures and electroencephalographic disturbances is the most accurate way of counting absence seizures and massive infantile spasms.

Prognosis

The determination of prognosis is becoming increasingly important in the intelligent application of therapy in such a manner as to minimize the potential abuse of anticonvulsant drugs, to the detriment of the patient. There are many epileptic syndromes, including febrile seizures, the absence seizure syndrome (Sato et al 1976), the infantile spasm syndrome, and massive epileptic myoclonus of adolescence, that contain at least two statistical populations of patients within the parent rubric. These populations include 1) those in whom the seizures under consideration are the only seizure type and who have a normal neurologic development, a normal neurologic examination, normal intelligence, and a good response to the appropriate anticonvulsant drugs; and 2) those whose neurologic findings, development, and intellectual capabilities imply structural neurologic disease and whose background abnormalities are considered to be abnormal compared with those of the first group. In the case of febrile seizures, this distinction will help to determine which seizures should be treated and which should be further observed. For absence seizures, this distinction will help to determine the duration of therapy and the choice of agent, ie, whether to proceed only with an antiabsence drug or whether also to cover other seizure types. For infantile spasms, it will aid in the prognostication regarding future intellectual attainment. Here again, particularly for absence seizures and infantile spasms, the simultaneous viewing of the seizures and the electroencephalogram greatly helps in the classification of the individual into the good-prognosis category or the high-risk category.

For all these reasons, intensive monitoring has become a technique that is now widely employed. It should be even more widely used in the evaluation of all seizures that are difficult to treat and that have not come under good control in a reasonable period of time (Sutula et al 1981).

CAUSES OF INTRACTABILITY OF EPILEPTIC SEIZURES

From the foregoing, it is evident that there are several causes of intractability.

Faulty Diagnosis

Faulty diagnosis is the result of incorrect identification of seizure types. Examples of faulty diagnosis include mistaking absence seizures with automatisms for complex partial seizures and employing inappropriate medication (Dreifuss 1975). Failure to distinguish epileptic seizures from nonepileptic seizures or pseudoseizures is a common cause for lack of seizure control, which leads to overmedication. It should be remembered that seizures and pseudoseizures frequently occur in the same individual, and the distinction between the individual seizure types is of the utmost importance. Failure to recognize underlying disease processes, such as acute intermittent prophyria, hypoglycemia, or hypocalcemia, may lead to apparent intractability. Failure to recognize precipitating factors that should be eliminated (eg, stimuli that produce reflex epilepsy in an individual) may lead to difficulty in obtaining seizure control. Again, an inappropriate amount of medication may be administered as a consequence of poor seizure control.

Faulty Administration of Medication

The administration of inappropriate drugs may result from incorrect diagnosis. In addition, the administration of phenobarbital in children with absence seizures sometimes leads to perpetuation of seizures, even if appropriate drugs such as ethosuximide or valproic acid are also given. Phenobarbital is frequently given to children with absence seizures, both because of the mistaken impression that it helps and to prevent the occurrence of generalized tonic-clonic seizures. This drug is probably completely inappropriate in this situation, and it may make absence seizure worse.

Incorrect dosage adjustments may lead to apparent intractability. Both insufficient and excessive doses of drugs may lead to seizure exacerbation. The latter is particularly true of phenytoin, where paradoxical increase in seizures may result from doses that produce blood levels in the toxic range. The possibility of drug interactions should be considered. Frequently, the introduction of a second drug may lead to diminished blood levels because of enzyme induction and other interactions.

Inappropriate treatment sometimes consists of prolongation of useless drug therapy instead of consideration of surgical treatment of an active localized focus in a surgically accessible part of the brain. Surgery should be considered for patients in whom drug therapy has failed.

Patient at Fault

Insufficient compliance is a very complex problem and may, to some extent, be the result of inadequate patient education on the part of the treatment team. Generally, patients should be informed about their medications, the potential side effects of medication, the need for medication compliance, the factors that increase medication requirements, and other complicating factors. Sometimes compliance is interfered with by sociological factors. For example, patients may feel that they are not normal while taking medication and that normality might be achieved again by discontinuing that which constantly reminds them that they are not normal. Some patients are frankly rebellious and others are potentially suicidal. Others are afraid that coming out into the open will jeopardize certain areas of normal existence, including the operation of motor vehicles. This is particularly bothersome in teenagers. These factors all serve to promote intractability.

Nonavoidance of precipitating factors, including sleep deprivation, emotional stress, bright lights (particularly flashing lights such as discotheque strobe lights), may lead to perpetuation of seizures that could be controlled if such precipitating factors were avoided.

The administration of competing medications, such as antihistamines or psychotrophic drugs (including phenothiazines), may promote apparent intractability.

The presence of intercurrent illnesses may precipitate seizures that might otherwise be reasonably controlled. These intercurrent illnesses include nonspecific febrile illnesses and conditions that interfere with organ systems responsible for anticonvulsant drug metabolism, such as the liver, the kidneys, and the gastrointestinal tract. Pregnancy frequently increases the anticonvulsant drug requirement.

The Patient's Social Predicament

Intractability may be the result of a person's coping style. Whether or not someone can cope with epilepsy depends on many factors, some of which are environmental and some of which are inherent. The latter include 1) the age of onset of seizures: the earlier seizures begin, the worse the prognosis for coping, for cessation of seizures, and for attainment of intellectual milestones; 2) the site of the lesion responsible for the seizures: seizures of temporal lobe origin and seizures with a site of origin in the left cerebral hemisphere carry a worse outlook for coping than seizures whose site of origin is elsewhere in the nervous system; 3) the type of medication employed: barbiturates, hydantoins, and primidone are more likely to interfere with cognitive function and, further, to lead to depression. Environmental factors that influence a person's ability to cope include the constraints on participating in large areas of normal activity and an exclusion from educational, competitive, and recreational activities. These factors lead to a crippling of the coping style, with ensuing social intractability.

TYPES OF SEIZURES THAT ARE PARTICULARLY INTRACTABLE TO THERAPY

1. Seizures associated with progressive neurologic disease. Progressive disease of the nervous system include inborn errors of metabolism, degenerative processes affecting the cerebral gray matter, and progressive inflammatory conditions, such as SSPE, phakomatoses, collagen vascular diseases, and tumors.

2. Specific diseases, such as a) infantile spasms and b) the Lennox-Gastaut syndrome. These epileptic encephalopathies are characterized by seizures that are very difficult to control. They are conditions in which mental retardation plays a major part in the clinical picture.

3. Epilepsia partialis continua and status epilepticus. These conditions are extremely difficult to treat in children. Epilepsia partialis continua may be caused by a chronic encephalitis of cerebral vascular disease or by a brain tumor. The condition may continue for days, weeks, or months and may defy treatment with anticonvulsant drugs and doses other than those that produce unconsciousness. Status epilepticus may at times be a recurrent complication of seizure disorders, particularly in those disorders in which there is severe frontal lobe involvement.

4. Delayed intervention in the control of seizures. Delayed intervention may result in "kindling" and the development of a self-perpetuating epileptic condition that appears to be particularly frequently encountered in patients with chronic complex partial seizures. Those who have had uncontrolled seizures for many years tend to prove extremely resistant to all forms of medication adjustment. This fact rein-

forces the need for early and adequate intervention aimed at ultimate prevention of the development of intractable epilepsy.

BIBLIOGRAPHY

Brown JK: Migraine and migraine equivalents in childhood. *Dev Med Child Neurol* 1977;19: 683–692.

Commission on Classification and Terminology, International League against Epilepsy: Proposal for revised clinical and electroencephalographic classification of epileptic seizures. *Epilepsia* 1981;22:489–501.

Commission for the Control of Epilepsy and Its Consequences: *National Plan for Action.* U.S. Department of Health, Education, and Welfare, Washington, DC, 1977.

Dement W, Guillemiault C, Zarzone V: The pathologies of sleep: A case series approach, in Tower D (ed): *The Nervous System.* New York, Raven Press, vol 2, 1975.

Douglas CF, White PT: Abdominal epilepsy: A reappraisal. *J Pediatr* 1971;78:59–67.

Dreifuss FE: Differential diagnosis of complex partial seizures, in Penry JK, Daly DD (eds): *Advances in Neurology.* New York, Raven Press, vol 11, 1975.

Dreifuss FE: The development of a comprehensive epilepsy program, in Robb P (ed): *Epilepsy Updated: Causes and Treatment.* Chicago, Year Book Medical Publishers, 1980.

Eviatar L, Eviatar A: Vertigo in childhood: Differential diagnosis and management. *Petriatrics* 1977;59:833–838.

Finlayson PE, Lucas AR: Pseudoepileptic seizures in children and adolescents. *Mayo Clin Proc* 1979;54:83–87.

Holmes G, Sackellares JC, McKiernan J, et al: Evaluation of pseudoseizures using EEG telemetry and videotape monitoring. *J Pediatr* 1980;97:554–558.

Lombroso CT, Lerman P: Breath-holding spells (cyanotic and pallid infantile syncope). *Pediatrics* 1967;39:563–581.

O'Donohoe NV: Abdominal epilepsy. *Dev Med Child Neurol* 1971;13:798–800.

Penry JK, Porter RJ, Dreifuss FE: Simultaneous recording of absence seizures with videotape and electroencephalogram: A study of 374 seizures in 48 patients. *Brain* 1975;98:427–440.

Roman C, Gemme G, Ponguiglione RL: Aritmic cardiache rare dell'eta'pediatrica. *Clin Pediatr* 1963;45:656–683.

Sato S, Penry JK, Dreifuss FE: Prognosis in absence, in Janz D (ed): *Epileptology.* Berlin, Georg Thieme Verlag, 1976.

Schiffman PL, Westlake RE, Santiago TV, et al: Ventilatory control in parents of victims of sudden infant death syndrome. *N Engl J Med* 1980;302:486.

Schneider S, Rice DR: Neurological manifestations of childhood hysteria. *Behav Pediatr* 1979; 94:153–156.

Sutula TP, Sackellares JC, Miller JQ, et al: Efficacy of prolonged hospitalization and intensive monitoring in refractory epilepsy. *Neurology* 1981;31:243–247.

Ward OC: A new familial cardiac syndrome in children. *J Irish Med Assoc* 1964;54:103–106.

CHAPTER **18**

Psychosocial Considerations in Childhood Epilepsy

Carol Appolone Ford, Patricia Gibson, and Fritz E. Dreifuss

The impact of having a child with epilepsy can be significant medically, socially, psychologically, and financially. It upsets the equilibrium of the family system, affecting everyone in some way. Because epilepsy usually begins in childhood, the patient's formative years may be drastically altered by the reactions of the family, school, and peer group to this disorder.

Epilepsy can be a frustrating disorder for the family. Between seizures most children are normal and healthy, leaving parents confused as to what to expect or to demand of their "afflicted" child. The parents nervously ask whether their child will have more seizures. At best, the physician can offer only a calculated guess. "Will the child outgrow these seizures?" the parents want to know. Many children spontaneously improve, but there is little assurance that this will happen and certainly no guarantees that can be offered. For most patients, epilepsy will be a mild affliction medically. For a few whose seizures cannot be controlled, it may be a catastrophic illness that drains the family of its resources.

Although the severity of epilepsy affects the child's psychosocial adjustment, it is only one factor in many (Shope 1980, Goldin et al 1971). Sometimes patients with well-controlled seizures adjust quite poorly, while those whose control is not as good adapt well (Hodgman et al 1979, Lennox and Mohr 1950). How disruptive the family perceives the disorder to be, regardless of whether their perception is accurate, is a key factor in their reaction. The age of the child at the onset of epilepsy is an important variable. The older the child, the better the psychosocial adjustment (Goldin et al 1971). How the family system functions prior to the diagnosis is important in how it copes with this crisis. The family's adjustment in turn has a profound impact on how the child reacts.

Children with epilepsy learn quickly that there is something wrong with their brain, and they often have fears and fantasies that transcend the reality. The anxiety of their parents frightens them. The tests, hospitalization, doctor's visits, and the strange symptoms they experience create an acutely stressful situation. If siblings are stand-offish and the school somewhat rejecting, the child has nowhere to turn for support and confirmation of his worth.

Society's response to the child's epilepsy affects and is affected by his or her personal adjustment. Those who have strong family support may actually make strides in altering the attitudes and behaviors of the less enlightened people in their community. Less assured patients will be greatly affected by the social slights, the cruel remarks, and the institutional prejudice they may encounter. These vulnerable ones may downgrade their ambitions, avoid competition, and be socially withdrawn. They become wary of society because it offers little security.

In terms of economic impact, epilepsy can be a very costly disorder. With the introduction of new and expensive drugs, the price of daily medication has escalated dramatically for many. Technology brings new diagnostic tests, but they have a high price tag. Within families the expense of this disorder may be one factor in causing parental anger toward the child (Goldin and Margolin 1975). When seizures are poorly controlled, one parent may have to forego employment and a badly needed second income to remain home with the sick child. On a national scale, epilepsy costs billions annually. In 1975, the figure was placed at $3 billion and it is, of course, much higher now (Commission for the Control of Epilepsy and Its Consequences 1977).

There is controversy regarding the use of the word "epilepsy." Some physicians think that the patient's adjustment would be easier if such a stigmatizing label were not applied. Epilepsy engenders many misconceptions, and physicians seek to avoid the misconceptions by avoiding the term. (The Japanese, in turn, eschew their word *Tenkan* in favor of *epilepsy.*) Other terms commonly used are *seizure disorder, spells, convulsions, attacks,* and *fits,* although the last one is distasteful to many patients in this country. There are those who object to the term *epilepsy* because it is too ambiguous, referring to a collection of different seizure types with many causes. Nevertheless, the word epilepsy is difficult to avoid. It crops up time and again on forms for insurance, camp, driving, and employment. It can be injurious to patients to be unaware that *epilepsy* is one term for their disorder. A woman referred to our center for counseling was quite depressed when such ignorance resulted in her being fired. Her complex partial seizures had always been referred to as "spells" by her doctor so she marked "no" beside epilepsy on the employment form. After she had a seizure on the job, her medical report came back stating that she had a long history of epilepsy. She was fired for falsifying her application form. Being a conscientious, religious person, she was mortified. She suffered much more from the humiliation of being fired than she did from the term *epilepsy.* It undermines the doctor/patient relationship when the patient learns from a form, a health fair, or a public service announcement on television that the condition he has is called epilepsy.

PARENTAL REACTION

Common parental reactions to this diagnosis are disbelief, shock, anxiety, shame, and embarrassment. Parental fears include realistic fears about injury, mental abnormality, social handicaps, cause, drug treatment, and future handicaps.

Lessman (1982) points out that although parental response varies, all experience some sense of grief. They mourn for the loss of the healthy child they have known. They go through the grief stages of denial, anger, and depression. Denial cushions the family against the shock and gives them time to adjust to the change. Denial may also lead to noncompliance and lack of medical follow-up. Many parents seek second opinions, in an attempt to find someone who will verify that a mistake in diagnosis has been made. Arangio (1973) found that many families he studied showed a chornic lack of acceptance of the condition. He noted that many parents feel that their social position is threatened by the presence of a child with epilepsy in the family. Depression is a natural stage in the grief process but should not continue indefinitely. Chronic sorrow as described by Olshansky (1962) in his classic article should not be a way of life for the parents of the child with epilepsy, regardless of the severity.

All parents experience some guilt. For a few, the guilt is excessive and becomes a major problem in the adjustment process. Such guilt can result in feelings of hostility toward the child. It may also cause insidious permissiveness. Lennox and Mohr (1950) classified as "rejecting" those families who expressed marked overconcern and overprotection and who imposed unreasonable limitations on the patient's activities.

Parents are usually quite confused about this disorder. Epilepsy has a bad connotation. It has been associated with mental retardation and mental illness for centuries. Parents' information may be out of date and totally erroneous. Tales they have heard from friends and relatives about someone who died with epilepsy are frightening. Grandparents have an especially significant impact on the parent's attitude and knowledge about epilepsy (Romeis 1980). Unfortunately, they often communicate archaic ideas that may be quite damaging.

One common parental reaction is overprotection and overindulgence, a combination that can be much more disabling than the seizures. Lerman (1977) describes a young adult who was mistakenly diagnosed in childhood as having epilepsy and then raised with crippling permissiveness. When he was induced into the military service, his father explained to the authorities that he was unfit for such responsibilities because he was hopelessly spoiled. All physicians who treat adults have seen similar examples of disabled persons who are perfectly healthy but poorly reared. This occurs to a lesser extent in those patients who never realize their full potential although they lead adequate lives. Most of this faulty upbringing is preventable.

Sometimes the parents need the physician's permission and encouragement to impose limits and dispense discipline. A good example of this occurred with a 14-year-old girl treated in our clinic. After her first grand mal seizure, she was given medication and told to return in a month. At the time of the follow-up visit, it came to light that she had only gone to school 2 days in the previous month. She complained each morning that she did not feel well, and her mother was afraid to push her for fear she might have a seizure. The girl did not like school and had quickly learned how to avoid it by using her seizure disorder. The doctor's insistence that the mother force the child to go to school was the impetus she needed to revert to her normal parental functioning.

There are many theories as to why parents respond in an overprotective manner. The more Freudian interpretation perceives this as a reaction formation to deal with unconscious feelings of rejection toward the child. Voeller and Rothenberg (1973) state that the increase in structure and limits set by the overprotective parent are efforts to compensate for the lack of control parents feel over this disorder. Livingston (1977) reports that parents may regard the epileptic child as a pitiful, unfortunate person and that, therefore, they should make no demands on the child. He also points out that some parents think excitement might precipitate a seizure. Therefore, they strive to provide a quiet, pressure-free atmosphere. In our experience, most parents fail to make demands on the child because they are confused and afraid. They worry that the child may have more seizures when emotionally upset, and they seek to avoid such upsets. They may feel guilty about the epilepsy in general. To precipitate a seizure by frustrating the child would leave them feeling overwhelmingly guilty and inadequate as parents. As long as seizures are perceived as being life threatening—and most parents believe they are—overprotection seems to be the only course. The constant vigilance that some parents apply to this task is exhausting. Parents may resent this and become angry with the child because they cannot discipline him or her. Many overprotective parents want to impose limits, but fear the consequences and need encouragement to treat the child normally.

Poor Compliance

Noncompliance in giving medicine is an all-too-common parental reaction and one that is especially frustrating for the physician. Kutt (1974) believes that it is the most common cause for poor seizure control in epilepsy patients. Assuming that parents understand the doctor's instructions, there are several prevailing reasons for noncompliance. Voeller and Rothenberg (1973) point out that poor compliance often reflects the parent's inability to accept the child's epilepsy. Denial of the disorder may indeed be manifested by noncompliance. Such denial is more likely to occur when the parents have not witnessed a seizure or when the seizures are very mild in appearance. It would be difficult to maintain denial when confronted with frequent generalized tonic-clonic seizures. In fact, denial and poor compliance that persist despite such poorly controlled seizures might be indicative of severe psychopathology in the family.

Side effects, especially of barbiturates, may cause parents to frequently forget or totally discontinue a drug. Wolf and Forsythe (1978), in a study on behavior disturbance and phenobarbital use in children with febrile seizures, found that 42% developed behavior problems after being started on the drug. In another paper, Wolf and co-workers (1977) reported that 32% of the mothers prematurely decreased the phenobarbital, mostly because of behavior problems.

Parents' failure to understand the nature of epilepsy and the role of medicine may lead to poor compliance. Some parents give medicine when they think a seizure is coming on or immediately after one ends. They have no concept of blood levels or of medicine "insulating" the brain cells against abnormal electrical discharges.

The cost of medication can create problems, especially for financially insecure families. They do not qualify for welfare programs but rarely have medical insurance that covers drugs. If compliance is a problem, it is worthwhile to ask parents how much the medicine costs per month. Those patients on several drugs or on newer drugs may spend a large amount, and in difficult financial times the families may try to "stretch" the medicine, which results in the child getting fewer doses than prescribed, especially when the child's seizure control has been good.

Most parents forget doses from time to time but do not know whether to give the medicine later when they remember it. Too many parents skip the dose when they should go ahead and give it. Guidelines for this should be covered when the prescription is given.

Because the *Physicians' Desk Reference* is available in book stores, the public is reading it. The side effects listed for some of the medications sound serious enough to discourage some parents from administering them. Unfortunately parents do not realize that most side effects occur rarely.

Disclosure

This is an issue that all parents must wrestle with in their adjustment process. Whom should they tell about the epilepsy? The child, the siblings, the extended family, the neighbors? What about the school? Too much secrecy is harmful because it conveys to the child the message that his disorder is too terrible to discuss. However, no discretion at all may create problems also. Parents should, of course, discuss epilepsy with the school-age child and the siblings at a level they can understand.

The school staff usually should be told. The teacher can be very helpful in assessing behavioral side effects of medicine. With information about the child's condition, the teacher would be much calmer if a seizure occurred in the classroom. A well-informed, supportive school staff is invaluable in enabling the child to adjust well to the epilepsy.

Parents are sometimes dismayed by the reactions of people whom they tell about the epilepsy. The problem may be in the way in which parents convey the information. Most people do not know much about epilepsy, and what they know may be frightening. Simply saying, "My child has epilepsy," conveys little. A parent should describe the appearance of the seizure and the appropriate first aid, as well as the likelihood of a seizure. The parents' own feelings about the epilepsy are transmitted. If parents are very frightened, they cannot expect their listener to be otherwise. They should be matter-of-fact, informative, and receptive to questions.

PATIENT REACTION
Children keenly perceive and incorporate the attitude of their parents toward this disorder. If the parents have difficulty adjusting, the child may become anxious, withdrawn, fearful, insecure, and may cease to compete. School underachievement may result (Hodgman 1979, Green and Hartlage 1971). If overprotected, the child may become irritable, angry, and manipulative. Parents often think they do a good job of hiding their feelings. They may confidentially tell the doctor that the child has no idea how terrifying these seizures are to them. Yet, the child can relate that he quit breathing, turned blue, and almost died during a seizure. He had overheard much and is as frightened as his parents about his condition.

Dependency is a problem for some patients. Parents foster this, and they may later regret the pattern they have established. When it begins early and continues to adulthood, it is sometimes irreversible. These dependent ones rail against their parents' smothering ways but fail to pursue an independent course when they reach the age and stage to do so.

Many children will try to use their seizure disorder to manipulate the home and school situation. One of our patients who showed a rapid weight gain convinced the school staff that she would have a seizure if not allowed to eat frequently. They fed her four times during her 6-hour school day. Children who do not like school may use epilepsy as a way to avoid attendance. Parents need to be forewarned that children may perceive the leverage that their disorder gives them and may use it to full advantage.

The teenager with epilepsy experiences a unique set of problems. The periodic, unpredictable loss of control threatens the autonomy that the adolescent is struggling to achieve. During this developmental stage there is also great pressure to conform in dress, talk, and thought. It is an age that forgives few differences. Epilepsy can be mortifying, especially when the onset occurs during adolescence. Even if peers are accepting, the patient may feel stigmatized. Denial of the condition and rebellion against the limits that epilepsy imposes are stages that a teenager may traverse. It is important to spend time counseling the adolescent whose epileptic condition has recently been diagnosed. There are several points in particular that should be covered.

Daily Medication

The adolescent needs to understand that medicine must be taken daily for at least several years, even if the seizures do not recur. He sometimes thinks that several months is adequate. Suddenly stopping the medicine can be dangerous. Explanation may include the fact that the medicine does not "cure" seizures but suppresses them and gives the brain an opportunity to "render" the electrical abnormalities harmless over time in maturation.

Drugs and Alcohol

Teenagers with epilepsy need to know that street drugs and alcohol can be dangerous by lowering the seizure threshold and by interacting with antiepileptic drugs. For street drugs, the interaction is not predictable because the content of the active agents may be variable. Teenagers need to know that it is dangerous to mix sedatives and alcohol with phenobarbital. Stimulants may increase the likelihood of seizures. (Research has not determined whether marijuana increases or decreases seizure frequency.) If the teenager is determined to try alcohol, he should do so in a controlled setting with friends who know about his condition. Under no circumstances should he drive at that time or place himself in any dangerous situation.

Driving

The driving laws vary in different states and countries with respect to how long a patient must be seizure free before driving is permitted and to whether epilepsy is a reportable disorder. The physician should discuss driving with the teenager, give medical advice, and interpret the regulations.

For noncompliant teenagers, the driver's license can be a strong incentive to cooperate in taking medication.

Precipitating Events

Teenagers need to be advised as to what factors might bring on a seizure and to be reassured about those that do not. Sleep deprivation, alcohol and drugs, and illness (especially febrile illness) may lower the seizure threshold. Flashing lights are known to precipitate seizures in some patients, but this does not apply to most patients or even to the majority of susceptible patients on medication. There is, therefore, rarely a need to avoid discos, roller rinks, fast food places, and other sources of flashing lights unless specified by the physician. Some activities that teenagers worry about are dieting, smoking cigarettes, and physical exertion. Within reasonable limits, none of these should be a problem. Stress may play a role in precipitating seizures in those whose seizures are poorly controlled, but generally it does not affect patients who are well controlled.

Employment and Marriage

Some teenagers want to know what impact this disorder will have on their future in limiting the range of occupational choices. There is no point in the patient getting his hopes set on being an Air Force pilot or a high-wire performer. However, there is a broad range of job opportunities, even after the dangerous ones are eliminated.

Adults with epilepsy can marry, have children, rear a family, and live normal lives. There are obviously a few exceptions, but most teenagers can be reassured that their lives can be as normal as they choose. Where childbearing is inadvisable on genetic grounds, adoption may assuage childlessness.

SIBLING REACTION

Siblings of children with epilepsy have an important impact on the patient's overall adjustment. Siblings who continue to act in a normal fashion provide a secure, stable training ground for social relationships. Goldin and Margolin (1975) have found that there was less disruption in the interaction between siblings if the epilepsy began after age 6, by which time the sibling relationship is usually well established. A factor found to significantly increase the likelihood of conflict between siblings was the presence of other significant disabilities in the epileptic child.

For children whose seizures are easily controlled and whose parents have adjusted well, the siblings' adjustment should not be an issue. However, if parents focus excessively on the epileptic child, caution the siblings not to upset him, and give preferential treatment, natural sibling rivalry may be heightened. Anger, resentment, and scapegoating may be displayed by some of the siblings. Others may adopt the attitude of their parents, become overprotective, and foster dependency in the epileptic child.

At the time of the diagnosis, parents sometimes ask what they should tell the siblings about the epilepsy or whether it should be discussed at all. They should talk with all school-age children in the family. First aid procedures, assurance that the epileptic child will be all right after a seizure, and reassurance that no one is to blame for this condition are issues that may need to be covered. For children with absence seizures, very little needs to be said. However, the fact that the epileptic child has been the focus of parental concern and that he has been to the doctor or hospital for medical tests may leave the siblings feeling left out and confused if no explanation is given. An atmosphere of secrecy in the home is harmful to the child and may do more to stigmatize him than society's response (Lennox 1960).

MYTHS AND MISCONCEPTIONS

Parents hear old wives' tales about epilepsy from a myriad of sources. Rarely do they check out the validity of these misconceptions with the physician. Arangio (1977) notes the "strange phenomenon" in which people do not explain their irrational fears and anxieties about the seizure(s) to the doctor and the physician does not inquire, a situation that results in a communication hiatus between the parents and the physician and that also results in heightened tension in the family and contributes to an erosion of confidence in the physician and ultimately to doctor shopping. These communciation problems may be ameliorated if the physician takes the initiative in addressing some of the most common of these fears and misconceptions.

Death from a Seizure

Parents need to know that death from a generalized tonic-clonic seizure is quite rare. The universal fear of parents who have witnessed a seizure is that the child almost died and he will surely do so if another one occurs. Therefore, parents do everything in their power to avoid bringing one on. If frustration, anger, excitement, or exertion are thought to precipitate a seizure, the parents may protect the child from these. Parents may not have the same expectations for this child as they have for the others. Discipline may be rarely given. The siblings may be cautioned to give in to the sick child. If the seizure occurred while the child was sleeping, the parents may take to sleeping with the child, a pattern that is hard to break. If it occurred while the child ate, the parents may be highly nervous at mealtime. Usually the parent's anxieties subside as time passes without further seizures. However, if dysfunctional patterns of interacting have been established, these do not necessarily cease.

The fear of death should be openly discussed at the time of the diagnosis. Parents should be warned not to treat the child differently, and the subject should be re-opened on subsequent visits. Parents are generally reliable in reporting whether they now spoil the child because of the seizures.

Swallowing the Tongue

The idea that it is literally possible to swallow the tongue is a common belief. Unfortunately, this is periodically reinforced by the news media as, for example, when comedian John Belushi died. The first reports released by Associated Press stated that he had "choked on food and had swallowed his tongue" and died (*Winston-Salem Sentinel* 1982).

The mother of a 10-year-old boy (followed in our clinic for nocturnal seizures) said she had a tongue check every morning to see if his was still there. To prevent swallowing of the tongue, people put fingers, pens, rulers, even golf clubs into the convulsing person's mouth. One of our patients almost died from the top of a Bic pen that lodged in his trachea when a well-meaning bystander used it to administer first aid during a seizure. Broken teeth from metal objects thrust into the convulsing person's mouth are too common. Many parents have their fingers chewed repeatedly as they attempt to save the tongue.

Parents need to be informed that it is impossible to actually swallow the tongue; therefore, no heroic measures should be taken. They do need to be instructed on appropriate first aid so that they do not overtreat the situation. They also need advice on when to call an ambulance and some reassurance that this is usually not necessary.

Causality

The need to know why their child has epilepsy seems to haunt parents. The explanation that "we just don't know why" offers little solace and may leave the parents to devise an explanation of their own. Tavriger (1966) discusses this issue and the parental fantasies that emerge to fill the conceptual void which answers the question "why." Here are some examples from our patient population.

One mother of a 14-year-old boy with generalized tonic-clonic seizures thought she remembered being told when he was an infant that he had a blood clot in his brain. She believed that his seizures occurred when the blood clot moved about his brain. She feared it might settle in a dangerous part and result in death or serious damage.

The mother of an 11-year-old whose generalized tonic-clonic seizures were of recent onset thought that they were caused by his watching "The Hulk," a television show. In this show an ordinary man turns into a huge green monster when he becomes enraged. Her son would voluntarily draw his muscles taut and shake while he imitated the Hulk during the show. She thought that these imitations had gotten out of control and caused the seizures. The fact that he never had a seizure during the show or immediately afterward did not seem to influence her belief.

Some children may become pale or flushed during the seizure, and the idea that not enough or too much blood reaches the brain is common. Some parents imagine a mechanism such as "a vein in the back of the head" that constricts or expands too much.

If someone important to the child died or some other emotional trauma occurred in the months preceding the initial seizure, the family may attribute the epilepsy to that.

It seems that every child has fallen at some time and sustained a blow to the head. As parents scour the history for possible causes, many come up with this one. They also fear that an additional blow to the head might precipitate more seizures.

Such parental fantasies may interfere with treatment, increase anxiety and guilt, and may promote dysfunctional parental behavior. To assist parents and children in understanding seizures, one should explain in a very simple way the physiological event.

PSYCHOSOCIAL PROBLEMS

The psychosocial problems accompanying epilepsy have long been recognized as being as important as the medical aspects of this disorder. Livingston (1977), Kaye (1951), Pond and Bidwell (1959), and Henriksen (1977) estimated that 25% of the patients with epilepsy will develop psychosocial problems that need remediation by a multidisciplinary team. Most of these problems can be avoided through preventive efforts and early recognition and intervention.

The pediatrician or family physician can be instrumental in helping the family make a good adjustment. By virtue of his established relationship with the family, he may employ psychodynamic skills to ease the adjustment process. The primary care physician in many ways is a counselor to the family and undoubtedly uses many of these skills already. They are not as time consuming as some would think and actually save much time in the long run.

The first is *ventilation*. At the time of the first convulsive seizure, the family is frightened and upset. Many parents say that seeing their child have this type of seizure is the most frightening experience of their lives. Simply recognizing these feelings and allowing the parents to talk briefly about them will alleviate stress and enhance communication between the physician and family and improve coping strategies.

If the physician is too busy to listen or the family's need to talk is excessive, the listening can be assumed by other staff members, such as the nurse or social worker. However, the doctor needs to be apprised of the family's main concerns and does need to talk with them because he is the one who will continue to follow the family, to advise them as issues arise, to assess their problems, and to refer them if further intervention is required. The family's cooperation depends on this understanding.

The next is *reassurance*. Although the physician may not have fully evaluated the seizure problem when he first talks with the family, he can usually reassure them that the child is not at death's door. When a convulsive seizure has occurred, the parents may fear that the child is in mortal danger. The following example from our medical center illustrates this.

Mary, a 7-year-old child, was hospitalized for a diagnostic workup after her first seizure; her discharge diagnosis was idiopathic epilepsy. Approximately 2 weeks later a Public Health nurse called to ask whether this child could attend school in her fragile condition. The mother had informed the school that her child had cardiac arrest during the seizure and almost died and that only through heroic means had her life been saved. She told the teacher to call an ambulance immediately if the child had another seizure. This information made the teacher quite nervous, and even the Health Department did not doubt its validity. This mother had not understood or was not explicitly told during the hospitalization that her child had not been in serious danger.

A high level of anxiety interferes with comprehension and retention of medical information and instructions given by the doctor (Ley and Spelman 1967). Reassurance will reduce anxiety so that parents will hear instructions and advice.

The next skill is *clarification*. In this situation it involves giving factual information about the disorder. The family needs to be well informed and wants to know as much as possible about epilepsy. If the doctor does not educate the relatives, they will rely on neighbors and relatives indiscriminately. Being well informed increases the likelihood that parents will make the correct choices in day-to-day living with the child. There will be fewer parenting problems, probably fewer compliance problems, and, we hope, fewer adjustment problems.

Repetition is important. Research indicates that the patients forget a third of what a physician tells them immediately upon leaving the examining room. Over time, further distortion takes place (Francis et al 1969). For this reason, written information is very helpful. Many pamphlets on epilepsy are available through the Epilepsy Foundation of America, through drug companies, and from private sources (see Appendix A). Pamphlets allow the families to review the information as often as they like, and they are an excellent adjunct to the physician's efforts.

Oliver Wendell Holmes (1892) once said,

> Your patient has no more right to all the truth you know than he has to all the medicine in your saddle bags, if you carry that kind of cartridge-box for the ammunition that slays disease. He should get only just so much as is good for him.

There are certainly some things that are better left unsaid. An eager resident at our center informed a young man, shortly after he regained consciousness from his first convulsive seizure, that he would lose his driver's license for a year. This abrasive thoughtlessness compounded his problems in adjusting to the diagnosis. Likewise, there is no need to tell the mother of an 8-year-old child about job problems that her child may face in the distant future.

Giving *advice* is another important task in establishing success when the patient has a trusting relationship with the physician. Parents who continue to be overly permissive, overly restrictive, or overly protective need to be disabused strongly by the physician. Citing his experience with many children who have had seizure disorders, he can point out that the seizures may never recur but that the child will be warped for life if the parenting continues to be unrealistic.

There may be a variety of symptoms indicating a family that fails to make a good adjustment to the child's illness. Serious marital problems are frequent in families where the marriage was already unstable. Poor medical compliance may be an indication of the family's poor adjustment. Behavior problems exhibited by the child may be a symptom of family stress.

Children with epilepsy have been found by some researchers to have significantly more academic problems than would be expected from children of their age and intelligence (Holdsworth and Whitmore 1974, Rutter 1970). Reasons for such poor performance are a matter of speculation, but poor attendance does not seem to account for it (Stores 1978). Medication may be one factor. For example, phenobarbital causes hyperactivity, irritability, emotional lability, and mental slowing in a significant proportion of children (Stores 1980, Wolf et al 1977). Lowered expectations for epileptic children by teachers and parents is also a factor (Bagley 1970, Hartlage and Green 1972). Margolin (1963) postulates that the school setting could produce a failure syndrome whereby children do not try because they fear failure and that this may account for underachievement in this population.

Dikmen (1980) reviewed the literature on organic causes of epilepsy and found that there was no cognitive deficit characteristic of epilepsy. However, for those whose seizure etiology was known to derive from a localized brain lesion, there was sometimes a relationship between the location of the lesion and the severity and type of psychological defects. There is also the possibility of subclinical seizures or undetected clinical seizures interfering with the child's schoolwork. Underachievement should be evaluated psychologically and socially and should be treated early, before the pattern is too firmly established. Otherwise these children will go through life never realizing their full potential.

Emotional problems also occur at a higher frequency in children with epilepsy than in the general population (Rutter et al 1970, Pond and Bidwell 1960, Stores 1978). However, many studies found that when epileptic patients were compared with patients with other chronic illnesses, there was no difference in the frequency of psychiatric problems (Whitman et al 1980). Boys seem to be at much greater risk than girls for behavior problems, as well as for academic problems (Stores 1978). Medication can cause or exacerbate existing behavior problems. Although phenobarbital especially has been blamed for this, other drugs may be responsible. Before a referral for counseling is made, a change in medicine should be seriously considered if there is any relationship between worsened behavioral symptoms and the medication regimen.

A multidisciplinary team is the optimum approach to evaluation of epileptic children with school behavior and/or social problems. Many medical centers now offer such a team approach (see Chapter 17).

There are many resources available to children with epilepsy, epecially to those who are handicapped by their condition. Many states have a Crippled Childrens Program that may help to pay for medicines and medical care. There are vocational services through the Division of Rehabilitative Services in most states. Several organizations offer summer camps for handicapped children. Respite care for families, group homes, Supplemental Security Income, and state and local epilepsy chapters are among the available resources. For those families for whom epilepsy is a significant burden, referral should be made to a social worker at the local Department of Social Services or medical center.

THE WELL-ADJUSTED FAMILIES
Just as there are families who adjust poorly to this disorder, there are some who

adjust unusually well. They reach a point where they not only accept the cloud of epilepsy but see a silver lining. Some perceive that this disorder has strengthened the family or the child. Some see ways that they might use their epilepsy to be of benefit to others. Adults with epilepsy since childhood may point out ways in which it has positively affected important life decisions such as career choices. Here are some examples.

A widowed mother said that her teenage son's severe epilepsy and developmental problems were important factors in the closeness of her family. Her other five children were compassionate individuals, which she saw as an extension of their relationship with the disabled brother. Even the financial strain, which was due in part to the handicapped child, was seen as somewhat positive in that it forced more responsibility and independence on the other children. The mother was proud that all of them had achieved education beyond the high school level and were productive young adults.

A professional basketball player, Bobby Jones, said that overall his epilepsy has had a positive effect on his life. Since it began he has been taking better care of himself physically, sleeping and eating regularly, avoiding alcohol, and generally being moderate in all things. As a result, his basketball performance has been more consistent.

Another patient with a long history of epilepsy entered the entertainment field as a young adult. Her epilepsy required of her a regular sleep pattern and strict avoidance of alcohol and drugs. She felt fortunate that there was no temptation to use these substances that had ruined many of her colleagues. She was also relieved that her epilepsy forced her to rest, ensuring that her voice and her health were not injured by a frantic pace.

It is not clear what factors enable some families to rise above the crisis of epilepsy and grow from it, while others bow under the burden.

LIVING ARRANGEMENTS FOR THE CHILD WITH EPILEPSY

There was a time in the history of epilepsy when persons who suffered from it were frequently confined to instutitions for the insane. In the late 18th century, separate wards in these institutions were set aside for persons with epilepsy, though probably more for the protection of the insane than of the epileptic (Temkin 1971). In the mid-19th century, specialized institutions were established in Europe, eg, the National Hospital for the Paralyzed and Epileptic at Queen Square in London, which opened its doors in 1860, and Bethel at Bielefeld in Germany, which was established in 1867. At the end of the 19th century, institutions were founded in the United States, the first of which was at Gallipolis, Ohio; and a series of such institutions particularly for the pediatric patients were subsequently established. Although most of the institutions contained patients with predominantly mental retardation, there were many that admitted patients whose predominant diagnosis was epilepsy. Many of the epileptic patients were not significantly retarded or in other ways neurologically impaired. Most of these institutions were situated in remote and rural locations, a condition that had the effect of further isolating children with epilepsy from adaptation to normal community interaction. The institutions also had the effect of concentrating large collections of handicapped people. Although this may have been helpful in terms of concentrating medical care, it had the detrimental dehumanizing effect inherent in any large instutition. With the improvement in the treatment of seizures and with the increased social consciousness of society in the second half of the 20th century, most persons who have epilepsy but who are not suffering from other major handicapping neurologic disorders no longer find themselves institutionalized. Children with epilepsy now constitute approximately one-third of the population of centers for the developmentally handicapped, all of whom are concomitantly mentally retarded or psychotic. Under Public Law 94-103, every citizen has the right to "maximize his developmental potential in the setting that is least restrictive of the person's personal liberty."

The Commission for the Control of Epilepsy and Its Consequences (1977) recommended that whatever the environment in which the individual with epilepsy was living, there were certain basic needs that would have to be filled. Such needs include the following:

1. Direct, assured and continued access to medical care provided by persons with specific knowledge about the diagnosis and treatment of epilepsy.
2. An educational–vocational program with clearly defined goals and objectives and target dates. This program would have as its ultimate objective a continued productive role with the maximum independence of which the individual could become capable.
3. Training in and opportunities for social, recreational and physical activities leading towards the most normal types of social intercourse.
4. A physical environment appropriate to the maintenance of physical and emotional health. Such an environment would recognize the special safety hazards of the person with epilepsy, but would accept balance of risk and relation to the principle of the least restrictive environment.

It is evident that these requirements can be met only with the provision of a series of services ranging from residential institutions through group homes with supervised living and sheltered working environments, and semi-independent living and training activities to foster-home placement or from placement in a normal residential environment with special educational and vocational facilities. Several European institutions have a long tradition of specialized medical, social, and educational programs for children with epilepsy. Such institutions include The Epilepsy Centre at Chalfont and the David Lewis Centre in England, Sandvika in Norway, Meer-en-Bosch in Holland, and Bethel in Germany. In addition, these centers have contributed to scientific progress and to the training of epileptologists. In the United States, the tendency has been to discourage the grouping of persons with epilepsy in segregated institutions, however, in view of the fact that almost one-third of persons in institutions for the retarded suffer from epilepsy, a recent study has recommended that medical services should be upgraded to meet minimal standards and to provide specialized care for persons with epilepsy, that such institutions should develop relationships with the neurologic departments of a teaching institution, that specialized staff of such institutions should receive salaries commensurate with the salaries of equivalent positions in the affiliated academic institution and that such institutions should provide in-service training for physicians and nurses. Such institutions should have access to serum anticonvulsant drug level monitoring with rapid turn-around time and up-to-date electroencephalographic and other diagnostic facilities. It was found that when these measures were instituted, epileptic morbidity such as status epilepticus, head injury and subdural hematomas, and uncontrolled seizures were markedly reduced within a short period of time (O'Neill et al 1977). In this study, nurses and attendants received special training to achieve competence in the nursing problems presented by persons with epilepsy, including the recognition of the nature and understanding of various types of seizures, their management, the uses and side effects of anticonvulsant drugs, and danger signals requiring more sophisticated methods of intervention. A physician with knowledge about epilepsy was available, and an EEG laboratory with well-trained electroencephalographers and an antiepileptic drug monitoring laboratory were established.

The Commission for the Control of Epilepsy and Its Consequences recommended the establishment of foster-home placement and of group homes and apartments for persons with epilepsy, with thoughtful consideration for transportation problems and needs for medical and vocational services. One of the disadvantages of deinstitutionalization is the danger of dispersion without adequate regard for the availability of such services. In some regions, a state-wide program dedicated to the care of children with epilepsy through a regional clinic structure has assured continuing up-to-date medical therapy (Dreifuss 1980). Among the recommendations of the Commission and among the responsibilities of existing Comprehensive Epilepsy Programs is the mandate to establish community–family training programs for parents of children with epilepsy, for persons with epilepsy, and for those who come in contact with them, such as teachers, public safety officials, nurses, and potential employers.

There continues to be an unmet need for special centers for management and study of patients with epilepsy who are also suffering from severe behavioral or psychiatric complications. These special centers would provide intermediate care with an emphasis on rehabilitation.

THE INFLUENCE OF EPILEPSY ON EDUCATION

Epilepsy frequently interferes with the normal educational process in a child. The recognition of this has led to specific programs for the education of those who come in contact with children with epilepsy, especially teachers, school nurses, and, of course, parents. The School Alert Program of the Epilepsy Foundation of America represents an educational endeavor of this type. Most Comprehensive Epilepsy Programs employ special education consultants who have studied epilepsy. These consultants evaluate the special needs of the children with seizure disorders and make recommendations to the child's school teacher. It is recognized that school age represents the age with the highest prevalence of epilepsy (Dreifuss 1949). Much epilepsy in schools continues to be unrecognized, and screening programs have brought to light a large number of children with hitherto unrecognized seizures. The area of recognition and management of seizures is important in terms of prevention. Unrecognized defective school performance may be caused by subclinical epileptic discharges (Aicardi and Chevrie 1973, Goode et al 1970). Behavioral aberrations such as inattentiveness, "daydreaming," and "fidgetiness" may represent events beyond the child's control. Poor school performance and reprimand may, therefore, be avoidable. As mentioned earlier, the consequences of epilepsy are sometimes more detrimental than the seizures themselves.

Many children suffering from epilepsy do not do well in school (Bagley 1970, Myklebust 1977). There appear to be many factors upon which this depends. Thus, patients with early-onset epilepsy do less well than those with late-onset epilepsy (Dodrill 1975). This is in keeping with the finding of lower intelligence quotients in the early-onset groups. This is probably not due to the duration of the condition but to the effects of early injuries to the brain, such as those received during difficult births or cerebral infections. In both the early-onset and the late-onset groups, the patients without evidence of cerebral lesions have intellectual quotients approximately ten points above those with a clinically evident lesion. Difficulties in memory and concentration in many cases vitiate otherwise adequate IQ and often lead children to a psychometrically unsound position. The side and the site of a cerebral lesion is an important determining factor (Ounsted et al 1966) with frontal and temporal abnormalities and left-sided lesions more deleterious than lesions in other sites. Children with epilepsy of nonfocal variety and without evidence of structural lesions do considerably better at school. Lesions in the dominant hemisphere are more likely to be associated with performance difficulties, particularly in the verbal and mathematical spheres, and with significant impairment of cognitive functioning. The frequency of seizures bears a relationship to school performance. Frequent absence seizures disrupt attention and reduce the child's ability to assimilate information. Frequent major seizures lead to more prolonged alterations of the conscious state and tend to occupy the attention of other children; therefore, they are more devastating. However, many children with generalized tonic-clonic seizures continue to do well in school. The most severely affected children are those with a combination of complex-partial seizures and generalized tonic-clonic seizures.

The degree to which seizures are controlled is an important determinant of scholastic achievement; so also is the nature of the medication used to treat the seizures. Phenobarbital has been implicated in reduction of learning ability, particularly when administered in a dose that produces drowsiness (Camfield et al 1979). In many children, barbiturates lead to an abbreviation of the attention span, hyperactive behavior, and inability to filter out extraneous stimuli; these effects lead to severe problems with concentration and consequent learning ability. Phenytoin has been associated with alteration in learning ability (Trimble and Reynolds 1976) and on occasion with a deterioration in school performance and the development of a progressive dementia (Vallarta et al 1974). Primidone and clonazepam have both been associated with deleterious behavioral change, diminution of concentration, and impairment of cognitive function. Carbamazepine, ethosuximide and valproic acid are relatively free of side effects involving school performance.

A major factor is the quality of instruction. In general, pupils attained a higher standard in schools known for excellence of teaching and individual attention. Even below-average children reached some proficiency in certain subjects in schools where the teachers maintained that ineducability is purely relative. It has been frequently noted that teachers' attitudes frequently determine the behavior of other children in the class. If the attitude of the teacher is free of anxiety and unnecessary fuss, the witnessing of occasional attacks does other children no harm. The seizure tends to arouse curiosity but is not frightening unless adults show alarm. The provision of instruction for children about epilepsy is important. In fact, association with handicapped persons, who are cheerfully and courageously bypassing their physical difficulties, can be an aid to education of normal individuals and films, and other educational materials about epilepsy are useful adjuncts.

An adequate education is particularly important for the epileptic where employment restrictions are such that success depends upon careful planning and thoughtful consideration of the vocational assets and liabilities. Any indication of a special ability or unusual interest from the school history may be a clue to prospective employment, and the maximum intellectual training that the patient can assimilate may help in developing the inner resource and insight necessary to withstand society's attitudes toward the condition. A sound academic background may open jobs that are often more suitable for a person with epilepsy than industrial employment or unskilled labor jobs. Psychometric evaluation by a trained examiner may be helpful in deciding how ambitious an academic program is advisable for a patient, and for a child who is not up to standard for his age the psychometric evaluation may determine whether this is due to limited mental ability or to interrupted education. In underprivilaged children suffering from malnutrition and deprivation, and in children who have other neurologic impairments including cerebral palsy, and in those in whom the epilepsy is associated with previously poor environmental conditions, parental neglect or abuse and lack of proper medical care, great progress may be made by intensive medical, social, psychological, and educational intervention in a rehabilitation center setting.

The role of the educational consultant in the evaluation of children with epilepsy is the early detection of educational handicaps (such as associated learning disabilities), the identification of epilepsy-related educational handicaps (which are potentially remediable by appropriate medical intervention), the modification of the child's educational environment (by furnishing education prescriptions appropriate to the child's needs), follow-up school contact to check on the implementation of the recommendations, in-service education for the classroom teacher about epilepsy and its consequences, and the identification of alternative educational resources for those children who cannot adequately function in the age-appropriate classroom setting by virtue of the epilepsy or the associated problems. As was noted by Myklebust (1977), "Some programs face serious circumstances both in health and learning. Most authorities think the school problems largely remediable. However, the task is a major one, requiring participation of parents, educators, psychologists, pediatricians, physicians, school nurses, counsellors, and other related professional workers."

Many of the problems have their origin in the setting of misunderstanding of the principles of child training, and at school the epileptic child may be terrified while playing with other children lest he or she have a seizure and become the butt of ridicule. Children with epilepsy must adjust themselves as best they can, or they will be excluded from educational and recreational opportunities. Exclusion may cause a forceful child to fight for his or her rights, sometimes to become disagreeable, domineering, and sullen, or withdrawn, silent, and solitary. At times, the epileptic child may secure success by conscientious effort in the absence of social interaction. These reaction patterns are neither unique to the epileptic child nor are they permanent or irreversible. Cutting short social and psychological handicaps avoids the main threat, which is not that of the attacks but of the handicap of being excluded from large areas of normal childhood life.

APPENDIX A

Epilepsy Foundation of America, 4351 Garden City Drive, Suite 406, Landover, Maryland 20785

The National Epilepsy Library and Resource Center of the Epilepsy Foundation of America is an up-to-date repository of epilepsy-related information at the professional and consumer levels. Comprehensive collections of medical and psychosocial literature, a directory of model programs, and a telephone information network are available with access to the national computerized data banks at the National Library of Medicine and the National Institutes of Health.

Many states have local chapters of the Epilepsy Foundation of America. These usually provide free literature and may have monthly group meetings for patients, their families and other interested individuals. Information about these chapters is available through EFA.

Ayerst Laboratories, New York, New York 10017

Handbook for Parents and *Handbook for Patients* are informative booklets written by Dr. Eli Goldensohn and designed for the more literate consumer. They are available through the local Ayerst drug representative and are free of charge.

Epilepsy Information Service, Department of Neurology, Bowman Gray School of Medicine, Winston-Salem, North Carolina 27103

A small selection of pamphlets is available: free in small quantities, at cost in large quantities. They include:

Dilantin and Gums
Febrile Convulsions
Medicine for People with Seizures
Petit Mal or Absence Epilepsy
Seizure Man: First Aid for Seizures (comic book)
Seizure Man: In the Classroom (comic book)
You and Your Seizures

BIBLIOGRAPHY

Aicardi J, Chevrie J: The significance of electroencephalographic paroxysms in children less than three years of age. *Epilepsia* 1973;14:47–55.

Arangio A: A systematic examination of the psychosocial needs of patients with epilepsy: The need for a comprehensive change approach, in Commission for the Control of Epilepsy and Its Consequences: *Plan for Nationwide Action on Epilepsy*. US Department of Health, Education, and Welfare, DHEW publication no 78276, 1977.

Arangio A: Epilepsy and attitudes: A review of the literature and the construction of an attitude measurement scale plan, in *Facts Not Fiction*. Evansville, IN, Tri-State Epilepsy Association, 1973.

Bagley CR: The educational performance of children with epilepsy. *Br J Educ Psychol* 1970; 40:82–93.

Camfield CS, Chaplin S, Doyle AB, et al:Side-effects of phenobarbital in toddlers: Behavioral and cognitive aspects. *J Pediatr* 1979;95:361–365.

Commission for the Control of Epilepsy and Its Consequences: *Plan for Nationwide Action on Epilepsy.* US Department of Health, Education, and Welfare, DHEW publication no 78276, 1977.

Dikmen S: Neuropsychological aspects of epilepsy, in Hermann B (ed): *A Multidisciplinary Handbook of Epilepsy.* Springfield, IL, Charles C Thomas Publisher, 1980.

Dodrill CB: Diphenylhydantoin serum levels, toxicity and neuropsychological performance in patients with epilepsy. *Epilepsia* 1975;16:593–600.

Dreifuss FE: The epileptic in the community, thesis. Otago University, Dunedin, New Zealand, 1949.

Dreifuss FE: Development of a comprehensive epilepsy program, in Robb P (ed): *Epilepsy Updated.* Chicago, Year Book Medical Publishers, 1980.

Francis V, Korsch B, Morris M: Gaps in doctor-patient communication: Patient's response to medical advice. *N Engl J Med* 1969;6:535–540.

Goldin G, Margolin R: The psychosocial aspects of epilepsy, in Wright GN (ed): *Epilepsy Rehabilitation.* Boston, Little Brown & Co, 1975.

Goldin G, Perry S, Margolin R, et al: *The Rehabilitation of the Young Epileptic.* Lexington, MA, DC Heath & Co, 1971.

Goode DJ, Penry JK, Dreifuss FE: Effects of paroxysmal spike-wave on continuous visual-motor performance. *Epilepsia* 1970;11:241.

Green J, Hartlage L: Comparitive performance of epileptic and non-epileptic children and adolescents on academic, communicative, and social skills, in *Proceedings of 3rd European Sympsoium on Epilepsy,* 1971.

Hartlage LC, Green JB: The relation of parental attitudes to academic and social achievement in epileptic children. *Epilepsia* 1972;13:21–26.

Henriksen O: The modifidication and rehabilitation of patients with epilepsy, in Penry J (ed): *Epilepsy, the 8th International Symposium.* New York, Raven Press, 1977, pp 225–233.

Hodgman C, McAnarney R, Myers G, et al: Emotional complications of adolescent grand mal epilepsy. *J Pediatrics* 1979;95:309–312.

Holdsworth L, Whitmore K: A study of children with epilepsy attending ordinary school. II. Information and attitudes held by their teachers. *Dev Med Child Neurol* 1974;16: 759–771.

Holmes OW: *Medical Essays, 1842–1848.* New York, Houghton Mifflin Co, 1892.

Kaye I: What are the evidences of social and psychological maladjustment revealed in the study of seventeen children who have idiopathic petit mal epilepsy? *J Child Psychiatry* 1951;2:115–160.

Kutt H: The use of blood levels of antiepileptic drugs in clinical practice. *Pediatrics* 1974; 4:557–560.

Lennox M, Mohr J: Social and work adjustment in patients with epilepsy. *Am J Psychiatry* 1950;107:257–263.

Lennox WG: *Epilepsy and Related Disorders.* Boston, Little Brown & Co, 1960.

Lerman P: The concept of preventive rehabilitation in childhood epilepsy: A plea against overprotection and overindulgence, in Penry JK (ed): *Epilepsy, the 8th International Symposium.* New York, Raven Press, 1977.

Lessman SE: Accepting epilepsy: Social and emotional issues for patients and their families, in Black RB, Hermann PP, Shope JT (eds): *Nursing Management of Epilepsy.* Rockville, MD, Aspen Systems, 1982.

Ley P, Spelman MS: *Communicating with the Patient.* St. Louis, Warren H Green, 1967.

Livingston S: Psychosocial aspects of epilepsy. *J Clin Child Psychol* 1977;6:12.

Margolin RJ: The failure syndrome and its prevention in the rehabilitation of the mental patient. *Rehabilitation Record* 1963;4:34–39.

Myklebust H: Educational problems of children with epilepsy, in Commission for the Control of Epilepsy and Its Consequences: *Plan for Nationwide Action on Epilepsy.* 1977;2,part 1: 474–490.

Olshansky S: Chronic sorrow: A response to having a mentally defective child. *Social Casework* 1962;4:190–193.

O'Neill BP, Ladon B, Harris LM, et al: A comprehensive interdisciplinary approach to the care of the institutionalized epileptic, in Penry JK (ed): *Epilepsy.* New York, Raven Press, 1977.

Ounstead C, Lindsay J, Norman C: Biological factors in temporal lobe epilepsy. *Clinics in Developmental Medicine.* London, William Heineman Medical Books, 1966, p 22.

Pond DA, Bidwell BH: A survey of epilepsy in fourteen general practices. Social and psychological aspects. *Epilepsia* 1960;1:285–299.

Romeis J: The role of grandparents in adjustment to epilepsy. *Social Work Health Care* 1980; 6(1):37–43.

Rutter M, Graham P, Yule W: *A Neuropsychiatric Study in Childhood. Clinics in Developmental Medicine.* Philadelphia, Lippincott, 1970, pp 35–36.

Shope J: Nursing in epilepsy: Focus on the patient's perspective, in Hermann B (ed): *A Multidisciplinary Handbook of Epilepsy.* Springfield, IL, Charles C Thomas Publisher, 1980.

Stores G: Children with epilepsy. Psychosocial aspects, in Herman B (ed): *A Multidisciplinary Handbook of Epilepsy.* Springfield, IL, Charles C Thomas Publisher, 1980.

Stores G: Schoolchildren with epilepsy at risk for learning and behavior problems. *Dev Med Child Neurol* 1978;20:502.

Tavriger R: Some parental theories about the causes of epilepsy. *Epilepsia* 1966;7:339–343.

Temkin O: *The Falling Sickness. A History of Epilepsy from the Greeks to the Beginnings of Modern Neurology,* ed 2. Baltimore, Johns Hopkins Press, 1971.

Trimble MR, Reynolds EH: Anticonvulsant drugs and mental symptoms. *Psychol Med* 1976;6: 169–178.

Vallarta JM, Bell DB, Reichert A: A progressive encephalopathy due to chronic hydantoin intoxication. *Am J Dis Child* 1974;128:27–34.

Voeller K, Rothenberg M: Psychosocial aspects of the management of seizures in children. *Pediatrics* 1973;51:1072–1082.

Whitman S, Hermann BP, Gordon A: Psychopathology in epilepsy. How great is the risk? Read before the American Epilepsy Society, annual convention, San Diego, 1980.

Winston-Salem Sentinel. Comedian Belushi dies of choking. March 6, 1982.

Wolf S, Forsythe A: Behavior disturbance, phenobarbital, and febrile seizures. *Pediatrics* 1978;61:728–731.

Wolf SM, et al: The value of phenobarbital in a child who has had a febrile seizure. A controlled perspective study. *Pediatrics* 1977;59:378–385.

INDEX